Gamebird Medicine and Management

Gamebird Medicine and Management

Edited by

Teresa Y. Morishita, DVM, PhD, DACPV
College of Veterinary Medicine
Western University of Health Sciences
Pomona, CA, USA

Robert E. Porter, Jr, DVM, PhD, DACVP, DACPV
College of Veterinary Medicine
University of Minnesota
St. Paul, MN, USA

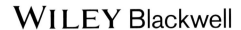

Registered Office
John Wiley & Sons, Inc., 111 River Street, Hoboken, NJ 07030, USA

Editorial Office
111 River Street, Hoboken, NJ 07030, USA

For details of our global editorial offices, customer services, and more information about Wiley products visit us at www.wiley.com.

Wiley also publishes its books in a variety of electronic formats and by print-on-demand. Some content that appears in standard print versions of this book may not be available in other formats.

Library of Congress Cataloging-in-Publication Data applied for

Paperback ISBN: 9781119712213, LCCN 2022029461 (print)

Cover Design: Wiley
Cover Images: Courtesy of Teresa Y. Morishita (Top-Left), MacFarlane Pheasants (Top-Middle; Top-Right), and Robert E. Porter (Bottom 3 Images).

Set in 9.5/12.5pt STIXTwoText by Straive, Chennai, India

Printed in Singapore
M108957_270622

This book is dedicated to my loved ones – my parents, dear P, SG1, and Capt. F, and my ohana-SFSGGBWCFMRPMPBPK-by blood or by choice, who provided me life-giving waters of love, wisdom, and kindness; fertilizing my life with curiosity, courage, and exploration; and providing protection from adversity and the patience, perseverance, and calmness to weather storms, and thereby allowing me to grow and be the person I am.

Teresa Y. Morishita

I dedicate this book to my loving wife Patty with whom all things are possible.

Robert E. Porter, Jr

Contents

List of Contributors

Douglas Anderson, DVM
Veterinary Director
Georgia Poultry Laboratory Network
Forsyth, GA, USA

Gen Anderson
General Curator
St Augustine Alligator Farm Zoological Park
St Augustine, FL, USA
AZA Galliformes TAG Vice-Chair

Elena Behnke, DVM, MAHM, DACPV
Senior Coordinator
National Poultry Improvement Plan
United States Department of Agriculture
Animal and Plant Health Insepction Services
Veterinary Services
Conyers, GA, USA

Steven E. Benscheidt, DVM
Veterinarian
Nelson Road Veterinary Clinic
Longmont, CO, USA

Mark C. Bland, DVM, MS, DACPV
Poultry Veterinarian
Cutler Associates International
Napa, CA, USA

Abigail Duvall, DVM, DABVP(Avian Practice)
Associate Veterinarian
Exotic Vet Care
Mount Pleasant, SC, USA

Linda G. Flores, BS
Professor
College of Veterinary Medicine
Western University of Health Sciences
Pomona, CA, USA

David D. Frame, DVM, DACPV
Associate Professor
Central Utah Veterinary Diagnostic Laboratory
Utah State University
Spanish Fork, UT, USA

Richard M. Fulton, DVM, PhD, DACPV
Professor
Avian Diseases
Michigan State University
East Lansing, MI, USA

Rodrigo A. Gallardo, DVM, PhD, DACPV
Associate Professor in Poultry Medicine
School of Veterinary Medicine
University of California-Davis
Davis, CA, USA

Kahina Boukherroub, PhD
Assistant Professor
Department of Animal Science
University of Minnesota
St Paul, MN, USA

Al Hollister, PhD
Technical Services Nutritionist
Dawe's Laboratories
Arlington Heights, IL, USA

Chris Holmes
Curator of Birds
Houston Zoo
Houston, TX, USA
AZA Galliformes TAG Chair

Jacqueline Jacob, PhD
Poultry Extension Project Manager
Department of Animal and Food Sciences
University of Kentucky
Lexington, KY, USA

Wael Khamas, BVM&S, MS, PhD
Professor of Anatomy and Histology
College of Veterinary Medicine
Western University of Health Sciences
Pomona, CA, USA

Bill MacFarlane
MacFarlane Pheasants, Inc.
Janesville, WI, USA
Past President of the North American
Gamebird Association (NAGA)

Tara Marmulak, PharmD, DICVP, FSVHP
Director of Pharmacy
Veterinary Teaching Hospital
College of Veterinary Medicine and
Biomedical Sciences
Colorado State University
Fort Collins, CO, USA

Krysta L. Martin, PharmD, FSHVP
Pharmacist
Food Animal Residue Avoidance and
Depletion Program
Department of Medicine and Epidemiology
School of Veterinary Medicine
University of California, Davis, CA, USA

Teresa Y. Morishita, DVM, PhD, DACPV
Professor of Poultry Medicine and Food Safety
College of Veterinary Medicine
Western University of Health Sciences
Pomona, CA, USA
AZA Galliformes TAG

Sally L. Noll, PhD
Professor
Department of Animal Science
University of Minnesota
St Paul, MN, USA

Anthony Pescatore, PhD, PAS
Extension Professor
Department of Animal and Food Sciences
University of Kentucky
Lexington, KY, USA

Robert E. Porter, Jr, DVM, PhD, DACVP, DACPV
Distinguished Teaching Professor
College of Veterinary Medicine
University of Minnesota
St. Paul, MN, USA

Casey W. Ritz, BS, MS, PhD
Professor and Extension Poultry Specialist
Department of Poultry Science
University of Georgia
Athens, GA, USA

Josep Rutllant, DVM, PhD
Professor of Anatomy and Embryology
College of Veterinary Medicine
Western University of Health Sciences
Pomona, CA, USA

Robert Sexton
Executive Director
North American Gamebird Association
Pierceville, KS, USA

Daniel P. Shaw, DVM, PhD, DACVP, DACPV
Professor Emeritus
College of Veterinary Medicine
University of Missouri
Columbia, MO, USA

Lisa A. Tell, ABVP(Avian), ACZM
Professor
Food Animal Residue Avoidance and
Depletion Program
Department of Medicine and Epidemiology
School of Veterinary Medicine
University of California, Davis, CA, USA

Eva Wallner-Pendleton, DVM, MS, DACPV
Clinical Associate Professor (retired)
Animal Diagnostic Laboratory
Department of Veterinary and
Biomedical Sciences
Pennsylvania State University
State College, PA, USA

Foreword

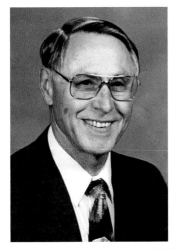

It is an honor to share a few thoughts on our father, Dr. L. Dwight Schwartz, as part of this new gamebird publication. In the late 1950s, Dad deliberately shifted the direction of his veterinary career following a short stint as a USDA Inspector at a poultry processing plant. Having to condemn so many diseased birds for human consumption, he suspected treatment and prevention of disease were far better alternatives for the producers and consumers. This idea led him to a Master's degree at the University of Georgia in the early 1960s followed by nearly three decades as an extension poultry veterinarian at Penn State and Michigan State Universities. However, as he provided veterinary services to poultry growers in both states, he also served the gamebird growers in many states, becoming a good friend to numerous gamebird growers throughout the United States and beyond.

One key accomplishment of Dr Schwartz's career was his authorship of the *Poultry Health Handbook* in 1972, which had three more editions released over the next 22 years. He had long wanted to compile a similar easy-to-use gamebird health handbook based on his vast knowledge and experience with gamebirds. He retired from university life in 1993 and used this new-found "free time" to sit at a desk instead of in a rocking chair and make that dream come true. After more than a year of hard work, with our mother, Wilma J. Schwartz, as his typist and editorial director, he authored and published the *Grower's Reference on Gamebird Health* in 1995.

Whether it was at a professional presentation, a local gamebird breeders association, a necropsy class of vet students, or even a 4-H club, Dr Schwartz had the ability to explain diagnostic and treatment information on diseases to anyone. No question was too simple. No group size was too small. He wanted those raising gamebirds to be successful. In that same light, his *Grower's Reference on Gamebird Health* was intended to be helpful to those raising only a few birds as well as to those raising large flocks. Dad wanted growers to be successful and birds to be healthy.

As it has been 26 years since publication of the *Grower's Reference on Gamebird Health*, we celebrate the efforts of the present team of avian veterinary professionals to bring the heart of that book up to date. The newly updated information and the wealth of photographs in this current publication will prove to be invaluable to numerous gamebird growers here in North America, and hopefully around the world as well. We are so very thankful to Drs Teresa Morishita and Robert Porter for spearheading this great effort, as well as to the host of contributing authors, for working to make the current publication the best and most valuable book ever written on the topic of gamebird health. We know our father would be honored and proud of all those who worked so hard to make this book a reality.

December 2021

Roger D. Schwartz, DVM, MAM
Vicki J. Schwartz, M.Ed

Preface

This book is a culmination of our years of working as an extension poultry veterinarian (Morishita) and as an avian pathologist (Porter) with Galliformes species and recognizing the need for such a resource. How did we get interested in gamebirds and exhibition Galliformes? For Teresa, her childhood memories include being intrigued with the beautiful peacocks and their shimmering tails; the ring-necked pheasant scurrying across the country roads; and finishing up every zoo visit with the exotic pheasant collections by peering into their cages to get a glimpse of the elusive and oh so colorful golden or Lady Amherst's pheasants as they hid among the foliage. Teresa then learned autogenous vaccine production working on marble spleen disease for pheasants and the first birds she learned blood collection on were chukar partridges and quails. The vulturine guineafowl necropsy was Teresa's most memorable, especially when she turned her back to get some additional equipment and when she returned to the bird's carcass, there, on the necropsy table, appeared multiple brown slug-like creatures. How creepy, yet exciting! The specimens were later identified as the air sac fluke with the scientific name *Morishitium*! What a fluke (of a coincidence)! Teresa realized that there was a lack of information on these species which often resulted in the need to extrapolate from the chicken and turkey. Teresa developed a mission to create such a resource for this diverse family of birds that were raised for their meat or eggs, or just for their pure beauty and conservation.

Rob's interest in avian pathology began with pet and wild birds, and domestic poultry. As he began his veterinary career, he soon learned that gamebirds, such as pheasants, partridges, and quail, were categorized as poultry and, in fact, could be considered as commercial poultry because of the millions of dollars that their production contributed to the agricultural economy of the US. Additionally, the breeding, husbandry, and management of these birds was quite different from that of other domestic poultry because the utility of these birds required that they maintain their wild characteristics as well as their distinctive, colorful plumage. They are fascinating birds!

At the same time, Rob, like Teresa, relied heavily on the text (*Grower's Reference to Gamebird Health*) written by L. Dwight Schwartz to diagnose the conditions in gamebirds that were submitted to his veterinary diagnostic laboratory. Upon directly purchasing a copy of this gamebird medicine book, Rob was honored to receive a personally inscribed, lengthy acknowledgment from the author on the first page. This book served as a useful reference and still sits on his office shelf. Rob remembers calling Dr Schwartz to glean his experience on various diagnostic cases.

Teresa is grateful to collaborate on this amazing book project with one of her first colleagues, and friend, Rob Porter, whom she met close to 30 years ago when she became an extension poultry veterinarian in Ohio. Little did she know that her mission of writing such a book was also one of his goals. For Rob, preparing a text dedicated to L. Dwight Schwartz and collaborating with his colleague and good friend Teresa has been a pleasure! We have both personally enjoyed working with the gamebird growers and exhibition pheasant and peafowl breeders these many years, Teresa serving as the veterinary advisor for the United Peafowl Association (2004–2014) after L. Dwight Schwarz. Since 2008, Teresa has also served as the veterinary advisor for the Galliformes Taxon Advisory Group of the Association of Zoos and Aquariums. It is great to work with a fantastic, enthusiastic group of knowledgeable individuals. Rob has served as an advisor to the National American Gamebird Association and continues to be an invited speaker at gamebird symposia to speak on diseases, diagnosis, and management.

We were fortunate to assemble a team of experts to share their knowledge and expertise on various aspects of gamebird health, physiology, nutrition, management, conservation, and regulations with the goal of providing the best care for these species. Special chapters on guineafowl and peafowl are included as well. Spanning over 30 years, we also hope that you enjoy Rob's expansive photo archive of gamebird diseases and disorders. This is a book dedicated to gamebirds!

There is a saying by the twelfth-century philosopher John of Salisbury: "We are like dwarfs sitting on the shoulder of giants. We see more and farther than our predecessors, not because we have keener vision or greater height, but because we are lifted up and borne aloft on their gigantic stature." With this in mind, we "stand on the shoulders" of L. Dwight Schwartz and his pioneering work on gamebird medicine and hope this book builds upon his legacy to increase the knowledge of gamebird medicine and management for all to benefit.

Teresa Y. Morishita
Robert E. Porter, Jr

Acknowledgments

Robert Frost's famous poem ends with…"Two roads diverged in a wood, and I, I took the road less traveled by, and that has made all the difference." When I reflect on my life journey, I can't help but thank my parents for instilling in me curiosity about the world around me; fostering the spirit of taking the initiative to fulfill my dreams and to be adventurous in new things and experiences; teaching me patience and perseverance to forge ahead when life gives me bumps in the road; helping me to have courage and always do the right thing; and to always be kind and generous as I travel my own road. They instilled in me the courage to pursue my dreams of becoming a veterinarian and to leave my home state of Hawaii where I spent my entire life and where all my family and friends resided. Their support and determination gave me the confidence and courage to make new friends and learn new cultures as I moved to California to embark on my veterinary career. Then again, to uproot like a migrating bird by moving to Ohio, and to again make new friends and colleagues. Yes, forging a new road, to go into the unknown and live in a new place is difficult as you leave familiarity behind, but as in the Frost poem, it has made all the difference… as it allowed me to grow. I would not have had the life I have if it wasn't for that spirit of adventure instilled by my parents whom I could always count on for support. I knew there was always a nest for me if I ever needed it. With this spirit of adventure, I learned new things; had novel experiences; visited new places; and met many new colleagues and friends. All this would not have been possible without the support of my parents, my loved ones, extended family and true friends, the friends who remain with you when the road darkens and when it brightens again, as it always does; and to all the new and welcoming individuals that I encountered along my way. I am so fortunate and for that I am grateful.

This book was also like a journey, a thought, a dream which I shared with one of my friends and colleagues only to find out that he too dreamed of such a book. The rest is history and we joined forces to create such a project. Thank you to my co-editor, colleague and I am lucky to count as a friend, Rob Porter who joined me on this effort. Thank you to all the gamebird breeders and exhibition Galliformes enthusiasts who entrusted me with the care of their flocks which allowed me to continue to work with these beautiful birds. I also thank the many chapter authors, experts in their own disciplines, who joined us to make this book a reality by sharing their knowledge and expertise. Much appreciation to Deborah Ann Harris and Chris Vander Veen for their technical assistance and advice in helping me with this project's organizational and developmental stages. A special thanks to Merryl Le Roux who assisted us in this book's organization and production and to Erica Judisch who believed in our dream to make this book a reality. Thank you all for choosing to take the same road to writing this book with us.

We hope that this book will help to provide better care for our gamebird and exhibition Galliformes species. We know the importance of experts from all disciplines working together to ensure better health for these birds in captivity and in conservation for future generations. Let us promote kindness and caring for the land and all its creatures, including each other, as we each walk our own road. Much Aloha!

Teresa Y. Morishita

The planning and creation of this book was more challenging than I had originally anticipated. I am grateful to my wife Patty for tolerating my absences this year as I toiled at the computer. You are the greatest! Additionally, I have had the opportunity to collaborate with Teresa Morishita, a genuine scholar who I have long admired. Thanks for your patience, Teresa. I must give credit to the many gamebird growers who have been willing to work with me. I would not have had the appropriate resources for this book without your cooperation. Finally, this gamebird medicine book is buttressed by a cadre of talented authors who represent a wide breadth of knowledge and expertise. Thanks to you all.

Robert E. Porter, Jr

1

Gamebird History

Robert Sexton, Robert E. Porter, Jr, and Teresa Y. Morishita

1.1 Origins of Gamebird Terminology

Before discussing the origin of the terminology of gamebirds, the term *gamebird* must be defined. This term has been written in many forms, from gamebird to game bird to "game" bird. The original term *gamebird* referred to a bird which was hunted and thus was the "game." In the broadest sense, gamebirds were those birds that were free living and were hunted primarily for food, and then later for sport. Hence, the collective term *gamebird* includes a variety of bird orders including the landfowl (primarily Galliformes), which mostly lived on the ground, and waterfowl (primarily Anseriformes), which spend their time associated with water bodies. There were also perching birds like the Columbiformes and Passerines which, while they also lived on land, could also roost above ground in trees. Because these birds were associated with different habitats, the hunting method used to capture this game varied.

Even before the use of the term *gamebird*, the term *fowl*, derived from the Old English *fugel*, was used to refer to a bird. The term was of Germanic origin from *fluglaz*, the general term for bird. The term *fowl* was replaced with the term *bird*. The first documented record of the use of the term *fowl* was in 1570. In recent times, the word *fowl* is more associated with the domesticated chicken and turkey. The terminology in the United States was also expanded to include domestic ducks and geese in this category. The word *fowl* can also be used as a verb, originated from the Old English *fuglian*, which means "to catch birds" as in the term *fowling*. The individual who caught birds for a living was known as a fowler and the fowling piece was the gun used to shoot wild fowl, as early as 1570s [1].

The interchangeable use of the terms *fowl* and *bird* led to many combinations such as gamebird/gamebird and game fowl/gamefowl. While we utilize the term *gamebird* to refer to those that were once hunted as game, the terms *gamebird* and *game fowl* have totally different uses and connotation. The term *game fowl* currently refers to roosters, known as "game cocks," trained for cockfighting. While cockfighting is illegal in many countries, its origins can be traced back to Greece where it was to stimulate warriors preparing for battle [2]. It was likely adopted from ancient Persia but many believe that its origins are rather from South-East Asia [2]. This pastime spread to Europe and England during the Middle Ages. It was brought to America by the English colonists. A Spanish variant of cockfighting was also introduced by Spanish settlers in the south-western United States. This Latino variant of cockfighting spread along migration routes from recent immigrants from Mexico and Central America [2].

Gamebird Medicine and Management, First Edition. Edited by Teresa Y. Morishita and Robert E. Porter, Jr.
© 2023 John Wiley & Sons, Inc. Published 2023 by John Wiley & Sons, Inc.

Because cockfighting is illegal, it is unfortunate that the term *gamebird* has a connotation with the illegal activity of game fowl and/or game cocks. Hence, it is extremely important to use the correct terminology. Many gamebird breeders want to ensure that the gamebird industry is not affiliated with illegal cockfighting activity so it is important to use the correct terminology.

While humans primarily hunted gamebirds, other closely related species that were hunted for game initially were also easily domesticated, including landfowl (chickens and turkeys) and waterfowl (ducks and geese). These birds were easily domesticated due to their docile nature, and they could be raised in large numbers to provide a constant supply of food for the home. Domestic fowl (birds) raised for meat and/or eggs are often referred to the collective term *poultry* [3]. The definition of *poultry* is any domesticated bird raised in captivity for meat, eggs, and feathers [3]. The word *poultry* originated in the late fourteenth century from *pultry*, a place where poultry is sold, from the thirteenth century Old French term *pouletrie* or "domestic fowl" [3]. In the broadest sense, gamebirds such as quail and pheasants that are commercially raised for meat and/or eggs can also be seen as part of the poultry industry but many such producers prefer to be called gamebird producers rather than poultry producers.

As humans depended less on subsistence hunting for food and agricultural farming became the predominant way of life, the domestication of poultry took place. The chicken and turkey, because of their docile nature, were now kept in larger numbers. As advances were made in raising birds in captivity, some gamebirds could also now be raised in captivity in large numbers, leading to the development of the modern gamebird industry.

According to the Agricultural Marketing Resource Center [4], gamebirds are either native or non-native birds that were historically either wild game or decorative fowl. Most of these birds are now raised commercially for their meat or eggs. Others are known as "flight-ready" which means that they are released on hunting preserves or by state wildlife agencies. In this book, only gamebirds of the Galliformes order will be discussed, including guinea fowl, partridge, peacocks, pheasants, and quail. While the wild turkey is a gamebird and belongs to the Galliformes order, it is not raised commercially, and diseases of turkeys are discussed in books covering the common domesticated turkey. Other orders that can be considered gamebirds are pigeons, including squabs, and doves (Columbiformes), and swans, geese, and ducks (Anseriformes).

Galliformes gamebirds are unique as some are raised as flight ready, such as pheasants, partridges, and quail, while the majority are ornamental and raised for the exhibition or hobby market [5].

1.2   Birds as Game

The concept of hunting birds is as old as the history of humankind [5, 6]. Hunting involved the seeking, pursuing, and killing of game. Hunting for birds and other animals was a means of survival to provide food for self, family, and the community. Throughout the world, different trapping methods were developed to capture birds, utilizing their entire bodies for meat for food, feathers for clothing, decorations and bedding material, and bones for tools. Every part of the bird was fully utilized.

Not only have humans hunted birds for food, but some Galliformes were eventually captured and domesticated, including the chicken and turkey. Those that were not as easily domesticated remained in the free-living state of forests and grasslands where they continued to be hunted. However, with increasing habitat destruction due to deforestation for farming and other agricultural purposes, the numbers of gamebirds have dwindled with resultant population declines. With these declines came conservation programs, some of the most successful being the greater prairie chicken of the great plains of the United States. Throughout history, gamebirds have been present [5].

Early documentation of hunting birds is found in all continents. The initial tools of hunting included sticks and stones, which later developed into specifically shaped clubs and throwing sticks [6]. Later, sharpened stone, bone, or metal were added to improve killing efficiency and effectiveness, as seen with the use of bows and arrows. Blowpipes or blow guns with poison darts were efficient for mammals as targets were larger. Because birds were smaller, such methods were only effective for the highly skilled hunter. Other techniques used during the hunt included camouflage to get the hunter as close to the prey as possible.

As agricultural production increased and the hunter mode of living decreased, the idea of hunting continued for different reasons. These reasons included the social activity aspect which gained prestige since land was only owned by individuals of power [6]. Hence, hunting became a sport for the wealthy and those who had time for leisure activity. Hunting has been documented in ancient Egypt with the hunter being a separate social class in society [6]. The use of hawks and falcons for hunting was first documented by the Assyrians before 700 BCE but it may have been established earlier in India and China. The horse was also used for the hunting of larger game but not for gamebirds. The sport of hunting became less popular during the time of the Romans where it was maintained only in the upper class and professionals. However, to the Franks and others of Germanic origin, hunting, especially falconry, and the thrill of the chase remained a popular activity [6].

From the earliest times, a distinction was made between hunting for food and hunting for sport. When hunting for food, the important factor was obtaining the most kills for the least effort [5, 6]. However, hunting for sport had a strict code of conduct based on the standard used by royalty and nobles [6]. For example, a noble taking gamebirds for sport used a falcon but a fowler who earned a living by selling gamebirds was able to use a net. Those who hunted for sport had a code to allow their quarry a fair chance to escape, which lead to the establishment of European game laws. In the sixteenth century, the use of guns in hunting was initiated and this allowed the hunter to kill from farther distances [6].

In North America, European settlers and explorers found a multitude of game, including gamebirds such as the wild turkey and waterfowl. Unfortunately, this was associated with uncontrolled hunting, as in the extermination of the passenger pigeon, and laws establishing kill limits and licensures were required for hunters. Hunting fees could then be used to provide revenue to promote the replenishment of stock. It should be noted that it was hunting that motivated the initiation of wildlife conservation [5, 6].

The basic methods of sport hunting are stalking, still-hunting, tracking, driving, sitting up and calling. While stalking, still-hunting, and tracking are used for large mammalian quarry, gamebirds and other landfowl usually go into cover and must be driven out into the open. Driving, also known as beating, the quarry out into the open can be done with the help of people or dogs [6]. The term *beating about the bush* had its origin in gamebird hunting, meaning to flush birds out of bush cover. This is in contrast to hunting waterfowl, which is performed via the sitting-up method, where a hunter is usually concealed in blinds, and is used for waterfowl with or without calling.

Since the times of the ancient Egyptians, dogs have been used for hunting gamebirds. Spaniels, setters, and pointers, which hunt by scent and sight, were called gun dogs as they retrieved the shot birds but also located birds for the hunters and flushed them out while the hunter was in the shooting position [6]. Shotguns were used for shooting waterfowl and gamebirds due to the possibility to kill multiple small quarry rather than using a single shot. Modern-day reserves try to recreate this type of hunting for sports enthusiasts by stocking birds raised under intensive conditions but still maintain their wild behaviors necessary for survival in the free-living state.

1.3 The "Professionalization" of the United States Gamebird Industry

The modern era of the gamebird industry began in the 1960s and expanded during the 1970s and 1980s. It was during this time that many farms that had been raising pheasants and quail as more of a hobby operation, sideline or small farm scale expanded into businesses with much greater capacities. But what makes this transition interesting is that this expansion did not come at the expense of the one common attribute that ties these farms together – the fact that businesses that make up the gamebird industry remain almost exclusively family farms. The family gamebird farm existed prior to this period of expansion and persisted during the 1990s when much was written about the loss of family farms in the mainstream media. It continues to thrive today, with many multigenerational farms continuing to expand capacity. Advances and developments in technology, equipment, and animal science covering all aspects of the gamebird business have significantly aided this expansion.

The history of the gamebird industry's trade association, the North American Gamebird Association (NAGA), is woven throughout this story as well. The nation's largest and most prominent gamebird farms underwrite the cost of the association which functions as a clearinghouse for vital information, as the tip of the spear in defending the industry before government, the public relations arm for the gamebird business, and finally as a gathering place where like-minded people can share their experiences in this business.

Despite the continued existence of family-owned and -operated gamebird farms, the gamebird industry has evolved into efficient farms that maximize bird production, improve overall bird health, decrease disease and mortality issues, and most importantly produce a high-quality sporting bird that is sought after by America's sporting public.

1.4 Advances in Disease Prevention and Treatment

A major factor in the successful evolution and expansion of gamebird production has been the ongoing partnership with university veterinary programs and extension programs. This partnership is literally nationwide and features some of the nation's most prestigious universities, including Auburn University, Clemson University, North Carolina State University, The Ohio State University, Pennsylvania State University, Texas A&M University, University of California-Davis, University of Georgia, University of Minnesota, and Washington State University.

Dr Thomas Eleazer was one of the early pioneers of gamebird medicine. Long fascinated with birds, he raised gamebirds as a youth. After completing his undergraduate studies at Clemson University, he earned his Doctor of Veterinary Medicine from the University of Georgia in 1958. After a stint in the US Air Force, Eleazer initially worked on swine disease issues for the North Carolina Department of Agriculture, but soon found that veterinary skills were far more in demand in the poultry business. It was then that he heard about a position at Clemson University and began working with gamebird farms. Over the next 31 years, Eleazar worked with gamebird producers, testing products and treatments that would gain USDA approval. He also worked to get gamebird producers interested in drug trials, understanding that there would need to be a large enough market for them to compel pharmaceutical companies to produce and sell them. Eleazer strongly encouraged gamebird producers to become involved in the USDA's National Poultry Improvement Plan (NPIP) to ensure that other poultry producers would recognize that this smaller, but growing, industry was producing a safe product. Notably, for the first time, gamebird farms now had their own subsection as part of NPIP.

Dr Gary Davis, former Executive Director of the NAGA and the Southeast Gamebird Association, described early breakthroughs for the gamebird industry. Like Eleazer, Davis grew up on a farm and hunted quail at a young age, which led him to the poultry science department at North Carolina State University. Dr Davis became a regular contributor to *Wildlife Harvest*, a trade journal, and often worked with Walter Walker, an extension specialist at Clemson University. Walker had served as the NAGA's Executive Director, and Davis succeeded him in leading the association. During the tenure of Dr Davis, there were marked improvements in disease treatment and prevention as well as gamebird nutrition that helped the industry to grow.

The country's most prominent pheasant and quail producers have long recognized the value of veterinarians and poultry scientists within academia and have relied on them during some of the biggest challenges facing the industry. The value of this collaboration was never more apparent than in 2015 when an outbreak of highly pathogenic avian influenza was spreading across upper midwestern states including Iowa, Missouri, Minnesota, and Wisconsin. The NAGA commissioned its Health Committee to guide the industry's response and recruited some of the nation's top veterinary disease specialists to address the outbreaks. For 3 months, the committee published guidance about disease prevention, identification, reporting, quarantining procedures, and the pathways to receiving compensation and resuming business operations once certified as clean. These published guidelines continue to be refined as the industry faced the avian influenza outbreaks of 2022 which also affected commercial gamebird operations.

1.5 Nutrition Advances Improve Bird Health and Quality

Disease prevention and treatment were not the only focus. Advances in bird nutrition have resulted in improvements in nearly every aspect of the industry. Companies including Star Labs and Dawe's Laboratories have long served as essential partners to farms for these types of products. The nutrition industry itself has greatly evolved, beginning with the post-World War II boom. Over the years, offerings that had previous been produced with naturally occurring vitamin and mineral supplements gave way to synthetically produced products that deliver dependable results. Specific diets are now utilized for different times in bird life cycles, including starter diets, grower diets, finishing or flying diets and maintenance diets for birds that are kept longer. Moreover, the development of breeder diets was a major advance to ensure continued production of hatching eggs for the development for future flocks. These research developments in nutrition now allowed for specific diets for chukar, quail or pheasant, an improvement from the days when all gamebirds were treated the same as chickens or turkeys.

1.6 Equipment Changes Eliminate Losses and Increase Efficiency

During this same period, advances in equipment contributed to make life easier and more profitable for gamebird farms. The industry has long been served by loyal suppliers such as New Jersey's 100+-year-old Kuhl Corporation, which makes everything from large-scale machinery, such as egg washers and feeders, to smaller products such as peepers. The Kuhl family had raised poultry since its beginnings, and Paul R. Kuhl raised gamebirds, which led him to work with the NAGA in the 1950s. In 2007, NAGA members and gamebird producers Troy and Todd Laudenslager created 3T

Products to provide niche equipment for gamebird producers. Drawing on their own needs, the brothers utilized their family gamebird farm as their own research and development laboratory to improve their products which included nets, feeders, crates, and blinders.

All these examples provide yet another area where innovations from NAGA members have improved many aspects of the gamebird industry, including decreasing bird loss, improving bird and egg health and survivability, and preventing predation.

1.7   Gamebird Entrepreneurs

While much emphasis has been devoted to the multigenerational family farms that make up the modern gamebird industry, the other common element of those involved in raising gamebirds is a strong entrepreneurial spirit. These people are problem solvers and risk takers. Gamebird producers have embraced emerging science, such as lighting management to reduce bird injuries and mortality. They learned how to eliminate or mitigate invasive problems such as mold, bacteria, water contamination, and predators. Off the farm, they have learned to navigate the halls of Congress and the labyrinth of government bureaucracies at state and federal levels, working with both agriculture and wildlife agency leaders.

The modern gamebird industry appears to have the best of both worlds. It is a segment of agriculture that remains true to the traditional family farm and remains largely devoid of the corporate atmosphere that permeates much of the agricultural world. Yet at the same time, the industry has evolved to operate as sophisticated businesses capable of meeting the same challenges experienced in the larger livestock industry.

References

1 Harper, D. (2021) Fowl. www.etymonline.com/word/fowl (accessed February 2022).

2 Oklahoma Historical Society (2021) Cockfighting. www.okhistory.org/publications/enc/entry.php?entry=CO012 (accessed February 2022).

3 Harper, D. (2021). Poultry. www.etymonline.com/word/poultry (accessed February 2022).

4 Agricultural Marketing Resource Center (2021) Gamebirds. www.agmrc.org/commodities-products/agritourism/game-birds (accessed February 2022).

5 Woodard, A., Vohra, P., and Denton, V. (1993). *Commercial and Ornamental Gamebird Breeders Handbook*, 19–30. Washington: Handcock House Publishers.

6 Anonymous (2021) Hunting Codes. www.britannica.com/sports/hunting-sport/Hunting-codes (accessed February 2022).

2

Gamebird Laws, Regulations, and the National Poultry Improvement Plan

Elena Behnke

2.1 Introduction

One of the most daunting undertakings in any complex industry associated with live animal production is to understand or, at the very least, to develop a familiarity with laws and regulations in order to ensure a more successful venture. No responsible business owner wants to incur fines or penalties from ignorance or negligence. The gamebird industry is no exception. Familiarity with laws and regulations is an arduous task because it takes time and energy, while demonstrating and documenting necessary steps to comply is an even greater time commitment, sometimes without immediate or even long-term tangible returns or incentive other than potential mitigated risk. Operations investing great amounts of time and money to produce a quality product or experience, and their owners, workers, and affiliates, must recognize the importance of knowing the limits within which facilities may legally operate. Not only can reputations be at stake, but violations of any laws at best may come with a verbal reprimand, fine, or other type of punishment, or at worst, with criminal consequences and/or a dissolution of the business itself.

Currently no central body governs gamebird operations in the United States of America. This reality can be viewed as both desirable and undesirable. It is good in that producers may operate with relative freedom, within reason, and most of the regulatory programs available are voluntary, and will be the major focus of this chapter. However, it may not be ideal in that consistency is not necessarily achievable on a national scale because different states have the ability and authority to manage their gamebird operations as they determine necessary, primarily either through the Department of Natural Resources or the Department of Agriculture or both.

Another consideration when discussing laws and regulatory aspects for the gamebird industry is that the intended purpose of the birds may lead producers down different paths for ensuring compliance with regulations. For instance, raised-for-release operations that primarily cater to hunters will have a different set of objectives and hence, potentially, a different set of regulations, from niche markets raising specialty birds for the purpose of meat or egg consumption. In this example, a gamebird meat processing plant will want to consider the benefits of having a facility that is inspected by the United States Department of Agriculture's Food Safety and Inspection Service (USDA-FSIS). This entity keeps a directory of meat, poultry, and egg inspection locations, with establishment

Gamebird Medicine and Management, First Edition. Edited by Teresa Y. Morishita and Robert E. Porter, Jr.
© 2023 John Wiley & Sons, Inc. Published 2023 by John Wiley & Sons, Inc.

number, location, phone and date granted (www.fsis.usda.gov/inspection/establishments/meat-poultry-and-egg-product-inspection-directory). Similarly, producers raising shell eggs for human consumption may need to familiarize themselves with the Food and Drug Administration (FDA) Egg Safety Rule, if they raise over a certain number of birds (www.fda.gov/food/eggs-guidance-documents-regulatory-information/egg-safety-final-rule).

While these entities are worthy of investigation for producers using their birds for the purpose of either meat or egg production, they will be of little value for the hunting preserve enthusiast, whose business focus is on hatching, breeding, and/or dealing with the terminal purpose of releasing birds. In the raise-for-release category, a gamebird producer may need to become more familiar with the Environmental Protection Agency (EPA) guidelines on establishing an erosion prevention and sediment control plan. Some states may require additional measures related to land usage, such that facilities that have animals which produce manure or apply manure to crop fields and pastures are required to have a written manure management plan.

Perhaps the most important lesson to be learned when engaging in the discussion of regulatory practices common in the gamebird industry is that laws, regulations, and ordinances vary widely by state and by region. Aside from the intended bird purpose governing which regulatory body may need to be consulted, the producer must take responsibility to contact his or her state and local authorities within the particular region where the business and birds are located in order to be successful in compliance. Additionally, because regulations are fluid and subject to change, the ongoing work of not only mastering an understanding of current applicable regulation but also staying up to date with any changes is part of the responsible gamebird owner's job. Several resources, however, such as the North American Gamebird Association, may be able to offer assistance in navigating the realm of rules. This organization may be a great place to consider starting in order to obtain pertinent information with appropriate contacts.

The remainder of the chapter will focus on another tremendous resource for the gamebird industry, which is the USDA National Poultry Improvement Plan (NPIP) and its voluntary programs. This organization is the one exception to the aforementioned lack of a central body governing gamebird operations in the United States. The NPIP is not truly a regulatory or governing body but its very essence is cooperative in nature, with a variety of groups and their collaborative efforts ensuring that it has been and continues to be a highly successful and extremely valuable program for the purposes of trade and movement of birds and bird products.

2.2 The National Poultry Improvement Plan

The National Poultry Improvement Plan, established in 1935, is a cooperative industry, state and Federal program for controlling certain poultry diseases. Its mission is to provide a cooperative program through which new diagnostic technology can be effectively applied for the improvement of poultry and poultry products throughout the country. The plan traces its roots to the early 1900s as it was responsible for the successful eradication of pullorum disease, a serious poultry disease caused by the organism *Salmonella pullorum*, which could be vertically transmitted from hen to egg. Pullorum disease was severely limiting the expansion of the rapidly growing poultry industry in the early part of the twentieth century. Pullorum disease, also known as white bacillary diarrhea, could cause greater than 80% mortality in baby poultry. Because the disease wreaked havoc on the ability of the poultry industry to continue expanding, an act of Congress based on recommendations from the International Baby Chick Association established the National Poultry Improvement Plan.

(a) 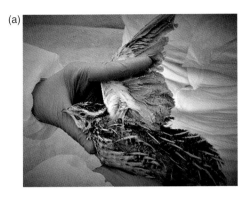 (b)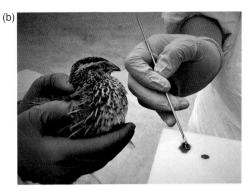

Figure 2.1 (a and b) Pullorum-typhoid testing a quail using stained antigen plate agglutination. The whole blood stained antigen rapid agglutination test, which is very effective, has not changed much in NPIP's history.

Over the years, the program has expanded to include other disease programs for *Salmonella*, *Mycoplasma*, low pathogenic avian influenza and, as of November 2020, Newcastle disease as well. Participants voluntarily sign up, and the program certifies states, flocks, hatcheries, dealers, and slaughter plants that meet disease control standards proven through testing, monitoring, and surveillance programs specified in the unique NPIP classifications (Figure 2.1).

The program is managed at state level, in which an official body administers the program. This body can be affiliated with a university, an NPIP authorized laboratory that conducts poultry testing, a state veterinarian's office, a Department of Agriculture or a poultry federation, to name a few. This entity is designated the Official State Agency. The Official State Agencies enter into Memoranda of Understanding, or MOU, with the USDA in order to carry out the provisions of the NPIP, which are the set of program rules located within Title 9 of the Code of Federal Regulations, Parts 145, 146, 147 and 56 as well as the NPIP Program Standards. The website www.poultryimprovement .org provides links to these rules and program specifications.

Within the NPIP provisions, certain classifications can be earned dependent on bird type. For example, in Part 145, currently the NPIP has nine subparts, each representing a different category of breeding poultry. Part 146 currently represents four categories of commercial poultry. Combined, there are 13 subparts, each with program descriptions for different testing regimes and certifications that can be earned specific to that particular subpart or bird type. Bear in mind that the NPIP began with the chicken breeding industry. In order to eradicate pullorum disease, efforts focused initially on a test and remove scheme. Later, as the program grew, it began to shift its focus onto certification of clean status. The chicken portion eventually merged with the National Turkey Improvement Plan in the 1950s. The NPIP was also originally a part of the USDA's Agricultural Research Service, or ARS, before becoming incorporated into the USDA's Animal and Plant Health Inspection Service agency. The first appearance of a Subpart E occurred in the early 1970s. This category represented not only gamebirds but also waterfowl, exhibition, and backyard poultry.

A primary factor in the NPIP's success is the event that occurs every 2 years, referred to as the Biennial Conference. These conferences bring together Official State Agencies, NPIP authorized laboratories, and official delegates that represent each of the 13 subparts within the program. These groups come together to review the proposed changes to the NPIP provisions found in Title 9 Code of Federal Regulations and the Program Standards, with the delegates' official vote as a key outcome from each conference. In the months leading up to the Biennial Conference, technical experts and poultry health experts in academia, government, and industry evaluate the proposed changes for

Table 2.1   Differences in Subpart E testing and Subpart J testing. For H5/H7 AI Clean, the programs vary in frequency of testing.

Disease classification	Subpart E	Subpart J
Pullorum-Typhoid Clean	Must be met before other classifications	Must be met before other classifications
H5/H7 AI Clean	30 every 180 days	30 every 90 days
Salmonella Monitored	Minimum of 5 environmental samples from the hatchery every 30 days	Minimum of 5 environmental samples from the hatchery every 30 days

their scientific merit. These experts then share their opinions, and the delegation discusses, debates, and votes on whether to accept, reject or modify the original proposals. The outcome is a critical component for the future direction of surveillance programs for *Salmonella*, *Mycoplasma*, avian influenza and Newcastle disease. The proposals that pass are then sent through the NPIP national office through regulatory and legalistic writing departments to codify the adopted segments, which are then published in the next version of the provisions, which is referred to as the Final Rule and can be accessed in the Federal Register online or through print copies. The Program Standards are also ratified and published.

At the time this chapter went to press, the most recent Final Rule that was published on October 5, 2020 contains the proposed changes that were voted on by the delegation and passed at the NPIP's 44th Biennial Conference in Franklin, TN, in 2018. Overall, this Final Rule incorporates 20 distinct changes from the conference, and the three biggest changes include the addition of a Newcastle Disease Clean Program and Newcastle Disease Clean Compartment Program, clarifications of regulations on low pathogenic avian influenza indemnity and compensation, and, importantly for this chapter, the creation of a new Subpart J for the gamebird industry.

The fact that the definitions and provisions within Subpart E did not really match the production methods and end uses for the gamebird industry led to a lot of confusion and frustration. Over time, gamebird producers expressed concerns that the size, complexity, and uniqueness of their industry indeed warranted separation from the hobby and exhibition poultry industry. This new separation now permits a distinction in gamebird testing protocols and classifications from other hobbyist, exhibitionist, and backyard flock testing. The newly created Subpart J allows the gamebird industry – the quail, partridge, pheasant, grouse and guinea fowl producers – to tailor their NPIP programs to meet their specific needs. Another important distinction that Subpart J allows for is clarification of terms. Those less familiar with the gamebird industry have at times conflated the terms "gamebird" and "gamefowl" or believed the terms to be synonymous. These mistakes occurred with regular frequency, in part enhanced by the fact that gamebird participants were combined into Subpart E with other athletic and ornamental birds that could more appropriately be labeled "gamefowl." Now that Subpart J has been created, less confusion should arise as Subpart J signifies with clarity that gamebirds, and not gamefowl, are the participants. Finally, Table 2.1 demonstrates that the requirements for H5/H7 AI testing for Subpart J are now more stringent than those requirements for Subpart E participants in terms of frequency of testing.

The advantages of participation are many. To begin with, participation in the NPIP can directly benefit producers in domestic movement of birds and bird products. Most states require that poultry imported across their state borders meet certain disease classification standards, which NPIP participation may satisfy. For example, states that require a pullorum test for entry may accept NPIP participants in lieu of a pullorum-typhoid test because the foundational requirement for participation includes demonstrating freedom from pullorum-typhoid by earning the Pullorum-Typhoid Clean classification. The Veterinary Services or VS 9-3 form (Report of Sales of Hatching Eggs, Chicks, and Poults), which is commonly referred to within NPIP as the "movement form," is an important part of documenting that birds and bird products that have met certain specifications and hold classifications deemed necessary by the importing state are transported correctly across state lines. The NPIP website keeps a directory of state importation requirements that can be accessed at www.poultryimprovement.org/documents/RequirementContactNumber .pdf. Once again, an important thing to note is that not all states require the use of a VS 9-3 form, and some states require permits or other documentation in addition to or in place of a VS 9-3 form; therefore, it is always best to call the state into which the birds will be moving to ensure that the requirements are met prior to that movement.

An indirect benefit of gamebird participation is associated with international movement. A VS 17-6 form (Movement of Poultry, Eggs, and Day Old Chicks) has a category for PT Clean. Also, many producers choose to type AI Clean or H5/H7 AI Clean in the box "Other," provided that the participant holds that categorization as well. Participation in the NPIP is highly respected and recognized as the gold standard and the minimum expected requirement for importation in many countries around the globe.

Besides movement of poultry, another advantage of NPIP participation is the reputation that the program carries for demonstrating freedom from certain diseases. Frequently potential buyers are encouraged to purchase from a clean source, or one in which the origins can be easily traced. NPIP participation again provides this structure by offering programs such as the Salmonella Monitored program that focuses on hatchery sanitation and efforts to reduce salmonella.

Finally, a major benefit of NPIP participation is offered through the H5/H7 Avian Influenza Clean program for gamebirds as well as the 14 Biosecurity Points program. The low pathogenic avian influenza programs have been in place since the 1990s and 2000s. For 6 months from December 2014 to June 2015, the United States suffered from the largest animal health emergency due to highly pathogenic avian influenza. More than 200 cases were documented in commercial and backyard poultry as well as wild birds, spread across the country but mostly concentrated in the upper Midwest. The event cost nearly $1 billion and 50 million birds were lost. In response to this catastrophic event, APHIS partnered with NPIP and the poultry industry to develop what are now referred to as the NPIP 14 Biosecurity Points. These points took nearly a year to develop and were discussed, debated, and voted on to adopt into the Program Standards at the 43rd Biennial Conference in Bellevue, WA.

Avian influenza is a constant threat to all poultry operations within the US and gamebird operations, even with extreme vigilance, are still vulnerable. A benefit of being an NPIP gamebird participant is indemnification eligibility. Should an avian influenza event strike a production facility, producers who are routinely testing for avian influenza and those that successfully document having a biosecurity plan in place, and that that plan was being followed at the time of an outbreak, are eligible to receive federal money for lost birds or eggs as well as compensation costs for cleaning and disinfection premises that have been contaminated and costs to defray activities associated with virus elimination. Having this safety net available if needed is a huge incentive and a reason that all gamebird producers should consider NPIP participation. Although participation does not guarantee that avian influenza will not strike, being a participant is an insurance plan of sorts, as the risks without it may lead to potential destruction of producers' livelihoods.

The NPIP will continue to evolve. Over the last 50 years, many changes have been made within the programs, with more changes on the horizon at each Biennial Conference. Active involvement at the Biennial Conferences is also a way for the gamebird industry to continue participating and adjusting to changes as industry dynamics change. The NPIP's General Conference Committee is an official federal advisory committee to the Secretary of Agriculture on matters pertaining to poultry health. The NPIP's Biennial Conference serves as the platform for participants to interact with this elected group of poultry experts and continue to raise concerns and issues which threaten their industry. Gamebird producers can benefit from forming relationships with their Official State Agents, who in turn can instruct them on things needed to enroll in the NPIP and become involved at the Biennial Conferences. The national office in Conyers, GA, can also be contacted for further information.

Additional References

Food and Drug Administration, https://www.fda.gov/food/eggs-guidance-documents-regulatory-information/egg-safety-final-rule. Accessed 6 November 2021.

Food Safety and Inspection Service, https://www.fsis.usda.gov/shared/PDF/MPI_Directory_Establishment_Name.pdf. Accessed 6 November 2020.

National Poultry Improvement Plan. www.poultryimprovement.org. Accessed 6 November 2020.

3

Galliformes: Species, Varieties, and Behavior
Gen Anderson and Chris Holmes

3.1 Introduction

Galliformes are robust, ground-dwelling birds with stubby, rounded wings adapted for short flights versus long distance dispersal. They are found nearly globally in a diverse variety of terrestrial habitats such as the ptarmigan (*Lagopus* sp.) living within the Arctic Circle, the cloud forest-residing horned guan (*Oreophasis derbianus*), and the desert-loving vulturine guineafowl (*Acryllium vulturinum*). Galliformes generally have a rotund body shape with stout legs and an anisodactyl toe arrangement ideal for scratching around in substrate, and are sexually dimorphic. Many species roost arboreally at night for safety. They typically are opportunistic omnivores, foraging on the ground for invertebrates, seeds, fallen fruits, tender leaves, and tubers. They serve an important role in the ecosystem as seed dispersers. Many species are highly valued economically for hunting and as a food source. Aside from humans, Galliformes are heavily preyed upon by most terrestrial carnivores.

3.2 Domestication and Hybridization

Multiple species within the order Galliformes have been domesticated for cockfighting, ornamental display and to supply meat, eggs, and feathers. Examples include helmeted guineafowl, Indian peafowl, wild turkey, bobwhite quail and the domestic chicken [1]. Recent genome sequencing analysis points to the red junglefowl, *Gallus g. spadiceus*, of China, Thailand and Myanmar as the primary source of origin for domestic chicken populations. The species split occurred roughly 9500 (±3300) years ago, with the domestication process progressing during the Holocene period. Wild populations of other *Gallus* species and subspecies have hybridized incrementally with free-ranging domestic birds [2]. Hundreds of chicken breeds are recognized worldwide. They are often used in zoological parks as animal ambassadors, for natural pest control, and incubation and rearing of exotic Galliformes when appropriate [1].

Gamebird Medicine and Management, First Edition. Edited by Teresa Y. Morishita and Robert E. Porter, Jr.
© 2023 John Wiley & Sons, Inc. Published 2023 by John Wiley & Sons, Inc.

Hybridization across species and color morphs within species of the Phasianidae family are abundant in private aviculture. Many were accidental crossings, but some were encouraged to increase ornamental appeal or economic profit through meat and egg production. Crossings of golden and Lady Amherst pheasants (*Chrysolophus pictus x amherstiae*) are far too common and unfortunately produce fertile offspring. Responsible breeders attempt to locate wild-type birds, but pure species of either of these are few and far between. Golden pheasants have historically also been crossed with silver (*Lophura nycthemera*) and ring-necked pheasants. Tragopan hens of differing species look nearly identical and have resulted in the production of hybrids by many a well-intentioned aviculturist. Vietnam pheasants (*Lophura edwardsi*) were historically hybridized with *L. nycthemera* and Swinhoe's pheasant (*Lophura swinhoii*). Indian and green peafowl crosses (*Pavo cristatus x muticus*) produce fertile hybrids referred to as Spalding peafowl. Domestic chickens, guineafowl, and other pheasant species are unfortunately still intentionally crossbred to this day [3].

3.3 Systematics

The taxonomic and phylogenetic relationships within the Galliformes order have been studied by numerous researchers, but remain debated and ever evolving. Referenced publications for this chapter analyze data from mitochondrial and nuclear DNA, known fossil calibrations, region of origin, and/or morphological characteristics. Dissimilar chronological results differ due to sample set variations, fossil placement, amount of data used, taxonomic sample sizes, mitochondrial vs nuclear data, etc. [4].

The ancestral Galloanserae (fowl clade) is universally accepted to have split into Galliformes and Anseriformes during the Cretaceous period roughly 76 million years ago [9]. The Cretaceous-Paleogene (K-Pg) mass extinction 66 million years ago devastated >75% of the planet's flora and fauna, including dinosaurs, arboreal vertebrates, and forests. Few avian species survived but among them were ground-dwelling birds, including Galloanserae and Palaeognathae (ratites), that went through massive adaptive radiation in the Paleogene period, resulting in the modern birds found today [5]. Jiang et al. estimated the family divergence of modern Galliformes to have occurred over 16–28 myr [6].

Cornell Lab of Ornithology's Birds of the World (BOW) was selected to use as the most up-to-date taxonomic source. This online resource was recently developed using a combination of *The Handbook of the Birds of the World Alive* (HBW Alive), *Birds of North America*, and *Neotropical Birds*. The following editorial note is stated: "Due to the merger of content from various sources, especially related to differing taxonomies, there are cases where the written text does not perfectly match up with the current taxonomy, or in the worst cases the two may contradict each other" [7]. Every effort has been made to use the most current accepted taxonomy here for reference. Differing taxonomies result from lumping species or subspecies into larger groups or splitting them into multiple small groups.

The living order Galliformes consists of two suborders, five families and 295 total species (Figure 3.1). The suborder Cracii is further divided into Megapodiidae (the megapodes, 22 species) and Cracidae (the chachalacas, guans, and curassows, 54 species). The suborder Phasiani is divided into Odontophoridae (the New World quails, 33 species), Numididae (the guineafowl, six species), and Phasianidae (pheasants, partridges, turkeys, and grouse, 180 species) [8].

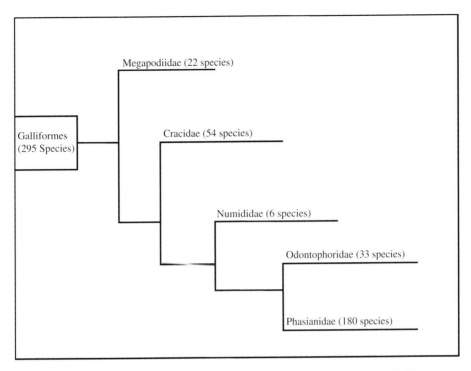

Figure 3.1   Galliformes cladogram displaying the relationships among families of the Galliformes. The taxonomic and phylogenetic relationships within this order remain debated and ever evolving.

3.4   Megapodiidae – Megapodes

This unusual family of extant Gallifomes contains 22 species within seven genera (Table 3.1). Morphologically large, stout birds from Australasian primarily inhabiting lowland tropical forests with the exception of the arid-adapted malleefowl. Numerous species are island endemics. Their reproductive techniques are unique in Aves, constructing nest mounds or burrows that depend on heat produced by the breakdown of organic material, geothermal sources or solar power for egg incubation. Lacking an eggtooth, the hatchlings burst out of their shells using powerfully kicking feet. Young are superprecocial, requiring no parental care, and fly away shortly after hatch [7].

Megapodiidae are estimated to have diverged during the late Cretaceous, around 66.8 million years ago (mya) [9] before increasing diversification around the Eocene–Oligocene period transition 33.9 mya [4]. They are a sister clade to Cracidae [6]. More species have gone extinct than exist today. Judging by fossil records, known extinctions and species sympatry preference, 45–55 species of Megapodes are presumed to have existed historically prior to human impact caused by colonization of Oceania during the past several millennia [10].

Per the Species360 Zoological Information Management System (ZIMS), few megapode species are managed in aviculture and none in genetically sustainable population sizes. The maleo (*Macrocephalon maleo*) (Figure 3.2) and Australian brush turkey (*Alectura lathami*) represent most of the birds in aviculture. Malleefowl (*Leipoa ocellata*) and a single Niuafoou scrub fowl (*Megapodius pritchardii*) are also maintained in insignificant numbers [11].

Table 3.1   Megapodiidae family with genera.

Family	Genus	Common name	Latin name	Number of subspecies	Described by	Date
Megapodiidae	*Alectura*	Australian brush turkey	*Alectura lathami*	2	J.E. Gray	1831
	Aepypodius	Wattled brush turkey	*Aepypodius arfakianus*	2	Salvadori	1877
		Waigeo brush turkey	*Aepypodius bruijnii*	Monotypic	Oustalet	1880
	Talegalla	Red-billed brush turkey	*Talegalla cuvieri*	2	Lesson	1828
		Yellow-billed brush turkey	*Talegalla fuscirostris*	4	Salvadori	1877
		Red-legged brush turkey	*Talegalla jobiensis*	2	A.B. Meyer	1874
	Leipoa	Malleefowl	*Leipoa ocellata*	Monotypic	Gould	1840
	Macrocephalon	Maleo	*Macrocephalon maleo*	Monotypic	S. Müller	1846
	Eulipoa	Moluccan scrubfowl	*Eulipoa wallacei*	Monotypic	G.R. Gray	1861
	Megapodius	Niuafoou scrubfowl	*Megapodius pritchardii*	Monotypic	G.R. Gray	1864
		Micronesian scrubfowl	*Megapodius laperouse*	2	Gaimard	1823
		Nicobar scrubfowl	*Megapodius nicobariensis*	2	Blyth	1846
		Tabon scrubfowl	*Megapodius cumingii*	7	Dillwyn	1853
		Sula scrubfowl	*Megapodius bernsteinii*	Monotypic	Schlegal	1866
		Tanimbar scrubfowl	*Megapodius tenimberensis*	Monotypic	P.L. Sclater	1883
		Dusky scrubfowl	*Megapodius freycinet*	3	Gaimard	1823
		Biak scrubfowl	*Megapodius geelvinkianus*	Monotypic	A.B. Meyer	1874
		Forsten's scrubfowl	*Megapodius forsteni*	2	G.R. Gray	1847
		Melanesian scrubfowl	*Megapodius eremita*	Monotypic	Hartlaub	1866
		Vanuatu scrubfowl	*Megapodius layardi*	Monotypic	Tristram	1879
		New Guinea scrubfowl	*Megapodius decollatus*	Monotypic	Oustalet	1878
		Orange-footed scrubfowl	*Megapodius reinwardt*	5	Dumont de Sainte Croix	1823

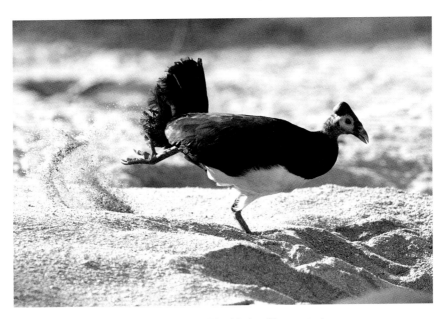

Figure 3.2 Maleo (*Macrocephalon maleo*). Source: Riza Marlon/Shutterstock.

3.5 Cracidae – Guans, Chachalacas, Curassows

Residing only in the New World, the chachalacas, guans, and curassows include 54 species in 11 genera (Table 3.2, Figure 3.3). Shared characteristics for this family include larger, heavy-bodied birds typically with elaborate head adornments in the form of crests, horns, wattles or casques. Though their wings are short and round, similar to other Galliformes, the tails of cracids are long and they are capable of strong flight. Prominent vocalizations include booming, hums, rattles, clucks, yelps, and whistles [7].

Cracidae are one of the earliest diverging families along with sister clade Megapodiidae, which together are sister clades to Numididae [6, 9]. Cracidae diverged either immediately prior to the Cretaceous–Paleogene boundary or in the early Paleogene 50–60 mya. All remaining Galliformes divergences occurred during the Paleogene period [9]. Early fossil records pointed to origins in North America when the region was tropical. Expansion into Central and South America occurred as ancient climates changed [12]. On the other hand, using a combination of mitochondrial and nuclear data with fossil calibrations, ancestral origins point to South America or dispersal from Africa when those continents were much closer than at present [9].

Cracids are fairly common in aviculture, though none of the species can be found in robust population sizes. In North America, most *Crax* sp. are maintained, but primarily only one guan species, the crested guan (*Penelope purpurascens*). All piping guan species (*Pipile* sp.) are extremely common in aviculture. Chaco chachalacas (*Ortalis canicollis*) are in greater numbers in Europe, but also are managed in the United States in very small numbers along with the plain chachalaca (*Ortalis vetula*). The distinctive horned guan (*O. derbianus*) and blue-billed curassows (*Crax alberti*) are only found within American Association of Zoos and Aquariums (AZA)-accredited zoological parks [11].

Table 3.2 Cracidae family with genera.

Family	Genus	Common name	Latin name	Number of subspecies	Described by	Date
Cracidae	*Ortalis*	Plain chachalaca	*Ortalis vetula*	4	Wagler	1830
		Gray-headed chachalaca	*Ortalis cinereiceps*	Monotypic	G.R. Gray	1867
		Chestnut-winged chachalaca	*Ortalis garrula*	Monotypic	Humboldt	1805
		Rufous-vented chachalaca	*Ortalis ruficauda*	2	Jardine	1847
		Rufous-headed chachalaca	*Ortalis erythroptera*	Monotypic	P.L. Sclater & Salvin	1870
		Rufous-bellied chachalaca	*Ortalis wagleri*	Monotypic	G.R. Gray	1867
		West Mexican chachalaca	*Ortalis poliocephala*	Monotypic	Wagler	1830
		Chaco chachalaca	*Ortalis canicollis*	2	Wagler	1830
		White-bellied chachalaca	*Ortalis leucogastra*	Monotypic	Gould	1843
		Colombian chachalaca	*Ortalis columbiana*	Monotypic	Hellmayr	1906
		Speckled chachalaca	*Ortalis guttata*	3	Spix	1825
		East Brazilian chachalaca	*Ortalis araucuan*	Monotypic	Spix	1825
		Scaled chachalaca	*Ortalis squamata*	Monotypic	Lesson	1829
		Variable chachalaca	*Ortalis motmot*	2	Linnaeus	1766
		Buff-browed chachalaca	*Ortalis superciliaris*	Monotypic	G.R. Gray	1867
	Penelope	Band-tailed guan	*Penelope argyrotis*	3	Bonaparte	1856
		Bearded guan	*Penelope barbata*	Monotypic	Chapman	1921
		Baudo guan	*Penelope ortoni*	Monotypic	Salvin	1874
		Andean guan	*Penelope montagnii*	5	Bonaparte	1856
		Marail guan	*Penelope marail*	2	Statius Müller	1776
		Rusty-margined guan	*Penelope superciliaris*	3	Temminck	1815
		Red-faced guan	*Penelope dabbenei*	Monotypic	Hellmayr & Conover	1942
		Spix's guan	*Penelope jacquacu*	4	Spix	1825
		Crested guan	*Penelope purpurascens*	3	Wagler	1830
		Cauca guan	*Penelope perspicax*	Monotypic	Bangs	1911
		White-winged guan	*Penelope albipennis*	Monotypic	Taczanowski	1878
		Dusky-legged guan	*Penelope obscura*	3	Temminck	1815

Table 3.2 (Continued)

Family	Genus	Common name	Latin name	Number of subspecies	Described by	Date
		White-crested guan	*Penelope pileata*	Monotypic	Wagler	1830
		Chestnut-bellied guan	*Penelope ochrogaster*	Monotypic	Pelzeln	1870
		White-browed guan	*Penelope jacucaca*	Monotypic	Spix	1825
	Pipile	Trinidad piping-guan	*Pipile pipile*	Monotypic	Jacquin	1784
		Blue-throated piping-guan	*Pipile cumanensis*	2	Jacquin	1784
		Red-throated piping-guan	*Pipile cujubi*	2	Pelzeln	1858
		Black-fronted piping-guan	*Pipile jacutinga*	Monotypic	Spix	1825
	Aburria	Wattled guan	*Aburria aburri*	Monotypic	Lesson	1828
	Chamaepetes	Black guan	*Chamaepetes unicolor*	Monotypic	Salvin	1867
		Sickle-winged guan	*Chamaepetes goudotii*	5	Lesson	1828
	Penelopina	Highland guan	*Penelopina nigra*	Monotypic	Fraser	1852
	Oreophasis	Horned guan	*Oreophasis derbianus*	Monotypic	G.R. Gray	1844
	Nothocrax	Nocturnal curassow	*Nothocrax urumutum*	Monotypic	Spix	1825
	Mitu	Crestless curassow	*Mitu tomentosa*	Monotypic	Spix	1825
		Salvin's curassow	*Mitu salvini*	Monotypic	Reinhardt	1879
		Razor-billed curassow	*Mitu tuberosa*	Monotypic	Spix	1825
		Alagoas curassow	*Mitu mitu*	Monotypic	Linnaeus	1766
	Pauxi	Helmeted curassow	*Pauxi pauxi*	2	Linnaeus	1766
		Sira curassow	*Pauxi koepckeae*	Monotypic	Weske & Terborgh	1971
		Horned curassow	*Pauxi unicornis*	Monotypic	J. Bond & Meyer de Schauensee	1939
	Crax	Great curassow	*Crax rubra*	2	Linnaeus	1758
		Blue-billed curassow	*Crax alberti*	Monotypic	Fraser	1850
		Yellow-knobbed curassow	*Crax daubentoni*	Monotypic	G.R. Gray	1867
		Black curassow	*Crax alector*	2	Linnaeus	1766
		Wattled curassow	*Crax globulosa*	Monotypic	Spix	1825
		Bare-faced curassow	*Crax fasciolata*	3	Spix	1825
		Red-billed curassow	*Crax blumenbachii*	Monotypic	Spix	1825

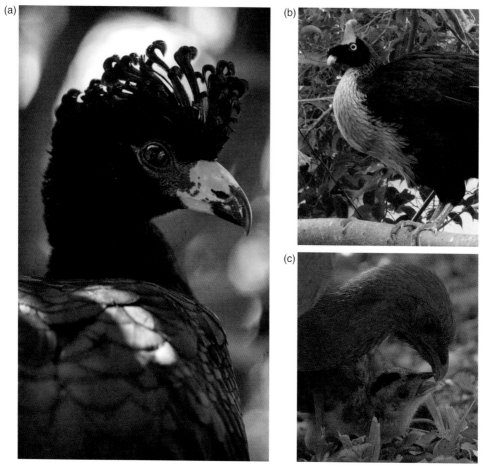

Figure 3.3   Cracidae. (a) Wattled curassow (*Crax globulosa*) hen. Source: Carolyn Atherton, Audubon Zoo. (b) Horned guan (*Oreophasis derbianus*). Source: JoEllen Toler, St Louis Zoo. (c) Plain chachalaca (*Ortalis vetula*). Source: Charles Alexander, Gladys Porter Zoo.

3.6   Numididae – Guineafowl

Composed of four genera and six species, this is one of the smallest Galliformes family groups (Table 3.3, Figure 3.4). All species reside in coastal and sub-Saharan Africa. Shared characteristics within Numididae typically include dark plumage with boldly distinctive spots and/or stripes. These taxa display brightly colored heads and facial wattles. All species are sexually monomorphic. Guineafowl were historically classified in Phasianidae, but were broken out by molecular phylogenetic studies [7].

Numididae diverged an estimated 45 million years ago in the Paleogene, although numerous phylogenetic trees have been developed and vary in time frame, but the geologic period is consistent [9]. The ancestral origin of the superfamilial clade (Numididae, Odontophoridae, and Phasianidae) may have been in Africa due to common geographic distribution patterns between the families [4].

Table 3.3   Numidae family with genera.

Family	Genus	Common name	Latin name	Number of subspecies	Described by	Date
Numididae	*Numida*	Helemeted guineafowl	*Numida meleagris*	9	Linnaeus	1758
	Agelastes	White-breasted guineafowl	*Agelastes meleagrides*	Monotypic	Bonaparte	1850
		Black guineafowl	*Agelastes niger*	Monotypic	Cassin	1857
	Acryllium	Vulturine guineafowl	*Acryllium vulturinum*	Monotypic	Hardwicke	1834
	Guttera	Plummed guineafowl	*Guttera plumifera*	2	Cassin	1857
		Crested guineafowl	*Guttera pucherani*	5	Hartlaub	1860

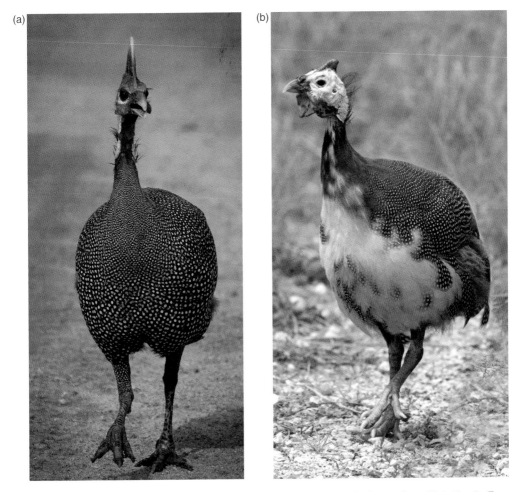

(a)   (b)

Figure 3.4   Helmeted guineafowl (*Numida meleagris*). (a) Wild form on left. Source: Larry Mah, Topeka Zoo & Conservation Center. (b) Domestic color morph form on right. Source: Karel Bock/Shutterstock.

The domestication of guineafowl (*Numida meleagris*) likely occurred around 2000 BP in western Africa, primarily for meat production, and then around the Mediterranean and into Europe [13]. Their high-quality protein is considered a delicacy and demand exceeds supply in most regions. Guineafowl also play an important cultural role in some countries as dowries, for the welcoming of guests, and as sacrificial entities [14]. Guineafowl have been domestically bred to produce jumbo-sized birds and numerous color varieties such as lavender, porcelain, sky blue, and royal purple. Most species are commonly maintained in aviculture except the two species of *Agelastes* [11].

3.7 Odontophoridae – New World Quail

The recent taxonomic reevaluation of the family Odontophoridae has resulted in 10 genera of 33 species, of which two are endangered, five are vulnerable, six are near threatened, and the remaining are categorized as least concern by the IUCN (Table 3.4, Figure 3.5). New World quail are a smaller, rotund species often with splendid crests; they exhibit various earthy plumage tones, with the males more vividly patterned. Sexual dimorphism in size is not well developed. They differ

Table 3.4 Odontophoridae family and their genera.

Family	Genus	Common name	Latin name	Number of subspecies	Described by	Date
Odontophoridae	*Ptilopachus*	Stone partridge	*Ptilopachus petrosus*	2	J.F. Gmelin	1789
		Nahan's francolin	*Ptilopachus nahani*	Monotypic	A.J.C. Dubois	1905
	Rhynchortyx	Tawny-faced quail	*Rhynchortyx cinctus*	3	Salvin	1876
	Oreortyx	Mountain quail	*Oreortyx pictus*	4	Douglas	1829
	Dendrortyx	Bearded wood-partridge	*Dendrortyx barbatus*	Monotypic	Gould	1846
		Long-tailed wood-partridge	*Dendrortyx macroura*	6	Jardine & Selby	1828
		Buffy-crowned wood-partridge	*Dendrortyx leucophrys*	2	Gould	1844
	Philortyx	Banded quail	*Philortyx fasciatus*	Monotypic	Gould	1844
	Colinus	Northern bobwhite	*Colinus virginianus*	21	Linnaeus	1758
		Black-throated bobwhite	*Colinus nigrogularis*	4	Gould	1843
		Crested bobwhite	*Colinus cristatus*	20	Linnaeus	1758
	Callipepla	Scaled quail	*Callipepla squamata*	4	Vigors	1830

Table 3.4   (Continued)

Family	Genus	Common name	Latin name	Number of subspecies	Described by	Date
		Elegant quail	*Callipepla douglasii*	5	Vigors	1829
		California quail	*Callipepla californica*	8	Shaw	1798
		Gambel's quail	*Callipepla gambelii*	7	Gambel	1843
	Cyrtonyx	Montezuma quail	*Cyrtonyx montezumae*	5	Vigors	1830
		Ocellated quail	*Cyrtonyx ocellatus*	Monotypic	Gould	1837
	Dactylortyx	Singing quail	*Dactylortyx thoracicus*	17	Gambel	1848
	Odontophorus	Marbled wood-quail	*Odontophorus gujanensis*	8	J.F. Gmelin	1789
		Spot-winged wood-quail	*Odontophorus capueira*	2	Spix	1825
		Black-eared wood-quail	*Odontophorus melanotis*	2	Salvin	1865
		Black-fronted wood-quail	*Odontophorus atrifrons*	3	J.A. Allen	1900
		Rufous-fronted wood-quail	*Odontophorus erythrops*	2	Gould	1859
		Chestnut wood-quail	*Odontophorus hyperythrus*	Monotypic	Gould	1857
		Dark-backed wood-quail	*Odontophorus melanonotus*	Monotypic	Gould	1861
		Rufous-breasted wood-quail	*Odontophorus speciosus*	3	Tschudi	1843
		Tacarcuna wood-quail	*Odontophorus dialeucos*	Monotypic	Wetmore	1963
		Gorgeted wood-quail	*Odontophorus strophium*	Monotypic	Gould	1844
		Venezuelan wood-quail	*Odontophorus columbianus*	Monotypic	Gould	1850
		Black-breasted wood-quail	*Odontophorus leucolaemus*	Monotypic	Salvin	1867
		Stripe-faced wood-quail	*Odontophorus balliviani*	Monotypic	Gould	1846
		Starred wood-quail	*Odontophorus stellatus*	Monotypic	Gould	1843
		Spotted wood-quail	*Odontophorus guttatus*	Monotypic	Gould	1838

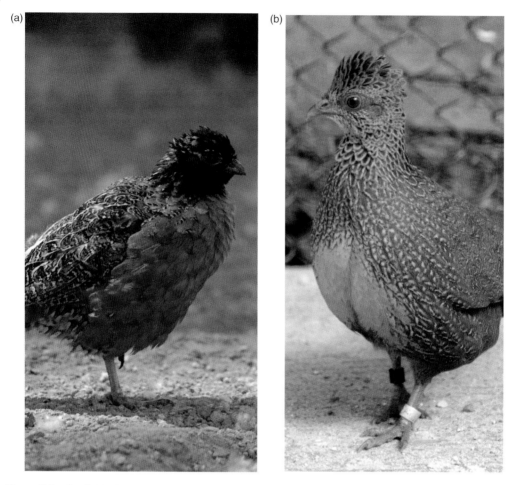

Figure 3.5 Quail. (a) Masked bobwhite (*Colinus virginianus ridgwayi*). Source: Phoenix Zoo. (b) Stone partridge (*Ptilopachus petrosus*). Source: Pinola Conservancy.

from Old World quail with unfeathered nostrils, jagged lower mandible margins ("tooth-beaked"), and lack of tarsus spur. Shared characteristics include rapid sexual maturity, large clutch sizes, and high mortality rates [15]. Odontophoridae are typically found in monogamous pairs or larger coveys foraging in the underbrush of forests, grasslands or arid scrub throughout the Americas. Most members of this family build simple depressions in the ground for egg disposition. Montezuma quail (*Cyrtonyx montezumae*) and some *Odontophorus* sp. are the exception, building domed nests with a side entrance [7].

Previously, this family, as its name suggests, only included species found in the "New World." Through recent taxonomic reevaluation, two African *Ptilopachus* sp. have been included in this family (stone partridge and Nahan's francolin). These two species are now considered an evolutionary link between the family Odontophoridae and the family Phasianidae [1]. New World quail diversified rapidly during the Paleocene–Eocene thermal maximum 55 mya, along with Numididae and Phasianidae [4]. Odontophoridae is behaviorally and morphologically distinct from its sister group Phasianidae [6] and not closely related to the Old World quail.

New World quail are popular with aviculturists due to their small size, mellow temperaments, and ease of breeding. The native quail are most commonly maintained, such as the scaled quails *Callipepla* sp., Montezuma quail *C. montezumae* and *Colinus* sp., especially *Colinus virginianus* [11]. The latter northern bobwhite has been domesticated for food and hunting purposes into larger size and color varieties, such as the Tennessee red, snowflake, and Georgia giant. Not only is *C. virginianus* one of the most economically important of all Galliformes, but it has also greatly bene-fited laboratory research studies [16]. The remaining genera are not maintained in North American aviculture or are in extremely small, nonviable population sizes [11].

3.8 Phasianidae – Pheasants, Partridges, Turkeys, Grouse

The recent taxonomic reevaluation of the family Phasianidae has decreased the described species from 187 to 180 species in 51 genera, 36% of which are rated as of conservation risk by the IUCN Redlist (Table 3.5, Figure 3.6). The inclusion of the former families Meleagrididae (turkeys) and Tetraonidae (grouse) into Phasianidae was justified after molecular phylogenic analysis [1]. By far the largest and most complex of all the Galliformes families, Phasianidae reside in every continent except South America and Antarctica and in nearly every terrestrial habitat. This highly variable, dynamic family contains birds of all sizes, bedazzling male plumage and adornments, and numerous courtship approaches. The sexual dimorphism of males is often very dramatic. The female is the decision maker in mate selection, then cares for the resulting chicks solo if a polygamous species, or with her male partner if a monogamous species [7].

A sister clade to Odonotophoridae, the Phasianidae diversified rapidly during the Paleocene–Eocene thermal maximum 55 mya along with New World quail. This combined clade is then sister clade to Numididae which also underwent adaptive radiation during the same time period [4]. Phylogenetic relationship studies focusing on this family group are intensive, conflicting, and often difficult to determine due to convergent morphological evolution and rapid species radiation [17].

Phasianidae includes species of high economic value as they are prized for game hunting. In North America, four Phasianidae species were successfully introduced in the twentieth century: chukar (*Alectoris chukar*), Himalayan snowcock (*Tetraogallus himalayensis*), gray partridge (*Perdix perdix*), and ring-necked pheasant (*Phasianus colchicus*) [15]. The latter is so ingrained in American culture that many incorrectly believe that this species is native to the US. It was even declared the state bird of South Dakota in 1943.

Heritage breed wild turkeys and domestic chickens are extremely popular in zoo farmyards along with the common ring-necked pheasant and Indian peafowl. Less commonly maintained species in aviculture that may occasionally be seen are Western capercaillie (*Tetrao urogal-lus*), ruffed grouse (*Bonasa umbellus*), *Alectoris* partridge species, the Madagascar partridge (*Margaroperdix madagarensis*), *Coturnix* sp., the transitional African stone partridge (*Ptilopachus petrosus*), bamboo partridge (*Bambusicola* sp.), Congo peacock (*Afropave congensis*), and francolins of any species. Far more abundant captive populations exist of crested wood partridge (*Rollulus rouloul*), most of the tragopans (Blyth's very rare, no Westerns), Himalayan monal (*Lophophorus impejanus*), the USFWS program Attwater's prairie chicken (*Tympanuchus cupido attwateri*) (see Chapter 20, Gamebird Conservation), green junglefowl (*Gallus varius*), all *Lophura* species except Bulwer's (*Lophura bulweri*) and Salvadori's (*Lophura inornata*), eared pheasants (*Crossoptilon* sp.), *Syrmaticus* pheasants, *Polyplectron* peacock pheasants, and great argus *Argusianus argus* [11].

Table 3.5 Phasianidae family and its genera.

Family	Genus	Common name	Latin name	Number of subspecies	Described by	Date
Phasianidae	*Xenoperdix*	Udzungwa forest-partridge	*Xenoperdix udzungwensis*	2	Dinesen et al.	1994
	Caloperdix	Ferruginous wood-partridge	*Caloperdix oculea*	3	Temminck	1815
	Rollulus	Crested wood-partridge	*Rollulus rouloul*	Monotypic	Scopoli	1786
	Melanoperdix	Black partridge	*Melanoperdix nigra*	2	Vigors	1829
	Arborophila	Hill partridge	*Arborophila torqueola*	4	Valenciennes	1825
		Sichuan partridge	*Arborophila rufipectus*	Monotypic	Boulton	1932
		Chestnut-breasted Partridge	*Arborophila mandellii*	Monotypic	A.O. Hume	1874
		White-necklaced Partridge	*Arborophila gingica*	2	J.F. Gmelin	1789
		Rufous-throated Partridge	*Arborophila rufogularis*	6	Blyth	1849
		White-cheeked Partridge	*Arborophila atrogularis*	Monotypic	Blyth	1849
		Taiwan Partridge	*Arborophila crudigularis*	Monotypic	Swinhoe	1864
		Hainan Partridge	*Arborophila ardens*	Monotypic	Styan	1892
		Chestnut-bellied Partridge	*Arborophila javanica*	2	J.F. Gmelin	1789
		Malaysian Partridge	*Arborophila campbelli*	Monotypic	Robinson	1904
		Roll's Partridge	*Arborophila rolli*	Monotypic	Rothschild	1909
		Sumatran Partridge	*Arborophila sumatrana*	Monotypic	Ogilvie-Grant	1891
		Gray-breasted Partridge	*Arborophila orientalis*	Monotypic	Horsfield	1821
		Bar-backed Partridge	*Arborophila brunneopectus*	3	Blyth	1855
		Oarnge-necked Partridge	*Arborophila davidi*	Monotypic	Delacour	1927
		Chestnut-headed Partridge	*Arborophila cambodiana*	3	Delacour & Jabouille	1928
		Red-breasted Partridge	*Arborophila hyperythra*	2	Sharpe	1879

Table 3.5   (Continued)

Family	Genus	Common name	Latin name	Number of subspecies	Described by	Date
		Red-billed Partridge	*Arborophila rubrirostris*	Monotypic	Salvadori	1879
		Scaly-breasted Partridge	*Arborophila chloropus*	7	Blyth	1859
		Chesnut-neckedlaced Partridge	*Arborophila charltonii*	3	Eyton	1845
	Rhizothera	Long-billed Partridge	*Rhizothera longirostris*	Monotypic	Temminck	1815
		Dulit Partridge	*Rhizothera dulitensis*	Monotypic	Ogilvie-Grant	1895
	Rheinardia	Crested Argus	*Rheinardia ocellata*	2	Elliot	1871
	Argusianus	Great Argus	*Argusianus argus*	2	Linnaeus	1766
	Pavo	Indian Peafowl	*Pavo cristatus*	Monotypic	Linnaeus	1758
		Green Peafowl	*Pavo muticus*	3	Linnaeus	1766
	Afropavo	Congo Peafowl	*Afropavo congensis*	Monotypic	Chapin	1936
	Haematortyx	Crimson-headed Partridge	*Haematortyx sanguiniceps*	Monotypic	Sharpe	1879
	Galloperdix	Red Spurfowl	*Galloperdix spadicea*	3	J.F. Gmelin	1789
		Painted Spurfowl	*Galloperdix lunulata*	Monotypic	Valenciennes	1825
		Sri Lanka Spurfowl	*Galloperdix bicalcarata*	Monotypic	J.R. Forster	1781
	Polyplectron	Palawan Peacock-Pheasant	*Polyplectron napoleonis*	Monotypic	Lesson	1831
		Malayan Peacock-Pheasant	*Polyplectron malacense*	Monotypic	Scopoli	1786
		Bornean Peacock-Pheasant	*Polyplectron schleiermacheri*	Monotypic	Brüggemann	1877
		Germain's Peacock-Pheasant	*Polyplectron germaini*	Monotypic	Elliot	1866
		Hainan Peacock-Pheasant	*Polyplectron katsumatae*	Monotypic	Rothschild	1906
		Moutain Peacock-Pheasant	*Polyplectron inopinatum*	Monotypic	Rothschild	1903
		Bronze-tailed Peacock-Pheasant	*Polyplectron chalcurum*	2	Lesson	1831
		Gray Peacock-Pheasant	*Polyplectron bicalcaratum*	4	Linnaeus	1758

(Continued)

Table 3.5   (Continued)

Family	Genus	Common name	Latin name	Number of subspecies	Described by	Date
		Sand Partridge	*Ammoperdix heyi*	4	Temminck	1825
	Synoicus	Brown Quail	*Synoicus ypsilophorus*	10	Bosc	1792
		Blue-breasted Quail	*Synoicus chinensis*	10	Linnaeus	1766
		Blue Quail	*Synoicus adansonii*	Monotypic	J.P. Verreaux & J.B.É. Verreaux	1851
	Anurophasis	Snow Mountain Quail	*Anurophasis monorthonyx*	Monotypic	van Oort	1910
	Margaroperdix	Madagascar Partridge	*Margaroperdix madagarensis*	Monotypic	Scopoli	1786
	Coturnix	Japanese Quail	*Coturnix japonica*	Monotypic	Temminck & Schlegel	1849
		Common Quail	*Coturnix coturnix*	Monotypic	Linnaeus	1758
		Harlequin Quail	*Coturnix delegorguei*	3	Delegorgue	1847
		Rain Quail	*Coturnix coromandelica*	Monotypic	J.F. Gmelin	1789
		Stubble Quail	*Coturnix pectoralis*	Monotypic	Gould	1837
		New Zealand Quail	*Coturnix novaezalandiae*	Monotypic	Quoy & Gaimard	1830
	Alectoris	Rock Partridge	*Alectoris graeca*	4	Meisner	1804
		Chukar	*Alectoris chukar*	14	J.E. Gray	1830
		Philby's Partridge	*Alectoris philbyi*	Monotypic	Lowe	1934
		Przevalski's Partridge	*Alectoris magna*	Monotypic	Przevalski	1876
		Red-legged Partridge	*Alectoris rufa*	3	Linneaus	1758
		Arabian Partridge	*Alectoris melanocephala*	Monotypic	Rüppell	1835
		Barbary Partridge	*Alectoris barbara*	4	Bonnaterre	1790
	Tetraogallus	Caucasian Snowcock	*Tetraogallus caucasicus*	Monotypic	Pallas	1811
		Caspian Snowcock	*Tetraogallus caspius*	2	S.G. Gmelin	1784
		Altai Snowcock	*Tetraogallus altaicus*	Monotypic	Gebler	1836
		Tibetan Snowcock	*Tetraogallus tibetanus*	4	Gould	1854
		Himalayan Snowcock	*Tetraogallus himalayensis*	5	G. R. Gray	1843
	Perdicula	Jungle Bush-Quail	*Perdicula asiatica*	4	Latham	1790

Table 3.5   (Continued)

Family	Genus	Common name	Latin name	Number of subspecies	Described by	Date
		Rock Bush-Quail	*Perdicula argoondah*	3	Sykes	1832
	Ammoperdix	See-see Partridge	*Ammoperdix griseogularis*	Monotypic	J.F. Brandt	1843
		Painted Bush-Quail	*Perdicula erythrorhyncha*	2	Sykes	1832
		Manipur Bush-Quail	*Perdicula manipurensis*	2	A.O. Hume	1881
	Ophrysia	Himalayan Quail	*Ophrysia superciliosa*	Monotypic	J.E. Gray	1846
	Pternistis	Hartlaub's Francolin	*Pternistis hartlaubi*	Monotypic	Bocage	1869
		Handsome Francolin	*Pternistis nobilis*	Monotypic	Reichenow	1908
		Cameroon Francolin	*Pternistis camerunensis*	Monotypic	Alexander	1909
		Chestnut-naped Francolin	*Pternistis castaneicollis*	Monotypic	Salvadori	1888
		Black-fronted Francolin	*Pternistis atrifrons*	Monotypic	Conover	1930
		Erckel's Francolin	*Pternistis erckelii*	Monotypic	Rüppell	1835
		Djibouti Francolin	*Pternistis ochropectus*	Monotypic	Dorst & Jouanin	1952
		Doube-spurred Francolin	*Pternistis bicalcaratus*	2	Linnaeus	1766
		Heuglin's Francolin	*Pternistis icterorhynchus*	Monotypic	Heuglin	1863
		Ahanta Francolin	*Pternistis ahantensis*	Monotypic	Temminck	1854
		Gray-stripped Francolin	*Pternistis griseostriatus*	Monotypic	Ogilvie-Grant	1890
		Scaly Francolin	*Pternistis squamatus*	3	Cassin	1857
		Red-billed Francolin	*Pternistis adspersus*	Monotypic	Waterhouse	1838
		Cape Francolin	*Pternistis capensis*	Monotypic	J.F. Gmelin	1789
		Natal Francolin	*Pternistis natalensis*	Monotypic	A. Smith	1833
		Hildebrandt's Francolin	*Pternistis hildebrandti*	Monotypic	Cabanis	1878
		Jackson's Francolin	*Pternistis jacksoni*	Monotypic	Ogilvie-Grant	1891
		Swierstra's Francolin	*Pternistis swierstrai*	Monotypic	Roberts	1929

(Continued)

Table 3.5 (Continued)

Family	Genus	Common name	Latin name	Number of subspecies	Described by	Date
		Clapperton's Francolin	*Pternistis clappertoni*	Monotypic	Children & Vigors	1826
		Harwood's Francolin	*Pternistis harwoodi*	Monotypic	Blundell & Lovat	1899
		Swainson's Francolin	*Pternistis swainsonii*	2	A. Smith	1836
		Yellow-necked Francolin	*Pternistis leucoscepus*	Monotypic	G.R. Gray	1867
		Gray-breasted Francolin	*Pternistis rufopictus*	Monotypic	Reichenow	1887
		Red-necked Francolin	*Pternistis afer*	7	Statius Müller	1776
	Francolinus	Black Francolin	*Francolinus francolinus*	6	Linnaeus	1766
		Painted Francolin	*Francolinus pictus*	3	Jardine & Selby	1828
		Chinese Francolin	*Francolinus pintadeanus*	2	Scopoli	1786
		Gray Francolin	*Francolinus pondicerianus*	3	J.F. Gmelin	1789
		Swamp Francolin	*Francolinus gularis*	Monotypic	Temminck	1815
	Dendroperdix	Crested Francolin	*Dendroperdix sephaena*	5	A. Smith	1836
	Bambusicola	Mountain Bamboo-partridge	*Bambusicola fytchii*	2	J. Anderson	1871
		Chinese Bamboo-partridge	*Bambusicola thoracicus*	Monotypic	Temminck	1815
		Taiwan Bamboo-partridge	*Bambusicola sonorivox*	Monotypic	Gould	1863
	Gallus	Red junglefowl	*Gallus gallus*	5	Linnaeus	1758
		Gray junglefowl	*Gallus sonneratii*	Monotypic	Temminck	1813
		Sri Lanka Junglefowl	*Gallus lafayettii*	Monotypic	Lesson	1831
		Green Junglefowl	*Gallus varius*	Monotypic	Shaw	1798
	Peliperdi	Coqui Francolin	*Peliperdix coqui*	4	A. Smith	1836
		White-throated Francolin	*Peliperdix albogularis*	3	Hartlaub	1854
		Schegel's Francolin	*Peliperdix schlegelii*	Monotypic	Heuglin	1863
		Latham's Francolin	*Peliperdix lathami*	2	Hartlaub	1854

Table 3.5   (Continued)

Family	Genus	Common name	Latin name	Number of subspecies	Described by	Date
	Scleroptila	Red-winged Francolin	*Scleroptila levaillantii*	2	Valenciennes	1825
		Ring-necked Francolin	*Scleroptila streptophora*	Monotypic	Ogilvie-Grant	1891
		Finsch's Francolin	*Scleroptila finschi*	Monotypic	Bocage	1881
		Orange River Francolin	*Scleroptila gutturalis*	4	Rüppell	1835
		Gray-winged Francolin	*Scleroptila africanus*	Monotypic	Stephens	1819
		Moorland Francolin	*Scleroptila psilolaema*	2	G.R. Gray	1867
		Shelley's Francolin	*Scleroptila shelleyi*	2	Ogilvie-Grant	1890
	Ithaginis	Blood Pheasant	*Ithaginis cruentus*	14	Hardwicke	1821
	Lophophorus	Himalayan Monal	*Lophophorus impejanus*	Monotypic	Latham	1790
		Sclater's Monal	*Lophophorus sclateri*	2	Jerdon	1870
		Chinese Monal	*Lophophorus lhuysii*	Monotypic	A. Geoffrey Saint-Hilaire	1866
	Lerwa	Snow Partridge	*Lerwa lerwa*	Monotypic	Hodgson	1833
	Tetraophasis	Verreaux's Partridge	*Tetraophasis obscurus*	Monotypic	J. P. Verreaux	1869
		Szechenyi's Partridge	*Tetraophasis szechenyii*	Monotypic	Madarász	1885
	Tragopan	Western Tragopan	*Tragopan melanocephalus*	Monotypic	J.E. Gray	1829
		Satyr Tragopan	*Tragopan satyra*	Monotypic	Linnaeus	1758
		Blyth's Tragopan	*Tragopan blythii*	2	Jerdon	1870
		Temminck's Tragopan	*Tragopan temminckii*	Monotypic	J.E. Gray	1831
		Cabot's Tragopan	*Tragopan caboti*	2	Gould	1857
	Syrmaticus	Reeve's Pheasant	*Syrmaticus reevesii*	Monotypic	J.E. Gray	1829
		Copper Pheasant	*Syrmaticus soemmerringii*	5	Temminck	1830
		Mikado Pheasant	*Syrmaticus mikado*	Monotypic	Ogilvie-Grant	1906

(Continued)

Table 3.5 (Continued)

Family	Genus	Common name	Latin name	Number of subspecies	Described by	Date
		Elliot's Pheasant	*Syrmaticus ellioti*	Monotypic	Swinhoe	1872
		Hume's Pheasant	*Syrmaticus humiae*	2	A.O. Hume	1881
	Chrysolophus	Golden Pheasant	*Chrysolophus pictus*	Monotypic	Linnaeus	1758
		Lady Amherst's Pheasant	*Chrysolophus amherstiae*	Monotypic	Leadbeater	1829
	Phasianus	Ring-necked Pheasant	*Phasianus colchicus*	34	Linnaeus	1758
	Crossoptilon	Tibetan Eared-pheasant	*Crossoptilon harmani*	Monotypic	Elwes	1881
		White Eared-pheasant	*Crossoptilon crossoptilon*	4	Hodgson	1838
		Brown Eared-Pheasant	*Crossoptilon mantchuricum*	Monotypic	Swinhoe	1863
		Blue Eared-Pheasant	*Crossoptilon auritum*	Monotypic	Pallas	1811
	Catreus	Cheer Pheasant	*Catreus wallichii*	Monotypic	Hardwicke	1827
	Lophura	Silver Pheasant	*Lophura nycthemera*	15	Linnaeus	1758
		Kalij Pheasant	*Lophura leucomelanos*	9	Latham	1790
		Siamese Fireback	*Lophura diardi*	Monotypic	Bonaparte	1856
		Bulwer's Pheasant	*Lophura bulweri*	Monotypic	Sharpe	1874
		Vietnam Pheasant	*Lophura edwardsi*	Monotypic	Oustalet	1896
		Swinhoe's Pheasant	*Lophura swinhoii*	Monotypic	Gould	1863
		Salvadori's Pheasant	*Lophura inornata*	2	Salvadori	1879
		Crestless Fireback	*Lophura erythrophthalma*	2	Raffles	1822
		Crested Fireback	*Lophura ignita*	3	Shaw	1798
	Perdix	Gray Partridge	*Perdix perdix*	7	Linneaus	1758
		Daurain Partridge	*Perdix dauurica*	2	Pallas	1811
		Tibetan Partridge	*Perdix hodgsoniae*	3	Hodgson	1856
	Pucrasia	Koklass Pheasant	*Pucrasia macrolopha*	10	Lesson	1829

Table 3.5   (Continued)

Family	Genus	Common name	Latin name	Number of subspecies	Described by	Date
	Tetrao	Black-billed Capercaillie	*Tetrao parvirostris*	3	Millendorff	1853
		Western Capercaillie	*Tetrao urogallus*	8	Linnaeus	1758
		Black Grouse	*Lyrurus tetrix*	7	Linnaeus	1758
		Caucasian Grouse	*Lyrurus mlokosiewiczi*	Monotypic	Taczanowski	1875
	Tetrastes	Hazel Grouse	*Tetrastes bonasia*	12	Linnaeus	1758
		Severtzov's Grouse	*Tetrastes sewerzowi*	Monotypic	Przevalski	1876
	Bonasa	Ruffed Grouse	*Bonasa umbellus*	14	Linnaeus	1766
	Centrocercus	Greater Sage-Grouse	*Centrocercus urophasianus*	Monotypic	Bonaparte	1827
		Gunnison Sage-Gouse	*Centrocercus minimus*	Monotypic	Young et al.	2000
	Falcipennis	Siberian Grouse	*Falcipennis falcipennis*	Monotypic	Hartlaub	1855
		Spruce Grouse	*Falcipennis canadensis*	6	Linnaeus	1758
	Lagopus	Willow Ptarmigan	*Lagopus lagopus*	19	Linnaeus	1758
		Rock Ptarmigan	*Lagopus mutus*	30	Montin	1781
		White-tailed Ptarmigan	*Lagopus leucurus*	5	Richardson	1831
	Dendragapus	Dusky Grouse	*Dendragapus obscurus*	4	Say	1823
		Sooty Grouse	*Dendragapus fuliginosus*	4	Ridgway	1873
	Tympanuchus	Sharp-tailed Grouse	*Tympanuchus phasianellus*	6	Linnaeus	1758
		Greater Prairie-chicken	*Tympanuchus cupido*	3	Linnaeus	1758
		Lesser Prairie-chicken	*Tympanuchus pallidicinctus*	Monotypic	Ridgway	1873
	Meleagris	Wild Turkey	*Meleagris gallopavo*	6	Linnaeus	1758
		Ocellated Turkey	*Meleagris ocellata*	Monotypic	Cuvier	1820

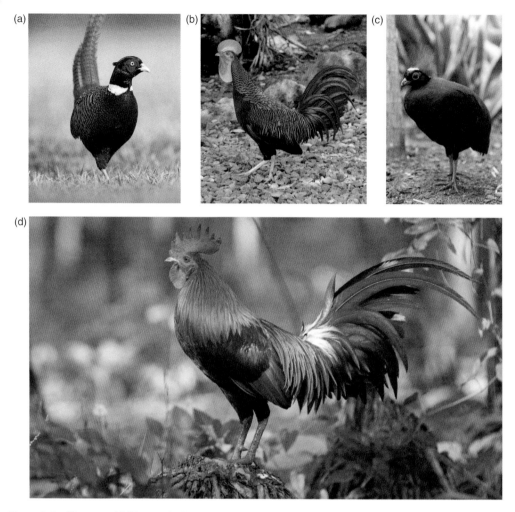

Figure 3.6 Pheasant. (a) Ring-necked pheasant (*Phasianus colchicus*). Source: Piotr Krzeslak/Adobe Stock. (b) Green junglefowl (*Gallus varius*). Source: Pinola Conservancy. (c) Crested partridge (*Rollulus rouloul*). Source: William Hinrichs, Lincoln Park Zoo. (d) Red junglefowl (*Gallus gallus*). Source: Suksamranpix/Adobe Stock.

References

1 Holmes, C. and Anderson, G. (2018). *Galliformes TAG Regional Collection Plan*. Houston Zoo: Houston, TX.

2 Wang, M.-S., Thakur, M., Peng, M.-S. et al. (2020). 863 genomes reveal the origin and domestication of chicken. *Cell Res.* 30: 693–701.

3 Vogelaar, E. and van Grouw, H. (2008). Hybrids. www.aviculture-europe.nl/nummers/08e06a07 .pdf (accessed February 2020).

4 Stein, R.W., Brown, J.W., and Mooers, A.Ø. (2015). A molecular genetic time scale demonstrates Cretaceous origins and multiple diversification rate shifts within the order Galliformes (Aves). *Mol. Phylogenet. Evol.* 92: 155–164.

5 Field, D.J., Bercovici, A., Berv, J.S. et al. (2018). Early evolution of modern birds structured by global forest collapse at the end-cretaceous mass extinction. *Curr. Biol.* 28 (11): 1825–1831.

6 Jiang, K., Fang, Z., and Zuhao, H. (2019). Inter-familial relationships of the Gamefowl (Aves: Galliformes) based on complete mitochondrial genome sequences. *Mitochondrial DNA Part B: Resour.* 4 (1): 723–724.

7 Billerman, S.M., Keeney, B.K., Rodewald, P.G., and Schulenberg, T.S. (ed.) (2020). *Birds of the World*. Ithaca, NY: Cornell Laboratory of Ornithology https://birdsoftheworld.org/bow/home.

8 Boyd, J. (2015). Galliformes – Landfowl. http://jboyd.net/Taxo/List2.html (accessed February 2022).

9 Wang, N., Kimball, R.T., Braun, E. et al. (2017). Ancestral range reconstruction of Galliformes: the effects of topology and taxon sampling. *J. Biogeogr.* 44: 122–135.

10 Steadman, D.W. (1999). The biogeography and extinction of megapodes in Oceania. *Zool. Verh.* 327: 7–22.

11 Species360 Zoological Information Management System (ZIMS) (2020) http://zims.Species360 .org (accessed January 2020).

12 López, R.R., Silvy, N.J., Peterson, M.J. et al. (2019). Curassows, guans, and chachalacas in Mexico. In: *Wildlife Ecology and Management in Mexico* (ed. R. Valdez and J. Ortega), 79. College Station, TX: Texas A&M University Press.

13 Boitard, S., Vignala, A., Thébault, N., et al. (2018). Guinea fowl domestication: new insights from the first whole genome assembly and the pool sequencing of wild and domestic populations. II Joint Congress on Evolutionary Biology, August 2018, Montpellier, France.

14 Houndonougbo, P.V., Bindelle, J., Chrysostome, C.A.A.M. et al. (2017). Characteristics of Guinea fowl breeding in West Africa: a review. *Tropicultura* 35: 222–230.

15 Johnsgard, P.A. (2017). The North American Quails, Partridges, and Pheasants. http:// digitalcommons.unl.edu/zeabook/58 (accessed February 2022).

16 Brennan, L.A., Hernandez, F., and Williford, D. (2020). Northern bobwhite (*Colinus virginianus*), version 1.0. In: *Birds of the World* (ed. A.F. Poole). Ithaca, NY: Cornell Lab of Ornithology.

17 Shen, Y.-Y., Dai, K., Cao, X. et al. (2014). The updated phylogenies of the Phasianidae based on combined data of nuclear and mitochondrial DNA. *PLoS One* 9 (4): e95786.

4

Gamebird Anatomy
Wael Khamas and Josep Rutllant

4.1 Introduction

The anatomy of gamebirds (quail, partridge, and pheasant) is briefly presented in this chapter. Any term not recognized by Nomina Anatomica Avium [1] will be avoided. Areas of clinical interest are emphasized, along with comparisons to other avian species, including the chicken, one of the most studied avian species. Both mature and immature animals will be described.

4.2 Body Regions

Body regions are used to describe the locations of certain structures and draw the attention of the clinicians to the site of infection or injury. Therefore, the body can be divided into head and neck, thoracic, wing, abdominal, pelvic, and pelvic limb regions.

4.2.1 Head and Neck Regions (Figure 4.1)

The natural orifices on the head are the eyes, external acoustic meatuses, nasal openings, and mouth. The ornamental structures on the head include cere, comb, wattles, and ear lobes when present. The appearance of orifices and ornamental structures is frequently used by clinicians to identify illness in birds. In chickens, the ornamental structures differ in size between sexes, being larger in males even at an early age. The same is true in pheasants. The regions of the head and neck include nasal, orbital, suborbital, forehead, crown, auditory, dorsal cervical, lateral cervical and ventral cervical (Figure 4.1a).

4.2.2 Thoracic Region and Wing

The ventral aspect of the wing region includes the chest, abdomen, shank, upper arm, propatagium, forearm, and hand (area of major and minor metacarpals) (Figure 4.2). This region can be used for examination of the bird to detect external parasites and determine feather conditions [2].

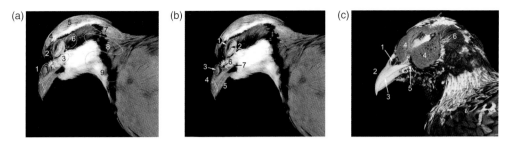

Figure 4.1 (a) Male partridge. 1. Nasal, 2. Orbital, 3. Suborbital, 4. Forehead, 5. Crown, 6. Auditory, 7. Dorsal cervical, 8. Lateral cervical, 9. Ventral cervical. (b) Male partridge, face and cervical regions. 1. Superior eyelid, 2. Inferior eyelid, 3. Operculum, 4. Superior (maxillary) beak, 5. Inferior (mandibular) beak, 6. External nares, 7. Maxillary rictus. (c) Male pheasant. 1. Nasal opening, 2. Culmen, 3. Tomium, 4. Periorbital wattle, 5. Mandibular rictus, 6. Auditory orifice.

4.3 Integument: Skin and Feathers

4.3.1 Ornaments

Ornaments vary among different gamebird species as well as between sexes of the same breed. These ornamental appendages, mentioned before, can be affected by the early nutritional status of the bird. Differences in growth conditions during early life have been suggested to cause long-lasting changes in the morphology and quality of adult birds, including their ornaments (Figures 4.1 and 4.2). Because of this factor, females may choose ornamented mates that are superior at handling early nutritional stress [3].

4.3.2 Skin

The skin of gamebirds is typically white in color, but pigmentation can change based on a variety of factors. For example, coloration of the shank and beak of the chukar partridge results from dietary pigments. The skin of birds is very thin and composed of two layers of epidermis and dermis. The epidermis is thin stratified squamous epithelium with different degrees of keratinization. Most notably, skin on the legs will form scales and is highly keratinized compared to other regions. The thin skin of birds is one of the modifications that aids in decreasing body weight for facilitation of flight.

4.3.3 Spur

The spur is a highly keratinized outgrowth of the hindlimbs of some birds. It is usually located at the distal tarsometatarsal region (Figure 4.3). It is well developed in mature males, and less so in female and immature birds. The main function of the spur is defense. Spurs are well developed in pheasants and are often used for aging. They are rudimentary in partridge and absent in quail. Spurs can be removed at an early age with electrocautery.

4.3.4 Uropygial Gland

Uropygial, preen, oil, rump, caudal, or perunctum gland are all names for the same gland. It is a bilobed gland situated above the caudal rump region. It is relatively large in pheasants (Figure 4.4). In rock partridge, the location varies from the first caudal vertebra or end of synsacrum to the last

(a)

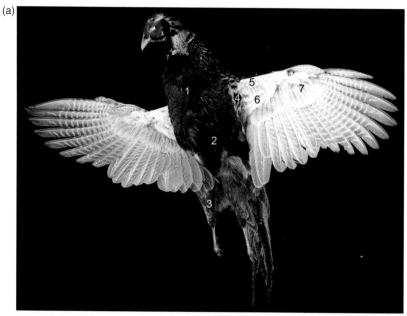

(b)

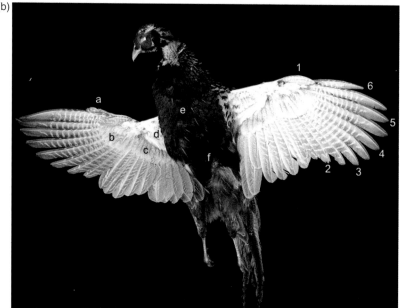

Figure 4.2   (a) Pheasant ventral view. 1. Chest, 2. Abdomen, 3. Shank, 4. Upper arm, 5. Propatagium, 6. Forearm, 7. Hand region (area of major and minor metacarpal). (b) External features showing wing feathers on adult pheasant. a. Alula, b. under covert primary feathers, c. under covert secondary feathers, d. under wing feathers, e. Contour feathers (chest), f. Contour feathers (abdomen). Primary feathers: 1. Alula, 2. II primary, 3. IV primary, 4. VI primary, 5. VIII primary, 6. X primary.

Figure 4.3 Male pheasant feet detail. 1. Tarsometatarsal, 2. Spur, 3. Digit I, 4. Metatarsal pad, 5. Digit II, 6. Digit III, 7. Digit IV, 8. Digital pads, 9. Claw.

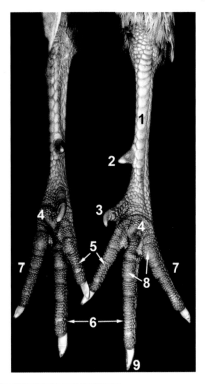

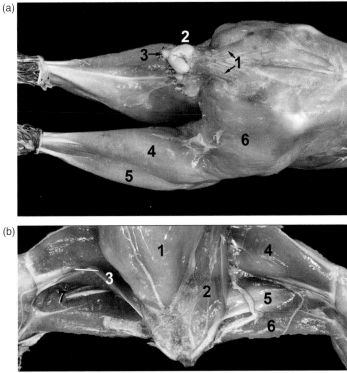

Figure 4.4 (a) Pheasant, caudal-dorsal region. 1. Levator caudae m., 2. Uropygial (bilobed) gland, 3. Papilla where the duct open, 4. Gastrocnemius m., 5. Fibularis longus m., 6. Iliotibialis lateralis m. (b) Pheasant, caudal-ventral region. 1. Pectoralis m., 2. Abdominal mm., 3. Puboischiofemoralis m. (reflected)., 4. Iliotibialis cranialis m., 5. Puboischiofemoralis m., 6. Flexor cruris medialis m., 7. Ischiadic vein, artery, and nerve.

3–4 caudal vertebra. The elevation at the tip of the gland is where the two lobes open and the oil can be accessed by the bird. The gland can be described as simple tubular with a holocrine mode of secretion. The gland in Japanese quail is elongated and described as heart-shaped, consisting of two active lobes. The gland has a very deep septum between the lobes [4].

4.3.5 Feathers

Feathers develop embryologically as buds from the skin during the early stages of embryonic development. Feathers do not cover the entire body of the bird but follow specific lines, depending on the region of the body. The line with feathers is called the pteryla (pl: pterylae) while the line without feathers is called the apteryla (pl: apterylae).

The feathers of birds have many classifications. The first classification discussed is flight. Flight feathers are either remiges or rectrices. Remiges are the flight feathers of the wing and rectrices are those of the tail. The remiges can be divided into primary, secondary, and tertiary. The wing has 10 primary, 13–21 secondary and 3–4 tertiary remiges. Birds typically have between 12 and 22 rectrices. Other feathers include the contour feathers, which are on the outer surface of the body. Contour feathers include the covert feathers, which cover the bases of flight feathers (Figure 4.2).

Although feathers have many different classifications, they have the same general structure. Feathers consist of a shaft, also known as the quill, and a vane (Figures 4.5–4.7). The shaft has two parts: the calamus and the rachis (Figure 4.7). The calamus is the proximal portion that is implanted into the skin. The rachis is the distal portion of the shaft. Barbs are singular strands of keratin that extend from the rachis. Barbs are either pennaceous or plumulaceous. Pennaceous

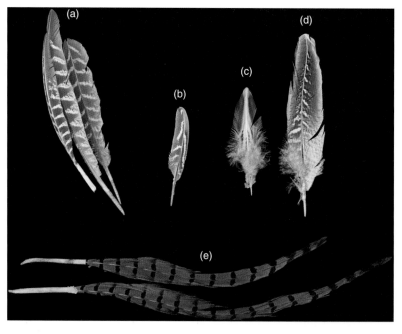

Figure 4.5 Pheasant feathers. (a) Primary, (b) Allula, (c) Secondary covert, (d) Secondary, (e) Tail.

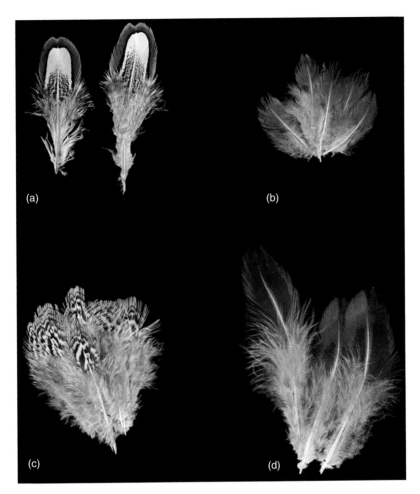

Figure 4.6   Adult pheasant contour feathers. (a) Lateral thoracic, (b) Neck, (c) Dorsal thoracic, (d) Ventral abdominal.

barbs have interlocking barbules, and plumulaceous barbs do not. Barbules are made by further branching of barbs. On either side of the shaft, the interlocking of the pennaceous barbs is known as the vane. The vane is what forms the smooth surface of the feather [5].

Primaries do not have any freedom of movement relative to the bones to which they are rigidly attached. Secondaries, on the other hand, are able to hinge up and down relative to the ulna through flexible attachment. When the elbow and wrist joints are fully extended, primaries spread out and secondaries are pulled downward by the tightening of the postpatagial tendon, which results in an increase in the camber of the wing [6].

Feathers are shed in intervals through a process called molting. Flight feathers are usually replaced annually while secondary feathers are replaced with less frequency. Many factors may affect the shedding of feathers including hormones, light, diet, and weather.

The male pheasant is one of the most colorful birds and has long tail feathers while the female has brown mottled plumage and a short tail. In contrast, male and female chukar partridges are

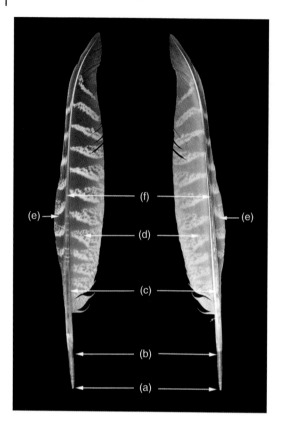

Figure 4.7 Pheasant primary feather of adult male. Dorsal view (left image), ventral view (right image). (a) Inferior umbilicus, (b) Remnant of feather sheath, (c) Calamus (quill), (d) Posterior barbs, (e) Anterior barbs, (f) Rachis.

almost identical in appearance of the feathers but differ in size, with males being larger. In bobwhite quails, males have white coloring of the head that is absent in the female.

4.3.6 Color of Feathers

The color of the feathers is due to pigments from three different groups: carotenoids, melanin, and porphyrine. Oxidation variability of a pro-pigment leads to the development of different types of melanin. For example, black and dark brown pigments are called eumelanin, while red, light brown, and yellow pigments are called phaeomelanin. Male and female birds differ in feather color because of the response of the feathers to hormones and genetic factors [7]. However, no details of this response are described in the literature.

4.4 Skeletal System

The skull of Aves has a number of fused bones and a larger orbit than that of mammals (Figure 4.8). The vertebral column also has many points of fusion, providing increased support for the entire body. The fusion of bones in the vertebral column, synsacrum, and unfused pubic bone allows for the passage of relatively large eggs. The fusion of the last few caudal vertebrae forms the pygostyle, which supports the tail feathers (Figure 4.9). Relative to body size, birds are lighter than mammals,

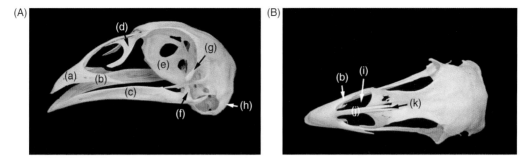

Figure 4.8 Pheasant skull. (A) Lateral view. (B) Dorsal view. (a) Maxillary bone, (b) Maxillary process, (c) Mandible, (d) Lacrimal bone, (e) Interorbital septum, (f) Quadrate bone, (g) Postorbital process, (h) Occipital bone, (i) External nares, (j) Intermaxillary process of the nasal bone, (k) Craniofacial hinge.

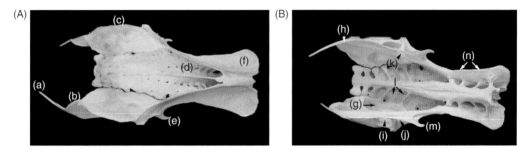

Figure 4.9 Synsacrum of an adult pheasant. (A) Dorsal view. (B) Ventral view. (a) Apex of pubis, (b) Wing of ischium, (c) Dorsolateral iliac crest, (d) Iliosacral canal, (e) Preacetabular tubercle, (f) Preacetabular wing of the ilium, (g) Caudal recess of renal fossa, (h) Shaft of pubis, (i) Ilio-ischiadic foramen, (j) Perforation of acetabulum, (k) Obturator foramen, (l) Iliosacral synostosis, (m) Preacetabular tubercle, (n) Lateral iliac crest.

and much of this is due to adaptations of the skeleton. This is done by the introduction of air into large bones such as the humerus, femur, coracoid, and sternum (Figures 4.10 and 4.11). These are known as pneumatic bones. Gamebirds are not highflyers, but their bones are similar to other birds with respect to pneumatization. Sexual dimorphism is obvious in pheasants, with the male being heavier than the female.

4.5 Muscular System

Aves have a large number of muscles in a unique and complex arrangement. Muscles of the chest and thoracic limb (wing) are enlarged to assist in flight. Since the primary function of the thoracic limb is flight, the musculature of the pelvic limb compensates by development of muscles specialized for walking, jumping, and hunting. A general view of the medial aspect of the wing and the thighs is presented in Figure 4.12. Additional major muscle groups, including the superficial group (major pectoral), help depress the wing and, although smaller than the pectoralis, the supracoracoideus muscle is the primary elevator of the wing. The supracoracoideus muscle is active during

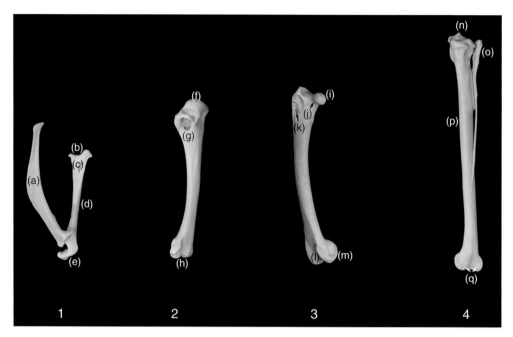

Figure 4.10 All bones are from an adult pheasant. 1. Scapula and coracoid: (a) Blade of scapula, (b) Coracosternal surface, (c) Pneumatic foramen, (d) Shaft of coracoid, (e) Coracohumeral surface. 2. Humerus: (f) Humeral head, (g) Pneumatic foramen, (h) humeral condyles. 3. Femur: (i) Head of femur, (j) Neck of femur, (k) Pneumatic foramen, (l) Intercondylar fossa, (m) Medial condyle. 4. Tibiotarsus and fibula: (n) Tibial plateau, (o) Fibula, (p) Shaft of tibia, (q) Fused proximal row of the tarsal bones with the tibia.

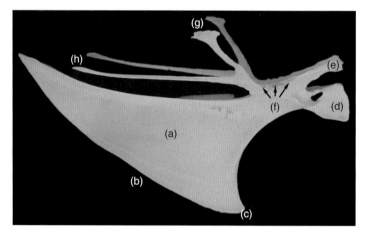

Figure 4.11 A pheasant sternum. (a) Lateral surface of keel, (b) Sternal keel (carina), (c) Carinal apex, (d) Rostrum of sternum, (e) Sternocoracoidal process, (f) Costal margin, (g) Thoracic process, (h) Caudal lateral process.

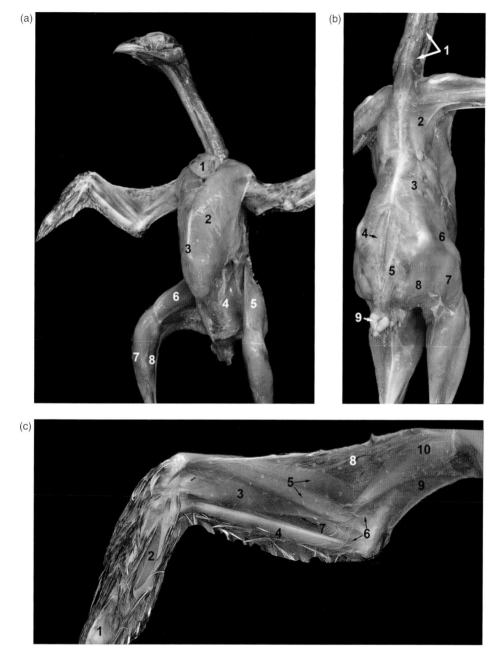

Figure 4.12 (a) Pheasant, ventral view. 1. Crop, 2. Pectoral m., 3. Keel (white line), 4. Abdominal m., 5. Iliotibialis lateralis m., 6. Iliotibialis cranialis m., 7. Fibularis longus m., 8. Gastrocnemius m. (medial). (b) Pheasant, dorsal view. 1. Thymus, 2. Scapulohumeralis m., 3. Latissimus dorsi m., 4. Longissimus dorsi m., 5. Levator coccygeus m., 6. Sartorius m., 7. Tensor fascia lata m., 8. Superficial part of biceps femoris m. (iliofemoralis caudalis), 9. Uropygial gland. (c) Pheasant, wing ventral muscles. 1. Alular mm., 2. Ventral interosseus m., 3. Deep digital flexor m., 4. Flexor carpi ulnaris m., 5. Superficial and deep pronator m., 6. Basilic vein, 7. Superficial ulnar vein, 8. Propatagium, 9. Triceps m., 10. Biceps brachii m.

upstroke, particularly at slow to moderate speeds and during hovering [8]. These muscles are best known as flight muscles and they originate on the keel bone (Figures 4.11 and 4.12a).

The breast muscles of most gamebirds are a mixture of red and white fibers, while chickens have mainly white.

In the pelvic limbs, the gastrocnemius and the peroneus longus (Figure 4.12) are strongly supported by the flexor muscles of the toes (three front and one hind). These muscles are actively involved in perching.

4.6 Respiratory System

The nasal openings (external nares) vary among birds. They are two oval openings at both sides of the base of the beak (Figure 4.1b,c). In some species they are covered by a soft flap of tissue (cere) to protect the entrance of the nasal cavity (Figure 4.1b). In some species, the flap is cartilaginous (operculum). During physical examination, increased or abnormal secretions can be observed in this region if the animal is unhealthy.

4.6.1 Nasal Cavity

The nasal cavity is divided into left and right cavities by the nasal septum. The nasal septum is perforated by a small opening at the level of the internal nares [9]. Rostral, middle, and caudal nasal conchae are described in birds. In the Japanese quail, the caudal nasal concha is the largest, while the cranial one is smallest. Caudally, the caudal nasal concha communicates with the single well-developed paranasal sinus (infraorbital) [10]. The caudal end of the nasal cavity communicates with the pharynx.

4.6.2 Larynx

There are three laryngeal cartilages: cricoid, procricoid, and arytenoid. The cricoid is the largest cartilage in the quail [11]. It is longer ventrally than dorsally. The glottis is a small slit-like opening supported by the arytenoid cartilage on both sides of the entrance into the larynx. Papillae are observed caudal to the tongue and caudal to the glottis in all gamebirds (Figure 4.13b). Generally, the pharynx and larynx in gamebirds are like other bird species.

4.6.3 Trachea

The windpipe or trachea is the tube that connects the laryngeal cavity to the lung. There are 83–91 complete tracheal rings which gradually narrow from cranial to caudal. No overlapping occurs between the rings. The last few tracheal rings do not fuse dorsally and form the tympanum. The trachea of birds is supported by three skeletal muscles: tracheolateralis, sternotrachealis, and cleidotrachealis. The pessulus is a cartilaginous structure connecting with the last tracheal ring and the first bronchial ring in Japanese quail [10]. In chukar partridge, there are 102–114 cartilaginous tracheal rings and the sternotrachealis muscles insert between the 90th and 102nd rings [12].

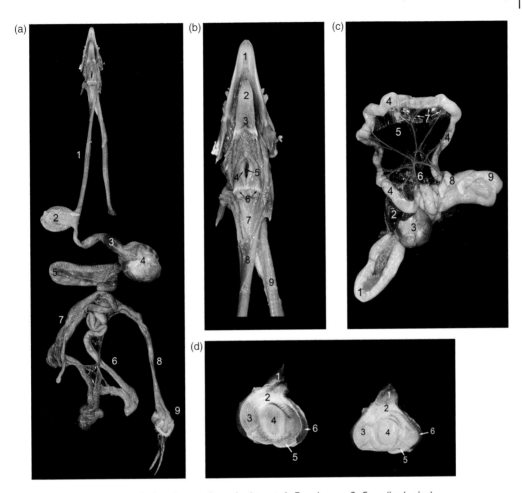

Figure 4.13 (a) Pheasant, isolated gastrointestinal tract. 1. Esophagus, 2. Crop (ingluvies), 3. Proventriculus, 4. Ventriculus (gizzard), 5. Duodenum and pancreas, 6. Jejunum, 7. Ileum and ceci, 8. Colorectum, 9. Cloaca. (b) Pheasant, floor of oral and pharyngeal cavities. 1. Lower mandible supporting lower beak, 2. Tongue, 3. Lingual papillae, 4. Laryngeal mound, 5. Glottis, 6. Pharyngeal papillae, 7. Pharyngo-esophageal junction, 8. Esophagus, 9. Trachea. (c) Pheasant. 1. Duodenum and pancreas, 2. Liver, 3. Ventriculus, 4. Jejunum, 5. Mesentery of jejunum, 6. Cranial mesenteric artery, 7. Intestinal vascular arcades (anastomosing arches), 8. Ileum, 9. Cecum. (d) Pheasant, stomach (gizzard) interior structures. Left: intact koilin layer. Right: koilin removed. 1. Proventriculus, 2. Intermediate zone (isthmus), 3. Cranial blind sac, 4. Body (fundus), 5. Caudal blind sac, 6. Thick muscle.

4.6.4 Syrinx

The bird's voice results from a structure called the syrinx, which is located where the trachea bifurcates into the two principal bronchi. It is positioned dorsal to the base of the heart within the thoracic cavity. The syrinx is formed by the paired, C-shaped, and incomplete bronchial syringeal cartilages. The tracheal rings produce the tympanum, which is the main component of the median part of the syrinx. The mucosa of the syrinx and trachea is lined with a pseudostratified columnar epithelium. Intraepithelial glands are reported to be numerous [13, 14].

4.6.5 Vocalization

All birds have a syrinx, but some are more structurally complex than others. The structure differs in the number of involved tracheal and bronchial cartilages and their level of ossification.

The syrinx is composed of ossified cartilages at the bifurcation of the trachea. The pessulus protrudes into the lumen of the trachea in the common quail [15, 16]. In adult partridges, the tympanum of the syrinx develops from the last two tracheal cartilages, whereas the caudal part of the syrinx is formed from eight pieces of bronchial and tracheal cartilages [17].

4.6.6 Air Sacs

Birds typically have nine air sacs: four paired (cervical, cranial thoracic, posterior thoracic, and abdominal), and one single (interclavicular). The air sacs are thin-walled structures and very difficult to demonstrate because of their transparency, fragility, and lack of vascularity. The low vascularity makes their contribution to gaseous exchange and thermoregulation negligible.

Cranial air sacs include paired cervical, unpaired clavicular, and paired cranial thoracic. The caudal group includes paired caudal thoracic and paired abdominal air sacs. The intrapulmonary bronchi connect to the abdominal air sac [18]. Cervical, clavicular, cranial thoracic, caudal thoracic, and abdominal sacs were identified in Japanese quail [19]. In rock partridge, the following air sacs are stated to be present: cervical, clavicular, cranial thoracic, caudal thoracic, and abdominal [20]. The humerus and clavicle are pneumatic in pheasants, as in several other birds (Figure 4.10). Abdominal air sacs medially produce a femoral diverticulum from a large extension above the kidney. This diverticulum does not enter the femur in Japanese quail, while it does in pheasant.

4.6.7 Lungs

Japanese quail and other gamebirds do not have a diaphragm, which is an important fact in understanding the mechanisms of respiration, and proper patient restraint. Avian lungs are rigid and closely attached to the dorsal aspect of the coelomic (thoracic) cavity and the ribs leave impressions on the lung when taken out. The ventral border is shorter than the dorsal border in Japanese quail lung. The ventral border line is located between the 3rd and 6th intercostal spaces. The principal bronchi connect to the lung and divide into primary, secondary, and tertiary bronchi. The primary bronchus enters the lung and exits to the ostium of the abdominal air sac. The cranial secondary bronchi [4, 5] are medioventral and the caudal bronchi [6–10] are mediodorsal [21]. The last division of the bronchi forms tertiary bronchi (parabronchi), where gaseous exchange takes place at the air and blood capillary interface. Breathing allows air to pass through the posterior air sacs. It then returns to the parabronchi inside the lung, followed by the cranial air sacs to the trachea. Air movement into the lung is continuous; therefore, active respiration occurs during both inspiration and expiration.

4.7 Excretory System

4.7.1 Kidneys

The kidney is the main excretory organ within the body. The characteristic features of the avian kidney are the lobation and the presence of large vessels on the ventral surface. Another important feature is the presence of the renal portal system. Under normal physiologic circulation, the blood drains from the hindlimb and caudal part of the body directly into the kidney. There is no renal pelvis in the kidney of birds. The ureter is relatively small and drains the urine into the middle compartment of the cloaca (urodeum).

Both kidneys consist of three lobes: cranial, middle, and caudal. The lobations are dictated by the presence of vessels passing over the kidney. The external iliac vein separates the cranial from the middle lobe, while the ischiatic artery and vein separate the middle from caudal lobes (Figure 4.14b,c).

The kidneys in Japanese quail and gamebirds are like those of chickens. The avian kidney has two types of nephrons; the cortical (reptilian) type, which are more numerous and lack a loop of Henle, and larger, medullary nephrons (mammalian) [22]. Other than the size and locations, no differences have been established between the two nephrons. Some researchers mentioned three types of nephrons in quail, and the presence of a brush border of interdigitating microvilli on the luminal surface of the collecting ducts [23]. The excretory product of the kidney appears as clear white-colored material (uric acid), which is visible in the feces of the birds.

4.8 Digestive System

The avian digestive system is reduced compared to mammals. Flight requires a lot of energy; therefore, food needs to be processed rapidly. The digestive system of the bird consists of the beak, pharynx, esophagus, crop, proventriculus, ventriculus (gizzard), small intestine (duodenum, jejunum, and ileum), and large intestine (cecum and colorectum). The colorectum opens into the coprodeum portion of the cloaca, which opens to the outside through the vent (Figures 4.14c and 4.15b). Figure 4.13a shows a labeled isolated digestive system of the pheasant.

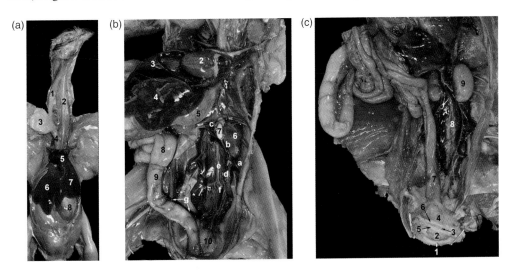

Figure 4.14 (a) Quail. 1. Cervical esophagus, 2. Trachea, 3. Crop, 4. Thoracic esophagus, 5. Heart, 6. Right lobe of liver, 7. Left lobe of liver, 8. Ventriculus. (b) Immature quail. 1. Lung, 2. Heart, 3. Liver left lobe, 4. Liver right lobe, 5. Proventriculus, 6. Kidney, cranial lobe, 7. Immature testis, 8. Ileum and ceci, 9. Colorectum, 10. Bursa of Fabricius, a. External iliac vein, b. Common iliac vein, c. Caudal vena cava, d. Caudal renal vein, e. Abdominal aorta, f. Ischiadic artery, g. Caudal mesenteric vein. (c) Adult male quail. 1. Vent (superior labium), 2. Proctodeum, 3. Urodeum, 4. Coprodeum, 5. Uroproctodeal fold, 6. Proctourodeal fold, 7. Colorectum, 8. Abdominal aorta, 9. Left testis.

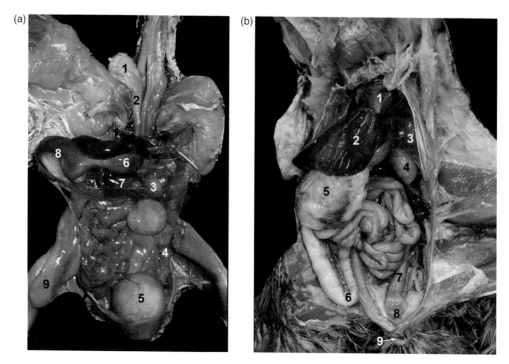

Figure 4.15 (a) Quail, adult female. 1. Crop, 2. Esophagus, thoracic, 3. Ovary, 4. Oviduct, 5. Egg inside the vagina, 6. Proventriculus, 7. Spleen, 8. Ventriculus (gizzard), 9. Duodenum and pancreas. (b) Pheasant, male. 1. Heart, 2. Liver, left lobe, 3. Lung, 4. Left testis, 5. Ventriculus, 6. Duodenum and pancreas, 7. Colorectum, 8. Cloaca, 9. Vent.

4.8.1 Beak

The beak size and shape dictate the size of the food particles a specific breed can consume. The beak is highly keratinized and covers the mandibular and maxillary jaws. The middorsal portion of the beak is called the culmen while the cutting edges are called tomia (singular: tomium) (Figure 4.1c). The jaw bones support the beak caudally. The beak of the partridge is curved, with a flattened and sharp extremity [24].

4.8.2 Tongue

Birds' tongue shape varies among species. The partridge tongue is triangular shaped with mechanical filiform papillae [24]. The tongue, like the mouth cavity, is lined with stratified squamous epithelium. The core or skeleton of the tongue is formed by hyaline cartilage and skeletal muscles.

4.8.3 Mouth Cavity

As with other avian species, the mouth cavity of gamebirds has two openings: choanal cleft and laryngeal mound (Figure 4.13b). In chukar partridge, the rostral aspect of the choanal cleft contains simple branched tubuloalveolar glands of both mucous and seromucous secretion, while the caudal aspect includes mucus-secreting simple branched tubular glands [25]. Salivary glands are present and secrete enzymes which assist in the digestion of carbohydrates.

4.8.4   Esophagus

The esophagus is a muscular distensible tube that starts at the pharynx and descends the cervical region (long portion) (Figure 4.14a). It is dilated at the entrance of the thorax, forming the crop. The short, most distal portion of the esophagus enters the thorax, runs dorsal to the trachea, and joins the proventriculus. The wall of the esophagus contains extensive mucous glands to facilitate lubrication and downward movement of food [26]. The lining epithelium is stratified squamous with varying degrees of keratinization, depending on the type of food the birds consume. Mucous glands decrease within the wall of the crop compared to the esophagus. The crop and esophagus in quail have longitudinal folds which allow them to distend further when filled with food [27].

4.8.5   Proventriculus

The esophagus leads into the stomach, which consists of the proventriculus and ventriculus. The proventriculus is considered the glandular portion of the avian stomach. The main function of the proventriculus is the production of gastric juices, such as hydrochloric acid and pepsinogen, for the initial digestion of proteins. This mixture is produced by oxynticopeptic cells. Openings of glands (papillae) are present on the mucosal surface. The glands are extensive and push the lamina muscularis mucosae close to the tunica muscularis, thus minimizing the thickness of the tunica submucosa. The lining epithelium is simple columnar in both proventriculus and ventriculus.

In the partridge, no clear line of demarcation exists between the lower esophagus and the proventriculus. In the caudal portion, the isthmus separates the proventriculus from the ventriculus [28]. The proventriculus is described in the partridge as a prolonged structure, with a fusiform shape toward craniocaudal. The proventriculus of Japanese quail is an elliptical-shaped organ and has typical histological tubular organ tunics [29].

4.8.6   Ventriculus (Gizzard)

The second compartment of the avian stomach is the ventriculus (biconvex). It is also known as the muscular stomach or gizzard. It lies in the left dorsoventral region of the thoracoabdominal cavity, partly between the liver lobes. The mucosa is formed by folds lined by simple columnar epithelial cells. These cells secrete a highly keratinized layer (koilin), above the epithelium to protect the cells from the acidic secretions of the proventriculus (Figure 4.13d). The gizzard is larger than the proventriculus and has a thick muscular wall. There are two pairs of opposing muscles: craniodorsal and caudodorsal. The asymmetry of these muscles aids in the contraction and grinding functions of the ventriculus. Aborally, the ventriculus is connected to the beginning of the duodenum. Bile may regurgitate from the duodenum into the ventriculus, resulting in green-colored mucosa.

4.8.7   Small Intestine

The ventriculus delivers the food to the beginning of the small intestine, the duodenum. The duodenum forms a loop and is in close association with the pancreas, which is positioned within the loop. The liver delivers bile to the duodenum. The second segment of the small intestine is the jejunum which has extensive mesentery. No clear line of demarcation from the duodenum can be identified in gamebirds. The ileum is the last segment of the small intestine, starting at the tips of the ceca and ending at the junction with the colorectum (Figure 4.13a,c). Some anatomists consider the starting point of the ileum to be at the Meckel's diverticulum, the remnant of the junction of the primitive gut with the yolk sac.

Characteristically, since the pheasant mainly eats grains which are difficult to break down, the small intestine is long while the large intestine is much shorter (Figures 4.13 and 4.14).

4.8.8 Ceca (Cecum)

The ceca are paired blind-end tubular structures which extend from the ileocolorectal junction into the abdominal cavity. They are attached by a mesenteric ligament to the ileum which lies in the middle of the two ceca (Figure 4.13a,c). They are almost 6 in. in length in the pheasant. In common quail, ceca are well developed and have a short proximal neck, a long middle thin-walled body, and a short apex [27]. The apices of the ceca have large aggregates of lymphoid tissue, and some anatomists consider these to be cecal tonsils. The ceca harbor large number of microflorae to help in digestion. Water reabsorption and vitamins synthesis are accepted functions for the ceca.

4.8.9 Colorectum

The short colon and rectum are merged, which makes it difficult to draw a line of demarcation between the two organs. Therefore, the term *colorectum* is most appropriate to use in birds. The colorectum starts at the junction of the two ceca and the terminal ileum. Absorption of water is one of the main functions (Figures 4.13 and 4.14).

4.8.10 Cloaca

The colorectum opens into the first cranial compartment of the cloaca, the coprodeum. The other two compartments of the cloaca are the urodeum, into which the ureters and genital system open (ductus deferens in male and left oviduct in female), and the proctodeum, which opens to the outside through the vent. There are two folds separating these cloacal compartments from each other: the coprourodeal and uroproctodeal folds (Figure 4.14c). The bursa of Fabricius is a relatively large pouch at the dorsal surface of the cloaca above the proctodeum in young birds (see section on immune system below).

4.8.11 The Vent

The vent is the external opening of the cloaca (Figures 4.14c and 4.15b). It consists of dorsal and ventral labia. There is an abrupt change in type of epithelium from simple columnar/cuboidal to stratified squamous as it joins the skin. There is a skeletal muscle sphincter at the opening that controls the vent.

4.8.12 Liver

The liver is the largest gland in the animal body, and birds are no exception. It is composed of two large lobes, with the right being larger than the left (Figure 4.14a,b). The ventriculus is usually lodged between the two lobes of the liver. The left lobe is divided in the black partridge [30]. The liver performs many vital functions such as bile production, red blood cell production, glycogen storage, plasma and protein synthesis, protein metabolism and transformation of proteinaceous waste into uric acid, hormone production, and detoxification. The avian liver is surrounded by a peritoneal layer of mesothelium. One characteristic feature of the liver is the absence of connective tissue septa between lobules except in the portal area [31].

4.8.13 Gall Bladder

The gall bladder is located on the visceral surface of the right lobe of the liver. It is a dilated sac that allows for the storage of bile prior to its secretion into the duodenum. The bile produced in the liver reaches the gall bladder through the hepatocystic duct. The bile can enter the duodenum in two different ways: through the hepatoenteric duct, bypassing the gall bladder, or through the cystoenteric duct, from the gall bladder to the duodenum [1, 9]. The gall bladder is present in the chukar partridge but has no lamina muscularis mucosa, glands, or goblet cells [32]. In the quail, the gall bladder is similar to that of the chukar partridge, except for the presence of goblet cells [33].

4.8.14 Pancreas

Like other animals, the pancreas of birds is located within the loop of the duodenum (Figure 4.13a,c). It is a compound tubuloacinar exocrine gland, with endocrine portions embedded throughout (islets of Langerhans). The pancreas of birds generally has two lobes, with the right lobe being larger than the left. However, some texts describe species with three lobes (ventral, dorsal, splenic) [9], or four lobes in the quail (dorsal, ventral, third, splenic). Much less connective tissue is present inside the avian pancreas compared to that of mammals. In species with two lobes, two ducts originate from the pancreas: ventral (main) and dorsal (accessory). These ducts correspond to the two embryonic origins of the pancreas. In quail, the pancreas is connected to the ascending duodenum by three main excretory ducts that open independently from each other into the wall of the duodenum separately from the bile duct (cystoenteric). The exocrine pancreas has intercalated ducts lined with simple squamous epithelium, intralobular ducts lined with cuboidal epithelium, and interlobular and interlobar ducts lined with columnar epithelium that display one or two layers of muscle and connective tissue [34].

The endocrine pancreas of the Coturnix quail consists of two major islet configurations. Islets containing B and D cells are found in all four lobes of the pancreas, but islets consisting of A and D cells occur with regularity only in the third and splenic lobes [35].

4.9 Immune System

A good immune system protects the bird from infection and disease. Primary lymphoid organs in birds are the thymus, bone marrow, and bursa of Fabricius. Spleen, lymph nodes (when present), and scattered tonsils in several organs act as secondary lymphoid organs/tissues. In birds, cecal tonsils (aggregate of lymphatic nodules at the apices of the two ceca) may harbor close to half the number of lymphatic nodules in the body [36]. In the chukar partridge, an age-dependent drastic change is observed in lymphoid tissue in general but is most prominent in the cloacal bursa and thymus. Involution occurs in the bursa and thymus of partridges around puberty rather than their juvenile stages. These changes are also appreciable in esophageal and pyloric tonsils, whereas the spleen keeps the same histological features before and during puberty [37].

4.9.1 Bursa of Fabricius (Cloacal Bursa)

The bursa of Fabricius is a relatively large pouch at the dorsal surface of the cloaca above the proctodeum in young birds (Figure 4.14b). It is a primary immune organ where B lymphocytes undergo maturation to become immunocompetent. If the bursa is removed at day 1 of age, no immunocompetent B lymphocytes will develop. The bursae of chukar partridges reach peak size at about 10 weeks of age, after which they abruptly regress. Bursal weights of pheasant males increased faster than those of females and the largest bursal weights are observed at 10 and 12 weeks for males and females, respectively. Thereafter, a sharp decline in bursal weight is also observed [38]. In contrast, the weight of the bursa in Chinese yellow quail increases from 0 to 5 weeks of age and then decreases rapidly from 5 to 9 weeks of age [39].

4.10 Spleen

The spleen of the Chinese yellow quail is located on the right dorsal side of the junction of the proventriculus and gizzard (Figure 4.15a). It is spherical and brownish red in color, similar to that of chicken. The spleen is covered by a connective tissue capsule containing smooth muscle. Trabeculae extend from the capsule into the spleen parenchyma. The parenchyma is composed of red and white pulp. The volume of the spleen gradually increases with age, reaching a peak at 14 weeks. Chinese yellow quail spleen is developed prior to hatching [40].

4.11 Circulatory System

4.11.1 Heart

The heart of birds has four chambers, similar to that of mammals. The heart has a tough fibroserous membrane, the pericardium. It is located within the thoracoabdominal (coelomic) cavity (Figures 4.14b and 4.15b). The size of the heart is inversely related to body size. Coronary blood flow increases due to hypoxia, as a result of low vascular resistance [41]. The heart is supplied with both sympathetic and parasympathetic nerve fibers.

4.11.2 Major Blood Vessels

There are several vascular anastomoses and plexuses in birds to facilitate blood flow during flight and aid in thermoregulation. Blood sampling is commonly performed using the basilic (wing) vein (Figure 4.12c). The vein is accompanied by a branch of the brachial artery. It is located on the ventral aspect of the wing. The wing vein resides between the biceps and triceps muscles. Some types of heavy pheasants are noted for weakness in this vessel. Erythrocytes are oval and nucleated. The number of erythrocytes varies with the activity level of the bird, such that increased activity leads to an increase in number. The opposite is true in less active species such as the ostrich. The male bird has more red blood cells than the female, which might be due to testosterone.

4.12 Endocrine System

4.12.1 Thyroid Gland

The thyroid gland of the bird is situated at the angle of the subclavian and common carotid arteries, which is more caudal than in mammals. The gland has several functions, among which are regulation of metabolism and assistance in adaptation to new environments. Thyroid gland activity varies according to the seasons. In summer, the pheasant thyroid is a relatively quiescent organ with reduced secretory activity; the follicular epithelium is low cuboidal, while the follicles are large and contain an increased amount of colloid [42]. The thyroid gland activity also correlates directly with body weight, as seen in male Korean pheasants [43].

4.12.2   Parathyroid Gland

The parathyroid gland is a small round organ found caudal to the thyroid gland. Most birds, like mammals, have four parathyroid glands that originate embryologically from the pharyngeal pouches III and IV. The Japanese quail is reported to have one pair of parathyroid glands located between the carotid artery and the jugular vein [44]. The gland functions in calcium homeostasis. This is a very important function, especially for chicken and quail because they lay eggs almost every day.

4.12.3   Ultimobranchial Body

The ultimobranchial body is present only in birds and reptiles. It is located close to the thyroid and parathyroid glands at the cranial celomic cavity, close to the major blood vessels. It is composed of adipose connective tissue and has two cell types. The organ produces calcitonin, the same hormone as that produced by C cells (parafollicular) in the thyroid gland in mammals. The ultimobranchial and carotid bodies share a close spatial relationship to the recurrent laryngeal nerve, resulting in heavy innervation of these two organs [45, 46].

4.12.4   Adrenal Glands

The adrenal glands of birds are yellow to orange, and triangular or pear shaped. An important feature of the avian adrenal gland is the intermixing of cortical and medullary components [47]. A mixture of medulla and cortex is observed in chicken and several other species. The adrenal gland is covered by a capsule composed of collagenous fibers. The capsule is infiltrated with nerves, as well as blood and lymphatic vessels. The partridge adrenal glands are small, ovoid, yellow, and found inside the abdominal (coelomic) cavity cranial to the respective kidney [48]. Interrenal tissue and chromaffin tissue are reported in the adrenal gland of juvenile Japanese quail, but this tissue was found to decrease during molting [49].

4.12.5   Pituitary Gland (Hypophysis Cerebri)

The pituitary gland has nervous and glandular portions. Embryologically, the nervous portion arises from the base of the diencephalon and descends distally. The glandular portion develops as a pouch (Rathke's pouch) from the dorsal surface of the pharyngeal wall. The portions migrate close together and become surrounded by a connective tissue capsule. The glandular portion has several secretory cells with different affinities for certain stains. These cells are very similar to those present in the mammalian pituitary gland.

4.12.6   Pineal Gland

The avian pineal gland functions to control the circadian and seasonal rhythms, and migration. It develops from the roof of the diencephalon. The jungle bush quail possesses a tubulofollicular type of pineal gland that is situated between the paired cerebral hemisphere and cerebellum [50].

4.13 Reproductive Systems

4.13.1 Male Reproduction

Birds have two testes situated inside the abdominal cavity close to the cranial lobe of the kidney. They retain their embryologic position and do not migrate caudally and distally, as in mammals. The testes vary in size, depending on the size of the bird and the season (Figure 4.14b,c). They are under the influence of pituitary hormones (FSH and LH). Partial removal of the hypophyses (hypophysectomy) will result in testicular involution in chickens [51] and Japanese quails [52]. Seasonal cycles elicit significant changes in weight, sperm production, and testosterone levels in pheasants [53] and quails [54]. The epididymis lies on the concave surface of the testis. It is followed by the ductus deferens which, in turn, connects to the urodeum of the cloaca.

In Japanese quail, the transport of sperm from the seminiferous tubules to the epididymis requires approximately 24 hours, with sperm being stored for a very short period in the ductus deferens. There is no long-term storage of sperm in gamebirds as there is in mammals [55, 56].

4.13.2 Female Reproduction

The left oviduct persists in adult birds while the right involutes early in development, and only a remnant persists close to the cloaca (Figure 4.15a). The functional female genital system in all birds consists of an ovary and an oviduct. Persistent right oviduct in ring-necked pheasant has been reported [57].

4.13.2.1 Ovary
The ovary has a grape-like structure with developing pedunculated ova (follicles) attached. It is located close to the respective kidney in the dorsal coelomic cavity (Figure 4.15a).

4.13.2.2 Oviduct
The oviduct is not directly connected to the ovary and consists of infundibulum, magnum, isthmus, uterus (eggshell gland), and vagina (Figure 4.15a). The oviduct attaches to the dorsal body wall by a double fold of peritoneum (mesotubarium). The infundibulum receives the developing ovum and conveys it to the magnum, which is long and convoluted. A relatively short and constricted segment, the isthmus, connects the magnum to the uterus. The egg passes most slowly through the uterus (eggshell gland), which is a dilated tube. Once the egg is inside the vagina, it will be delivered through the opening of the female genital system to the urodeum of the cloaca to the outside. Egg binding usually happens when the egg stops at the uroproctodeal fold and fails to be released. Under optimal conditions of temperature and humidity, the embryo continues to develop for 23–24 days for pheasants, chukars, and bobwhite quail.

In birds, spermatozoa can be stored within the female genital system in the uterovaginal junction and within the infundibulum. This storage capacity enables the hen to lay a sequence of fertile eggs for extended periods of time. Sperm survival inside the female genital tract of chicken and turkey is dependent on the sperm storage tubules found in the vagina, causing the difference in duration of fertility that ranges from 2–3 weeks in domestic fowls to 10–15 weeks in turkeys [56].

4.14   Nervous System

The central nervous system consists of the brain, cerebellum, and spinal cord. All three are surrounded by the meninges for protection and nutrition. Projections from the lateral surface of both sides of the diencephalon are the optic lobes, which are large relative to the brain of the bird. Birds have well-developed tectum and rostral colliculi. The spinal cord continues caudally from the medulla oblongata and decreases in size toward the coccygeal vertebrae. A significant difference from the mammalian spinal cord is the presence of specialized cells filled with glycogen, resulting in the formation of the glycogen body in the lumbar region.

References

1 Baumel, J.J., King, A.S., Breazile, J.E. et al. (1993). *Handbook of Avian Anatomy: Nomina Anatomica Avium*, 2e. Cambridge, MA: Nuttall Ornithological Club.

2 Lucas, A.M. and Stettenheim, P.R. (1972). *Avian Anatomy Integument: Part I and II*. Washington, DC: US Government Printing Office.

3 Ohlsson, T., Smith, H.G., Råberg, L. et al. (2002). Pheasant sexual ornaments reflect nutritional conditions during early growth. *Proc. Biol. Sci.* 269 (1486): 21–27.

4 Atalgin, H. and Kürtül, I. (2008). Arterial vascularization of the uropygial glands (gl. Uropygialis) in the Japanese quail (*coturnix coturnix japonica*) and silver polish (*gallus gallus domesticus*). *Anat. Histol. Embryol.* 37 (3): 177–180.

5 Thompson, M. (2014). *Everything you Need to Know about Feathers*. Bird Academy: Cornell Lab https://academy.allaboutbirds.org/feathers-article. (accessed February 2022).

6 Pennycuick, C.J. (2008). *Modelling the Flying Bird*, vol. 5, 105–134. Cambridge, MA: Elsevier.

7 Ralph, C.I. (1969). The control of color in birds. *Am. Zool.* 9 (2): 521–530.

8 Biewener, A.A. (2011). Muscle function in avian flight: achieving power and control. *Philos. Trans. R. Soc. B* 366 (1570): 1496–1506.

9 Konig, H.E., Korbel, R., and Leibich, H.G. (2006). *Avian Anatomy: Textbook and Color Atlas* (trans. C. Klupiec). Sheffield, UK: 5m Publishing.

10 Cevik-Demirkan, A., Kürtül, I., and Haziroglu, R.M. (2007). Gross morphological features of the nasal cavity in the Japanese quail. *Ank. Üniv. Vet. Fak. Derg.* 54: 1–5.

11 Cevik-Demirkan, A., Haziroğlu, R.M., and Kürtül, İ. (2007). Gross morphological and histological features of larynx, trachea and syrinx in Japanese quail. *Anat. Histol. Embryol.* 36 (3): 215–219.

12 Mobini, B. (2016). Histological and anatomical study of trachea of native partridges (chukar chukar). *Vet. Res. Biol. Prod.* 29: 2–9.

13 Frappier, B.L. (2006). Digestive system. In: *Dellmann's Textbook of Veterinary Histology* (ed. J. Eurell and B. Frappier), 208–211. Hoboken, NJ: Wiley Blackwell.

14 Bacha, W.J. and Bacha, L.M. (2012). *Color Atlas of Veterinary Histology*, 3e, 205–208. Hoboken, NJ: Wiley Blackwell.

15 Fitzgerald, T.C. (1969). Respiratory system. In: *The Coturnix Quail* (ed. T. Fitzgerald), 239–253. Ames, IA: Iowa State University Press.

16 Frank, T., Walter, I., Probst, A. et al. (2006). Histological aspects of the syrinx of the male mallard (Anas platyrhynchos). *Anat. Histol. Embryol.* 35: 369–401.

17 Erdogan, S., Sagsoz, H., and Paulsen, F. (2015). Functional anatomy of the syrinx of the Chukar partridge (*alliformes: alectoris chukar*) as a model for phonation research. *Anat. Rec.* 298: 602–617.

18 Maina, J.N. (2005). *The Lung-Air Sac System of Birds – Development, Structure, and Function*, 34–35. Berlin: Springer-Verlag.

19 Cevik-Demirkan, A., Kürtül, I., and Haziroglu, R.M. (2006). Gross morphological features of the lung and air sac in the Japanese quail. *J. Vet. Med. Sci.* 68 (9).

20 Kürtül, I., Aslan, K., Aksoy, G. et al. (2004). Morphology of the air sacs (sacci pneumatici) in the rock partridge (*alectoris graeca*). *Vet. Res. Commun.* 28 (7): 553–559.

21 Powell, F.L. (2000). Respiration. In: *Sturkie's Avian Physiology*, 5e (ed. G.C. Whittow), 233–241. London: Academic Press.

22 Bacha, W.J. and Bacha, L.M. (2012). *Color Atlas of Veterinary Histology*, 3e, 193–194. Hoboken, NJ: Wiley Blackwell.

23 Mobini, B. and Abdollahi, M.H. (2016). Effect of sex on histological and histochemical structures of different parts of the kidney in Japanese quail. *Poult. Sci.* 95: 2145–2150.

24 Rossi, J.R., Baraldi-Artoni, S.M., Oliveira, D. et al. (2005). Morphology of beak and tongue of partridge *Rhynchotus rufescens*. *Ciênc. Rural* 35 (5): 1098–1102.

25 Hakan, S., Erdoğan, S., and Akbalık, M.E. (2012). Histomorphological structure of the palate and histochemical profiles of the salivary palatine glands in the Chukar partridge (*Alectoris chukar*, gray 1830). *Acta Zool.* 94: 382–391.

26 Rossi, J.R., Baraldi-Artoni, S.M., Oliveria, D. et al. (2006). Morphology of oesophagus and crop of the partridge *Rhynchotus rufescens* (Tiramidae). *Acta Sci. Biol. Sci.* 28: 165–168.

27 Zaher, M., Ghareeb, A., Hamdi, H. et al. (2012). Anatomical, histological and histochemical adaptations of the avian alimentary canal to their food habits: I-Coturnix coturnix. *Life Sci. J.* 9 (3): 253–275.

28 Rossi, J.R., Baraldi-Artoni, A.M., Oliveira, D. et al. (2005). Morphology of glandular stomach (ventriculus glandularis) and muscular stomach (ventriculus muscularis) of the partridge rhynchotus rufescens. *Ciênc. Rural* 35 (6): 1098–1102.

29 Dahekar, N.M., Mamde, C.S., Ahmad, M. et al. (2014). Gross anatomical and histomorphological studies on proventriculus of Japanese quail. *Indian J. Vet. Anat.* 26: 62–63.

30 Khadhim, I.A.A., Mnati, I.M., and Mutlak, B.H. (2018). Morphological and histological study of liver in Iraqi black partridge, *Francolinus francolinus* (*linnaeus*, 1766). *Biochem. Cell. Arch.* 18 (1): 1055–1058.

31 Ozüdoğru, Z., Balkaya, H., Kara, H. et al. (2019). Morphologic and histologic observation of red-legged partridges (Alectoris Chukar) liver. *Van. Vet. J.* 30 (3): 159–161.

32 Mobini, B. (2012). Microscopic study of the gall bladder of the chukar partridge (*Alectoris chukar*). *Bulg. J. Vet. Med.* 15 (2): 73–78.

33 Mobini, B. (2014). Histological study of the gall bladder of the common quail (*Coturnix coturnix*). *Vet. Med.* 59 (5): 261–264.

34 Simsek, N. and Alabay, B. (2008). Light and electron microscopic examinations of the pancreas in quails (Coturnix coturnix japonica). *Rev. Med. Vet.* 159 (4): 198–206.

35 Smith, P.H. (1974). Pancreatic islets of the coturnix quail. A light and electron microscopic study with special reference to the islet organ of the splenic lobe. *Anat. Rec.* 178: 567–585.

36 Rezaian, M. and Hamedi, S. (2007). Histological study of the caecal tonsil in the cecum of 4-6 months of age white leghorn chicks. *Am. J. Anim. Vet. Sci.* 2: 50–54.

37 Arugh, A. and Hamedi, S. (2019). A histomorphometric study on age-related changes in selected lymphoid structures of Chukar partridge (*Alectoris chukar*). *Iran. J. Vet. Res.* 20 (3): 186–191.

38 Mercer-Oltjen, S.L. and Woodard, A.E. (1986). Development of the bursa of Fabricius in the partridge and pheasant. *Poult. Sci.* 66: 418–421.

39 He, M., Liang, X., Wang, K. et al. (2015). Age-related development and histomorphological observation of bursa of Fabricius in yellow quails. *Can. J. Anim. Sci.* 95 (3): 487–491.

40 Piao, Z., Min, H., Lv, Y., et al. (2018). Age-related histomorphological studies on the spleen of Chinese yellow quail. *Indian J. Anim. Res. B*: 985. https://doi.org/10.18805/ijar.B-985

41 Orosz, S. (2013). Anatomy of the avian heart. https://lafeber.com/pet-birds/anatomy-of-the-avian-heart (accessed February 2022).

42 Velický, J., Titlbach, M., Rychter, Z. et al. (1977). Light and electron microscopy observations in the thyroid gland of the pheasant (*Phasianus colchicus L.*). *Z. Mikrosk. Anat. Forsch.* 91 (3): 460–474.

43 Harclerode, J. and Dropp, J. (1966). Seasonal variation in thyroid gland activity in pheasants. *Ohio J. Sci.* 66 (4): 380–386.

44 Clark, N.B. and Sasayama, Y. (1981). The role of parathyroid hormone on renal excretion of calcium and phosphate in the Japanese quail. *Gen. Comp. Endocrinol. J.* 45 (2): 234–241.

45 Velický, J., Titlbach, M., and Rychter, Z. (1980). Fine structure of the ultimobranchial body of the pheasant (*Phasianus colchicus L.*). *Z. Mikrosk. Anat. Forsch.* 94 (1): 96–104.

46 Kameda, Y. (2017). Morphological and molecular evolution of the ultimobranchial gland of non-mammalian vertebrates, with special reference to the chicken C cells. *Am. Assoc. Anat.* 246 (10): 719–739.

47 Vestergaard, K. and Willeberg, P. (1978). Video scanning for determination of the proportion of cortical tissue in the avian adrenal gland. *Acta Vet. Scand.* 19: 331–340.

48 Ahmed, N.A. and Dauod, H.A.M. (2016). Morphological description and histological structure of adrenal gland in black Iraqi partridge *Francolinus francolinus*. *Iraqi J. Sci.* 57 (1B): 330–337.

49 Ghosh, A., Carmichael, S.W., and Mukherjee, M. (2001). Avian adrenal medulla: cytomorphology and function. *Acta Biol. Szeged.* 45 (1–4): 1–11.

50 Haldar, C. and Ghosh, M. (1990). Annual pineal and testicular cycle in the Indian jungle bush quail, Perdicula asiatica, with special reference to the effect of pinealectomy. *Gen. Comp. Endocrinol.* 77: 150–157.

51 Tanaka, S. and Fujioka, T. (1981). Histological changes in the testis of the domestic fowl after partial adenohypophysectomy. *Poult. Sci.* 60 (2): 444–452.

52 Brown, N.L. and Follett, B.K. (1977). Effects of androgens on the testes of intact and hypophysectomized Japanese quail. *Gen. Comp. Endocrinol.* 33 (2): 267–277.

53 Kim, I.S. and Yang, H.H. (2001). Seasonal changes of testicular weight, sperm production, serum testosterone, and in vitro testosterone release in Korean ring-necked pheasants (*Phasianus colchicus karpowi*). *J. Vet. Medical Sci.* 63 (2): 151–156.

54 Artoni, S.M., Orsi, A.M., Carvalho, T.L. et al. (1999). Seasonal morphology of the domestic quail (Coturnix coturnix japonica) testis. *Anat. Histol. Embryol.* 28 (4): 217–220.

55 Clulow, J. and Jones, R.C. (1982). Production, transport, maturation, storage, and survival of spermatozoa in the male Japanese quail, *Coturnix coturnix*. *Reprod. Fertil. J.* 64: 259–266.

56 Bakst, M.R., Donoghue, A.M., Yoho, D.E. et al. (2010). Comparisons of sperm storage tubule distribution and number in 4 strains of mature broiler breeders and in Turkey hens before and after the onset of photostimulation. *Poult. Sci.* 89 (5): 986–992.

57 Purohit, V.D., Basrur, P.K., and Reinhart, B.S. (1977). Persistent right oviduct in ring-necked pheasant. *Br. Poult. Sci.* 18 (2): 177–178.

5

Avian Physiology
Kahina Boukherroub and Sally L. Noll

5.1 Muscle Development and Growth

5.1.1 Skeletal Muscle Development and Growth

The musculoskeletal structure of birds can vary tremendously based on whether they fly or not. The majority of the muscles can be concentrated on the torso for birds that rely primarily on flight to move, as is the case in grouse, whereas birds that rely mostly on running, such as the pheasant and quail, have larger leg muscles [1]. Skeletal muscle cells are elongated, multinucleated cells, called myofibers. At hatch, chicks possess fully differentiated skeletal muscle cells, and muscle growth that occurs thereafter is due to an increase in muscle fiber size [2].

5.1.2 Embryonic Development of the Skeletal Muscle

During early stages of embryonic development, the primordial muscle cells, called myoblasts, concentrate in a block called the myotome. As development progresses, the myoblasts migrate from the myotome into their muscle beds where they continue to proliferate. Some myoblasts fuse with each other to form primary multinucleated muscle fibers, others continue to proliferate and eventually fuse into secondary muscle fibers. The formation of muscle fiber is complete at hatch and subsequent muscle growth is due to the enlargement of existing fibers in a process called hypertrophy [2, 3].

Chicks, for most common gamebirds, are precocial and possess relatively well-developed leg muscles at hatch. This is due to high levels of circulating maternal thyroid hormone during embryonic development and highly active thyroid during the perinatal period [4, 5].

5.1.3 Muscle Growth Post Hatch

Muscle hypertrophy occurs by the fusion of satellite cells located between the basement membranes of muscle fibers [6, 7]. The proliferation potential of satellite cells is higher in younger animals and diminishes as the animal gets older. Much of what is known about factors regulating the proliferation of satellite cells is derived from *in vitro* studies in cultured chicken and turkey embryonic myoblast satellite cells [1]. Among these factors, insulin-like growth factor (IGF) was found to enhance chicken myoblast differentiation and turkey myoblast proliferation [8]; fibroblast growth factor (FGF) was found to enhance turkey myoblasts and satellite cell proliferation [9, 10]; platelet-derived growth factor (PDGF) was found to enhance chicken myoblast proliferation [11, 12]; hepatocyte growth factor (HGF) was found to activate and enhance proliferation of dormant chicken and turkey satellite cells [13, 14]; transforming growth factor beta (TGF-beta) was found to inhibit both proliferation and differentiation of turkey satellite cells [15] but when added with FGF, it leads to chicken myoblast differentiation [16]; and myostatin was found to inhibit turkey and chicken myoblast and satellite cell differentiation [17, 18].

5.1.4 Maternal Inheritance of Muscle Growth Property

Muscle morphology is an important determinant of meat quality, and focusing on fast growth rates and muscling alone results in poor meat quality that displays pale, soft, exuding meat – PSE. When cooked, PSE results in soft, poor water binding and poor juiciness. Muscle morphology defined as extracellular matrix spacing and muscle fiber size was determined to be inherited from the mother in turkeys [19]. Although these studies were done in turkeys, maternal inheritance of muscle morphology could be a contributing factor in muscle morphology in gamebirds, so selection of sires and dams during breeding should be carefully considered.

5.2 Bone Development and Growth

The avian skeleton evolved to support flight, locomotion, and protection of the organs. It is a dynamic tissue that responds and adapts to physical stressors and is constantly undergoing remodeling. It also serves as a reservoir for calcium, phosphate, and other ions. The two main tissues of the skeleton are bone and cartilage. Cartilage is capable of growing quickly and that is why it is abundant in embryos and young individuals. Bone is more rigid and strong and predominant in the adult skeleton. Bone and cartilage parts are interconnected by joint structures, including synovial joints that connect between limb elements, intervertebral discs that confer pliability on the vertebral column, and fibrous joints to minimize movement between skull bones [20].

5.2.1 Bone Modeling

Bone acquisition during growth is referred to as bone modeling. It occurs in one of two ways: endochondral ossification or intramembranous ossification. During endochondral ossification, a cartilage anlagen is first formed, in a process referred to as chondrogenesis, followed by its replacement by bone. During embryonic development, progenitor cells that undergo chondrogenesis derive from the ectoderm and mesoderm. These mesenchymal cells condense and differentiate into cartilage-secreting cells known as chondroblasts. The resulting cartilaginous primary skeleton anlagen grows quickly and is subsequently turned into bone, during prenatal and postnatal growth. This process, referred to as endochondral ossification, is mediated by the activity of chondroclasts, that resorb the cartilage, and osteoblasts, that deposit bone [21].

The second process by which bone modeling occurs is intramembranous ossification, in which bones grow through a mesenchymal template without having to go through the cartilage state first. During this process, condensed mesenchymal cells differentiate directly into osteoblasts at a number of different sites simultaneously and start depositing bone [22].

5.2.2   Long Bone Growth

Long bones grow in both thickness and length. Increase in bone thickness (appositional growth) occurs through the formation of new bone on the outer surfaces of existing bone; increase in bone length (longitudinal growth) is achieved through the activities of the cartilaginous growth plates. Growth plates can be divided into several distinct zones: resting, proliferating, maturing, and terminally differentiated chondrocytes Appositional growth is the result of osteoblast activity on the outer layer of the bone where bone is deposited in successive laminar patterns. This process is coupled with osteoclast activity that causes the resorption of the inner surface of the bone.

5.2.3   Medullary Bone

Medullary bone is a secondary bone tissue that is exclusive to birds [23]. It deposits in spicules in the cavities of long bones and serves as a labile calcium reservoir to support the formation of eggshell in the uterus of the female. The contents of the medullary bone fluctuate with the ovulatory cycle and the position of the egg in the oviduct [24, 25]. When the egg is in the infundibulum, isthmus, or magnum, the bone-building osteoblasts, under the action of estrogen, actively deposit medullary bone; when the egg transitions to the uterus (eggshell gland), osteoblasts cease depositing bone, while the bone-resorbing osteoclasts, under the activity of parathyroid hormone, start their bone resorption activity to release calcium. The freed Ca is then deposited on the eggshell, which in turn serves as a reservoir for the developing embryo. The amount of Ca in each eggshell typically represents about 10% of the total body Ca stores in the bird [26]. In avian species that lay a lot of eggs, such as the commercial laying hen, the calcium demand for eggshell formation can get too high and result in the mobilization of calcium from cortical bone. This leads to thinning of the bone and osteoporosis [27].

5.3   Osmoregulation

Osmoregulation refers to the various mechanisms organisms use to regulate the levels of water and electrolytes in their bodies. Unlike in mammals, where osmoregulation is solely regulated by the kidneys, birds have three organs that play a role in osmoregulation: the kidneys, the lower gastrointestinal tract, and salt glands [28]. In this section, only kidney function will be discussed. For more on adaptive strategies for postrenal handling of urine in birds, see the review by Laverty and Skadhauge [29].

5.3.1   Metanephric Kidney Development and Osmoregulation in the Embryo

Osmoregulation in the avian embryo involves a balance between water loss, due to evaporation though the eggshell, and water gain through increased metabolic activity as development advances. Maintaining a balance between water loss and water gain is crucial for avoiding osmotic stress, dehydration, and embryonic death [30]. The metanephric kidney and the chorioallantoic membrane (CAM) work together to regulate water and electrolyte balance [31]. Early in embryonic development, the CAM is the major regulator of water and ion balance [32]. As development progresses, the mesonephros, which is then replaced by the metanephric kidneys, takes over osmoregulation as well as nitrogen secretion. During this time, nitrogen secretion switches from urea to uric acid [31].

5.3.2 The Urinary System in the Adult

The urinary system in birds consists of paired kidneys and ureters that empty into the urodeum of the cloaca. The role of the kidney is to filter blood, excrete waste products and ions, and reabsorb needed substances like glucose. The avian kidney is divided into three divisions: the anterior, middle, and posterior lobes [33]. Each lobe is a collection of units referred to as lobules. The outer part of the lobule is called the cortex, which constitutes about >75% of the lobule, and the inner part of the lobule is called the medulla, which constitutes <15% of the lobule; the rest is blood vessels. The functional unit in the kidney is a long convoluted tubule called the nephron [34]. Because birds do not have a urinary bladder, the output of the kidneys is emptied into the cloaca. It then moves in a retrograde fashion toward the large intestine where more water, sodium, and potassium are reabsorbed [35, 36].

In birds, the cloaca and lower intestine serve a similar function to that of the distal nephron in mammals, making fine adjustments in water and sodium reabsorption from the urine.

5.3.3 Urine Concentration and Response to Dehydration

Unlike mammals, the ability of birds to produce hyperosmotic urine is limited. Domestic chickens, for instance, can produce urine that is only twice the osmolality of their plasma [37]. This limited ability is attributed to the fact that the majority of the nephrons in their kidney (85%) are reptilian type nephrons, meaning they lack a loop of Henle, which is the part of the nephron that gives mammalian type nephrons the ability to excrete salt. When birds are subjected to extreme dehydration that results in acute osmotic load, the kidneys respond by slowing down their glomerular filtration rate (GFR) [38] and by reducing the number of functioning reptilian type nephrons [34]. When the bird is severely dehydrated, GFR can be reduced as much as 65%. GFR is controlled by the pituitary-secreted antidiuretic hormone arginine-vasotocin (AVT). AVT affects the GFR by decreasing the number of filtering loopless nephrons, by constricting the vasculature around the nephrons [34] and epithelium of renal tubules [39].

5.4 Respiratory System

As in other animals, the respiratory system functions to exchange oxygen (O_2) and carbon dioxide (CO_2) in the lungs. Oxygenated blood supplies the various tissues and organs with O_2 to support metabolic demands including maintenance, growth, and activities such as flight. Carbon dioxide is produced as the result of these metabolic processes and enters the bloodstream. Gases in the blood are expressed in terms of partial pressure (PO_2 or PCO_2) and in arterial blood as PaO_2 and $PaCO_2$. Besides exchange of gases, the respiratory system is involved in acid–base balance, thermoregulation, and water balance [40]. Further detail is available on the avian respiratory system [40, 41].

5.4.1 Gaseous Exchange

The function and anatomy of the respiratory system of gamebirds are not much different from other birds [42]. Cycles of inspiration and expiration bring air into the respiratory tract where the gaseous exchange occurs in the paleopulmonic parabronchi of the lung in a humidified environment. Gas exchange does not occur in the air sacs; however, the air sacs act as a bellows to move the air through and out of the respiratory tract. Breathing is an active process as the lung is not expansible and birds do not have a diaphragm. Muscle contraction is needed for both inspiration and expiration to create pressure differences for airflow. Contraction with inspiration moves the sternum forward and down, and the vertebral ribs move to expand the sternal ribs and abdominal cavity, creating negative pressure. During expiration, contraction with a different set of muscles decreases abdominal volume [40, 41].

The pattern of airflow through the respiratory tract means that two cycles of inspiration and expiration need to occur to move an initial volume of air into the tract and then its subsequent exit through the upper part of the tract [41, 43]. With both inspiration and expiration, airflow through the paleopulmonic parabronchi is unidirectional from caudal to cranial. Upon inspiration, airflow is to the cranial and caudal air sacs and air leaves the paleopulmonic parabronchi to the cranial air sacs; with expiration, air leaves the cranial air sacs for exhalation through the trachea and air from the caudal air sacs passes cranially to the parabronchi of the lung.

5.4.2 Ventilation Control

Ventilation changes in response to blood pH or arterial gases (PaO_2 and $PaCO_2$) can be species dependent. In response to changes from normal, ventilation frequency and/or tidal volume will adjust. Sensing is done by chemoreceptors with central, arterial and intrapulmonary receptors located in the brain, carotid artery, and lung, respectively. The arterial chemoreceptors detect changes in PaO_2, $PaCO_2$, and blood pH. Intrapulmonary receptors are very sensitive to PCO_2, assessing on a breath-by-breath basis. Overall, the system is more sensitive to changes in CO_2 than O_2 [44]. Under conditions of increased CO_2 in inspired air, frequency and tidal volume increase. When a decrease in $PaCO_2$ or intrapulmonary PCO_2 occurs, ventilation frequency is decreased. With hypoxia (low O_2), while typically not experienced, ventilation is initially increased, although once $PaCO_2$ starts to decrease, ventilation frequency will also decrease.

5.4.3 Respiration and Acid–Base Balance

Shifts in blood pH can have a number of negative effects on the animal's system. The respiratory system is able to respond quickly to these shifts. By changing ventilation frequency, blood pH can be modified through $PaCO_2$ adjustments [40]. Circulating levels of CO_2 are a primary determinant of blood pH. In the blood, CO_2 is present in different forms, about 5% as dissolved in arterial blood, combined with hemoglobin, and the majority in the form of bicarbonate ion ($HCO3^-$). To produce bicarbonate, CO_2 combines with water to form carbonic acid that dissociates to bicarbonate and hydrogen ions under enzymatic action as demonstrated in the following equation:

$$CO_2 + H_2O \leftrightarrow H_2CO_3 \leftrightarrow HCO_3^- + H^+$$

Under conditions that result in CO_2 accumulation, formation of bicarbonate is predominant along with production of hydrogen ions, which decreases blood pH (acidosis). Lowering of CO_2 results in alkalosis as production shifts toward carbonic acid removing H+ from the blood. Increased or decreased ventilation will be the result, respectively, for acidosis and alkalosis to return to normal blood PCO_2.

Disturbances in the respiratory system can directly influence blood pH [45]. An example would be the impact of panting due to heat stress, in which respiratory alkalosis develops. The decreased PCO_2 reduces bicarbonate. For female birds in egg production, mineralization of the eggshell occurs with the deposition of calcium carbonate. The calcium carbonate is formed from calcium and bicarbonate [25]. The shortage of bicarbonate because of panting can affect eggshell formation, especially if producing eggs at a high rate [46].

5.4.4 Respiration and Thermal Regulation

The respiratory system plays a major role in body temperature (Tb) control under conditions of heat stress. Slight increases in body temperature are sufficient to elicit a respiratory response with increased respiration [44]. Birds lack skin sweat glands and depend on heat loss through the latent heat of evaporation (evaporative cooling). While some cutaneous evaporation can occur, evaporative cooling is the main method of heat loss as ambient temperatures approach body temperature.

Evaporative cooling occurs as inspired air passes through the upper respiratory system [45, 47, 48]. As ambient temperature increases, birds will increase ventilation frequency by panting. Compound ventilation has been observed in older turkeys under heat stress [49] where panting is superimposed over a pattern of slower and deeper breathing [50]. The efficacy of heat loss through evaporation is influenced by both temperature and relative humidity (RH). Maximal respiration rates in turkeys were influenced more by higher RH under increasing temperature conditions [49], indicating that the combination of both temperature and RH should be considered. Hence, temperature–humidity indexes are more useful for identifying heat stress conditions [51].

While panting is an important part of combating hyperthermia, it has disadvantages. One limitation is that the respiratory system needs to balance sensory inputs regarding $PaCO_2$, pH, and the need for heat loss [45]. Panting reduces $paCO_2$ and then ventilation is lowered as a reflex. However, with the lowered rate of ventilation, the amount of heat loss through evaporative cooling is reduced. Depending on the temperature stress level, Tb will continue to rise while the respiratory system responds to the lowered $PaCO_2$ [44]. Another disadvantage with panting, besides respiratory alkalosis, is that water is lost from the body via evaporation. Water loss in some species can be substantial, with the loss nearing the amount that the bird would drink in a similar time, putting the bird at risk for dehydration [52]. Additionally, prolonged panting produces more heat from the respiratory muscles, disrupts feeding and drinking activities, and potentially overheats naturally incubated eggs [53].

5.5 Digestive System

The digestive system in terms of form and function shows variety in the gastrointestinal anatomy depending on the type of food ingested and how food is obtained [54] but is relatively similar within the order Galliformes [55]. Compared to mammals, organs of the digestive system in birds are more numerous [54]. Gallinaceous birds are omnivores so the gizzard and ceca are of particular importance due to processing of seeds with hulls and high fibrous content as part of their natural food source [55]. Reviews of digestive processes are available in more detail elsewhere [54, 56–58] with a brief overview presented here.

5.5.1 Form and Function

After food has been swallowed and has entered the esophagus, it reaches the crop. Food can bypass the crop depending on how long the bird has been fasting [56]. Digestion does not occur in the crop, but it is important for food storage in foraging birds. The food passes to the stomach, which is composed of the proventriculus (glandular stomach) and the ventriculus (gizzard). The proventriculus secrets mucus, acid (HCl), and pepsin. The low pH in combination with the pepsin denatures proteins and starts the hydrolysis process. Material then flows to the gizzard where mechanical forces are applied to grind material to a finer particle size while mixing contents with gastric secretions. Gizzard size and grinding capacity are related to food type, with coarse materials causing an increase in size and muscularity [54]. The gizzard selectively releases smaller size particles to the small intestine.

The small intestine is divided into three segments, the first being the duodenum. The pancreas sits in the duodenal loop. Ducts from the pancreas secrete bicarbonate to buffer the intestinal pH for enzyme activity. The pancreas secretes numerous digestive enzymes into the duodenal lumen. The gall bladder releases bile through the bile duct in the duodenum for fat emulsification. Digesta moves to the next section of the intestine, which is the jejunum. Most of the digestion and absorption of nutrients occurs here. Proteins, fats, and starch continue to be broken down enzymatically to smaller units such as amino acids and glucose for absorption. Mineral absorption occurs in the upper part of the jejunum. Remaining digesta enters the ileum with digestion and absorption continuing.

Water absorption occurs in the lower part of the tract, including the ileum, colon, and ceca. Ceca are filled with fine particle-sized material or smaller molecules from the ileum and colon. The ceca have several functions including water resorption, fiber digestion, and nitrogen homeostasis. For some Galliformes such as turkeys and quail, the ceca are large in comparison to other species and contain lymphoid tissue [54]. Similar to the gizzard, size increases with high-fiber food sources [59]. Cecal contents are different in color and consistency from the rectal feces. In the cloaca, openings for the digestive and urinary tracts empty into the cloaca.

5.5.2 Digestive Secretions

Enzymes are secreted from both the pancreas and intestines. Enzyme activity is highest in the jejunum, most likely due to the location of the pancreatic ducts near the anterior jejunum. Intestinal enzymes are found in the epithelial cells of the intestine. Secretion of gastrointestinal hormones occurs primarily from the pancreas, proventriculus, and upper small intestine. These hormones stimulate secretion of enzymes and bicarbonate from the pancreas and intestine, and secretion of gastric acid and pepsin from the proventriculus. Some of the secreted hormones can have an inhibitory effect, such as somatostatin which inhibits secretion of other gastrointestinal hormones [56].

5.5.3 Digestion and Nutrient Absorption

The internal layer of the intestine is lined with villi and crypts. The villi are finger-like projections lined with epithelial cells called enterocytes which absorb nutrients. Enzymatic digestion continues at the brush border of the enterocyte. Through different transport systems, nutrients enter the enterocytes and eventually transfer to the capillary bed for transport. Crypts serve as a source of replacement cells for the enterocytes [56].

5.5.4 Digestion and Gut Motility

Motility in the gut is necessary to move food/digesta through the tract or into the crop and ceca [54]. While most of the movement of contents is aboral (moving away from the mouth), unique to birds are refluxes that move material orad (moving toward the mouth) in order to mix contents with digestive secretions.

After swallowing food, peristaltic waves move undigested food through the esophagus to the crop while contractions of the crop move the undigested food to the proventriculus. The gastrointestinal cycle then moves contents from the proventriculus to the small intestine with a reflux of duodenal materials to the gizzard. The cycle starts with thin muscle contraction of the gizzard that closes the isthmus between the proventriculus and gizzard. The pyloris (between the gizzard and duodenum) opens with movement of digesta from gizzard to the duodenum. The duodenum then contracts, the isthmus opens, and the thick muscles of the gizzard contract, moving the gizzard materials into the proventriculus. The proventriculus then contracts to end the cycle. Recurrence of the cycle is controlled by a pacemaker located in the isthmus.

The ceca fill because of waves of ileal peristalsis and colonic antiperistalsis coming together at the ileal–cecal junction. Contractions of the ceca move material aborad and orad. Antiperistalsis occurs almost continually in the colon to reflux contents to the ceca and small intestine for resorption of intestinal water and renal water. Colonic antiperistalsis stops when defecation occurs. The ceca empty a couple times of day separately after rectal evacuation has occurred [56].

Food passage rate is relatively quick in domestic fowl, with the upper part of the gastrointestinal tract having a mean retention time of 1–2 hours. For the rest of the tract, the mean retention time is approximately 4 hours. Material in the ceca remains for a longer time even after 24 hours of fasting [56, 58].

5.6   Integument

The integument is the external surface of the bird composed of skin, feathers, and other derivatives. Appendages such as the beak (bill), head ornaments, and claws are derived from the skin along with oil glands of the outer ear and the uropygial gland. Physiologic functions of the skin include sebaceous production and its action as a somatosensory system [60].

5.6.1   Skin as a Somatosensory System

The skin contains nerve endings and sensors for responding to surrounding environments [61]. The surface of the skin, especially areas of feathered skin, beak or bill, toes and claws, contain cutaneous nerve receptors. The receptors are located in the dermis layer and recognize mechanical, thermal, and noxious stimuli. The most common mechanoreceptors are the Herbst corpuscles in the deep dermis which are widely distributed in the skin and are associated with the feather follicles and muscular association with feathers. These receptors are important in flight for sensing skin contact and changes in the air stream. Merkel cell receptors occur in the dermis, associated with the beak and tongue, toes, and feathered skin. In aquatic birds, Gandry corpuscles are present in the bill tip. Mechanosensors recognize ground vibration and abnormalities in plumage condition. For the beak and bill, the sensors are important for birds to select and manipulate a variety of food sources. Thermal receptors are important in body temperature regulation, recognizing changing temperature, and are present in the beak and tongue. Nociceptors react to things such as pain that could be the result of injury.

5.6.2   Skin as a Sebaceous Gland

Avian skin, along with the uropygial gland and the ear canal, produces lipids [60, 62]. The secretions vary by skin location or thickness, tending to be greater in thin skin areas and in association with skin derivatives such as combs and wattles. The secretions are hydrophobic and help keep the skin supple and serve as a moisture barrier. These secretions, along with those of the uropygial gland (preen gland in most avian species), keep feathers conditioned by preventing brittleness and moisture uptake. The preen oil is spread from the gland and is applied to the feathers and feet by the action of the beak/bill [63]. The gland has other functions such as production of pheromones [64], contribution to plumage color, antibacterial and antifungal properties including protection against keratin-degrading bacteria, maintaining thermal insulation, defense against predators, and whole-body detoxification through collection of pesticides in preen oil [65].

The preen oil is a combination of esters (fatty acids and wax alcohol chains) which vary in composition with age, species, and breeding status [64, 66]. Age-related shifts in composition have been hypothesized to occur in order to minimize odors in young birds or toward pheromones in breeding adults. Endocrine control of the preen gland composition is associated with gonadal steroids (estrogen/androgens), thyroxine, and corticosteroids.

5.6.3 Feathers

Feathers vary in type, form, and function. Functions include flying, gliding, insulation, water resistance, and communication. In gamebirds, quality feathering is especially important for insulation and protection from the elements when reared or released outdoors. Quality is also important for bird appearance and ease of feather removal for carcass processing.

Feathers are composed primarily of a protein called beta-keratin [60], making the feathers strong but with some flexibility. Once feathers stop growing, they are considered dead tissue and are not able to repair themselves. Replacement is then necessary to maintain functionality. Thus, there are cycles of new feather growth (anagen) and rest (telogen). New growing feathers push out the old feather (molt); new feather growth can also be stimulated after feather loss from plucking.

5.6.4 Feather Growth and Loss

Formation of the first set of feathers (natal, downy) begins during embryonic development. The second set of new feathers (juvenal) start forming before hatch occurs. The molt of juvenal plumage (prebasic) leads to overwintering or nonbreeding plumage. Depending on species, there may be intermediate molts in the first year of life and a lack of a prealternate molt (prenuptial, before breeding). After the first breeding season, annual molt cycles are prebasic (postnuptial, after breeding) and in some species, prealternate (prenuptial) prior to breeding. Mature birds undergo at least one complete molt per year [67–69].

Feather growth occurs in the feather follicle, which appears as a pocket or socket visible on the skin surface. Detailed descriptions of follicle development and feather growth have been previously published [60, 62, 70]. Feather follicle formation only occurs during embryo development, resulting in a permanent structure associated with the feather tract (pterylae). The follicle is an invagination of the skin's epidermal layer, which surrounds the developing feather cylinder. The epidermal and dermal layers of the feather follicle contribute to cell growth, cell differentiation, and keratinization of the new feather.

At the base of the follicle is the dermal papilla. The dermal papilla and its covering of epidermis form the blastema for future growth. Once activated, the cells start mitosis and form an epidermal ring or collar at the follicle base above the dermal papilla. The collar contains stem cells to initiate new feather growth. The stem cells are positioned differently in rings depending on feather type [62]. When feather growth is completed, the papilla regresses and a rest phase is entered. Remaining cells at the base of the papilla contribute to growth of a new collar for future new feathers after activation. The next set of feathers from the same follicle can differ in appearance, suggesting that these cells can be reprogrammed for each generation of feathers [71].

The dermis contributes to the core of pulp that is vascularized to deliver nutrients for feather growth. The cells from the three epidermal layers form the basis for the feather sheath, which encloses the developing feather, and for differentiation into barb ridges, rachis, and barbules. Keratin-producing cells populate the growing feather and eventually fill with keratin. As the feather grows, the pulp regresses and is resorbed. The last portion of the feather to grow is the calamus so that the feather remains seated in the follicle through follicle smooth muscle attachments and keratin bridges. The follicle has nearby nerve sensors that sense feather position and pressure. Nerve connections exist with other follicles.

Coordination of the growth of the different feather parts in the follicle is very complex and not well understood. Some cell signaling protein factors that guide cell differentiation have been identified. Bone modeling protein (BMP) plays a role in the spacing of follicles in the feather tract during embryo development [72]. Other cell signaling proteins such as SHH and Noggin have been identified; interference with their activity results in abnormal feather formation with effects on the rachis, barb, or barbules.

Endocrine influence on cycles of feather growth and molt in mature birds is primarily related to photoperiod, where exposure to long daylengths results in the eventual development of photorefractoriness and subsequent regression of the reproductive tract. Other environmental factors such as environmental temperature can modify molt times as well [69]. In mature birds, molt (prebasic) occurs after breeding. Hormones with the most involvement are thyroid hormone, gonadal steroids, and prolactin [69, 73, 74]. Receptors for gonadal steroid hormones are located in the feather follicle [73]. Estrogens and androgens appear to inhibit molt, while thyroid hormone, progesterone, and prolactin are correlated with occurrence of molt.

References

1 Velleman, S.G. and McFarland, D.C. Skeletal muscle. In: *Sturkie's Avian Physiology*, 6e (ed. C.G. Scanes), 379–396. San Diego, CA: Elsevier.

2 Smith, J.H. (1963). Relation of body size to muscle cell size and number in the chicken. *Poult. Sci.* 42 (2): 283–290.

3 Scaal, M. and Marcelle, C. (2018). Chick muscle development. *Int. J. Dev. Biol.* 62: 123–132.

4 McNabb, F.M.A., Stanton, F.W., and Dicken, S.G. (1984). Post-hatching thyroid development and body growth in precocial vs altricial birds. *Comp. Biochem. Physiol. Part A Physiol.* 78 (4): 629–635.

5 Darras, V.M. (2019). The role of maternal thyroid hormones in avian embryonic development. *Front. Endocrinol.* 10 (65).

6 Mauro, A. (1961). Satellite cell of skeletal muscle fibers. *J. Biophys. Biochem. Cytol.* 9 (2): 493–495.

7 Moss, F.P. and Leblond, C.P. (1971). Satellite cells as the source of nuclei in muscles of growing rats. *Anat. Rec.* 170 (4): 421–435.

8 Schmid, C., Steiner, T., and Froesch, E.R. (1983). Preferential enhancement of myoblast differentiation by insulin-like growth factors (IGF I and IGF II) in primary cultures of chicken embryonic cells. *FEBS Lett.* 161 (1): 117–121.

9 McFarland, D.C., Pesall, J.E., and Gilkerson, K.K. (1993). The influence of growth factors on Turkey embryonic myoblasts and satellite cells in vitro. *Gen. Comp. Endocrinol.* 89 (3): 415–424.

10 Wilkie, R.S., O'Neill, I.E., Butterwith, S.C. et al. (1995). Regulation of chick muscle satellite cells by fibroblast growth factors: interaction with insulin-like growth factor-I and heparin. *Growth. Regul.* 5 (1): 18–27.

11 Yablonka-Reuveni, Z. (1995). Development and postnatal regulation of adult myoblasts. *Microsc. Res. Tech.* 30 (5): 366–380.

12 Yablonka-Reuveni, Z. and Seifert, R.A. (1993). Proliferation of chicken myoblasts is regulated by specific isoforms of platelet-derived growth factor: evidence for differences between myoblasts from mid and late stages of embryogenesis. *Dev. Biol.* 156 (2): 307–318.

13 Gal-Levi, R., Leshem, Y., Aoki, S. et al. (1998). Hepatocyte growth factor plays a dual role in regulating skeletal muscle satellite cell proliferation and differentiation. *Biochim. Biophys. Acta, Mol. Cell. Res.* 1402 (1): 39–51.

14 Zeng, C., Pesall, J.E., Gilkerson, K.K., and McFarland, D.C. (2002). The effect of hepatocyte growth factor on turkey satellite cell proliferation and differentiation. *Poult. Sci.* 81 (8): 1191–1198.

15 Yun, Y., McFarland, D.C., Pesail, J.E. et al. (1997). Variation in response to growth factor stimuli in satellite cell populations. *Comp. Biochem. Physiol. A Physiol.* 117 (4): 463–470.

16 Schofield, J.N. and Wolpert, L. (1990). Effect of TGF-β1, TGF-β2, and bFGF on chick cartilage and muscle cell differentiation. *Exp. Cell. Res.* 191 (1): 144–148.

17 McFarland, D.C., Velleman, S.G., Pesall, J.E., and Liu, C. (2007). The role of myostatin in chicken (Gallus domesticus) myogenic satellite cell proliferation and differentiation. *Gen. Comp. Endocrinol.* 151 (3): 351–357.

18 McFarland, D.C., Velleman, S.G., Pesall, J.E., and Liu, C. (2006). Effect of myostatin on turkey myogenic satellite cells and embryonic myoblasts. *Comp. Biochem. Physiol. Part A Mol. Integr. Physiol.* 144 (4): 501–508.

19 Velleman, S.G. and Nestor, K.E. (2004). Inheritance of breast muscle morphology in turkeys at sixteen weeks of age. *Poult. Sci.* 83 (7): 1060–1066.

20 Lefebvre, V. and Bhattaram, P. (2010). Vertebrate skeletogenesis. *Curr. Top. Dev. Biol.* 90: 291–317.

21 Pechak, D.G., Kujawa, M.J., and Caplan, A.I. (1986). Morphology of bone development and bone remodeling in embryonic chick limbs. *Bone* 7 (6): 459–472.

22 Thompson, T.J., Owens, P.D., and Wilson, D.J. (1989). Intramembranous osteogenesis and angiogenesis in the chick embryo. *J. Anat.* 166 (1): 55–65.

23 Bloom, W., Bloom, M.A., and McLean, F.C. (1941). Calcification and ossification. Medullary bone changes in the reproductive cycle of female pigeons. *Anat. Rec.* 81 (4): 443–475.

24 González, M.S. (2019). Skeletal bone structure and repair in small mammals, birds, and reptiles. *Vet. Clin. North Am. Exot. Anim. Pract.* 22 (2): 135–147.

25 Dacke, C.G., Sugiyama, T., and Gay, C.V. (2015). The role of hormones in the regulation of bone turnover and eggshell calcification. In: *Sturkie's Avian Physiology*, 6e (ed. C.G. Scanes), 549–553. San Diego, CA: Elsevier.

26 Kenny, A.D. (1986). Parathyroid and ultimobranchial glands. In: *Avian Physiology*, 4e (ed. P.D. Sturkie), 466–478. New York: Springer-Verlag.

27 Whitehead, C.C. and Fleming, R.H. (2000). Osteoporosis in cage layers. *Poult. Sci.* 79 (7): 1033–1041.

28 Braun, E.J. (2015). Osmoregulatory systems of birds. In: *Sturkie's Avian Physiology*, 6e (ed. C.G. Scanes), 285–295. San Diego, CA: Elsevier.

29 Laverty, G. and Skadhauge, E. (2008). Adaptive strategies for post-renal handling of urine in birds. *Comp. Biochem. Physiol. Part A Mol. Integr. Physiol.* 149 (3): 246–254.

30 Davis, T.A., Shen, S.S., and Ackerman, R.A. (1988). Embryonic osmoregulation: consequences of high and low water loss during incubation of the chicken egg. *J. Exp. Zool.* 245 (2): 144–156.

31 Bolin, G. and Burggren, W.W. (2013). Metanephric kidney development in the chicken embryo: glomerular numbers, characteristics and perfusion. *Comp. Biochem. Physiol. Part A Mol. Integr. Physiol.* 166 (2): 343–350.

32 Gabrielli, M.G. and Accili, D. (2010). The chick chorioallantoic membrane: a model of molecular, structural, and functional adaptation to transepithelial ion transport and barrier function during embryonic development. *J. Biomed. Biotechnol.* 2010: 940741.

33 Johnson, O.W. (1968). Some morphological features of avian kidneys. *Auk.* 85 (2): 216–228.

34 Braun, J. and Dantzler, H. (1972). Function of mammalian-type and reptilian-type nephrons in kidney of desert quail. *Am. J. Phys* 222 (3): 617–629.

35 Nechay, B.R., Boyarsky, S., and Catacutan-Labay, P. (1968). Rapid migration of urine into intestine of chickens. *Comp. Biochem. Physiol.* 26: 369–370.

36 Anderson, G.L. and Braun, E.J. (1985). Postrenal modification of urine in birds. *Am. J. Phys* 248 (1pt 2): 93–98.

37 Korr, I.M. (1939). The osmotic function of the chicken kidney. *J. Cell. Comp. Physiol.* 13 (2): 175–193.

38 Dantzler, W.H. (1966). Renal response of chickens to infusion of hyperosmotic sodium chloride solution. *Am. J. Phys* 210 (3): 640–646.

39 Stallone, J.N. and Braun, E.J. (1986). Contributions of glomerular and tubular mechanisms to antidiuresis in conscious domestic fowl. *Am. J. Phys* 250 (6): 842–850.

40 Powell, F.L. (2015). Respiration. In: *Sturkie's Avian Physiology*, 6e (ed. C.G. Scanes), 301–330. San Diego, CA: Elsevier.

41 Casteleyn, C., Cornillie, P., Van Cruchten, S. et al. (2018). Anatomy of the lower respiratory in domestic birds, with emphasis on respiration. *Anat. Histol. Embryol.* 47 (2): 89–99.

42 Coles, B.H. (2009). Galliformes. In: *Handbook of Avian Medicine* (ed. T. Tully Jr., G. Dorrestein and A. Jones), 309–334.

43 Fedde, M.R. (1980). Structure and gas-flow pattern in the avian respiratory system. *Poult. Sci.* 59 (12): 2642–2653.

44 Burger, R.E. (1980). Respiratory gas exchange and control in the chicken. *Poult. Sci.* 59 (12): 2654–2665.

45 Yahav, S. Regulation of body temperature: strategies and mechanisms. In: *Sturkie's Avian Physiology*, 6e (ed. C.G. Scanes), 869–900. San Diego, CA: Elsevier.

46 Leeson, S., Diaz, G., and Summers, J.D. (1995). Electrolyte imbalance. In: *Poultry Metabolic Disorders and Mycotoxins* (ed. S. Leeson, G. Diaz and J.D. Summers). Guelph, Ontario.: University Books.

47 Dawson, W.R. (1982). Evaporative losses of water by birds. *Comp. Biochem. Physiol.* 71 (4): 495–509.

48 Menuam, B. and Richards, S.A. (1975). Observations on the sites of respiratory evaporation in the flow during thermal panting. *Resp. Physiol.* 25 (1): 39–52.

49 Brown-Brandl, T.M., Beck, M.M., Schulte, D.D. et al. (1997). Physiological responses of tom turkeys to temperature and humidity change with age. *J. Thermal. Biol.* 22 (1): 43–52.

50 Dawson, W.R. and Whittow, G.C. (2000). Regulation of body temperature. In: *Sturkie's Avian Physiology*, 5e (ed. G.C. Whittow), 344–379. San Diego, CA: Academic Press.

51 Xin, H. and Harmon, J.D. (1998). Livestock industry facilities and environment: heat stress indices for livestock. In: *Agriculture and Environment Extension Publications*, 163. Ames, IA: Iowa State University.

52 Leeson, S., Diaz, G., and Summers, J.D. (1995). Water imbalance. In: *Poultry Metabolic Disorders and Mycotoxins* (ed. S. Leeson, G. Diaz and J.D. Summers). Guelph, Ontario: University Books.

53 Marder, J. and Arad, Z. (1989). Panting and acid-base regulation in heat stress birds. *Comp. Biochem. Physiol.* 94a (3): 395–400.

54 Klasing, K.C. *Comparative Avian Nutrition*. Wallingford, UK: CAB International.

55 Schales, C. and Schales, K. (1996). Galliformes. In: *Avian Medicine: Principles and Application*, 1218–1236. Lakeworth, FL: Wingers Publishing.

56 Denbow, D.M. (2015). Gastrointestinal anatomy and physiology. In: *Sturkie's Avian Physiology*, 6e (ed. C.G. Scanes), 337–366. San Diego, CA: Elsevier.

57 Klasing, K.C. (1999). Avian gastrointestinal anatomy and physiology. *Sem. Av. Exot. Pet. Med.* 8 (2): 42–50.

58 Svihus, B. (2014). Function of the digestive system. *J. Appl. Poult. Res.* 23 (2): 306–314.

59 Svihus, B., Choct, M., and Classen, H.L. (2013). Function and nutritional roles of the avian caeca: a review. *World's Poult. Sci. J.* 69 (2): 249–264.

60 Stettenheim, P.R. (2000). The integumentary morphology of modern birds – an overview. *Am. Zool.* 40 (4): 461–477.

61 Necker, R. (2000). The somatosensory system. In: *Sturkie's Avian Physiology*, 5e (ed. C.G. Whittow), 57–67. San Diego, CA: Academic Press.

62 Pass, D.A. (1995). Normal anatomy of the avian skin and feathers. *Sem. Av. Exot. Pet. Med.* 4 (4): 152–160.

63 Moreno-Rueda, G. (2017). Preen oil and bird fitness: a critical review of the evidence. *Biol. Rev.* 92 (4): 2131–2143.

64 Sandilands, V., Powell, K., Keeling, L., and Savory, C.J. (2004). Preen gland function in layer fowls: factors affecting preen oil fatty acid composition. *Br. Poult. Sci.* 45 (1): 109–115.

65 Giraudeau, M., Duval, C., Guillon, N. et al. (2010). Effects of access to preen glad secretions on mallard plumage. *Naturwissenschaften.* 97 (6): 577–581.

66 Salibian, A. and Montalti, D. (2009). Physiological and biochemical aspects of the avian uropygial gland. *Braz. J. Biol.* 69 (2): 437–446.

67 Howell, S.N.G., Corben, C., Pyle, P., and Rogers, D.J. (2003). The first basic problem: a review of molt and plumage homologies. *Condor.* 105 (4): 635–653.

68 Gill, F.B. (2007). *Ornithology*, 3e. New York: W.H. Freeman.

69 Dawson, A. (2015). Avian molting. In: *Sturkie's Avian Physiology*, 6e (ed. C.G. Scanes), 907–914. San Diego, CA: Elsevier.

70 Yu, M., Yue, Z., Wu, P. et al. (2004). The developmental biology of feather follicles. *Int. J. Dev. Biol.* 48: 181–191.

71 Chen, M.J., Xie, W.Y., Jiang, S.G. et al. (2020). Molecular signaling and nutritional regulation in the context of poultry feather growth and regeneration. *Front. Physiol.* 10: 1609.

72 Noramly, S. and Morgan, B.A. (1998). BMPs mediate lateral inhibition at successive stages in feather tract development. *Develop.* 125 (19): 3775–3787.

73 Peczely, P. (1991). Hormonal regulation of feather development and moult on the level of feather follicles. *Ornis. Scand.* 23: 346–354.

74 Decuypere, E. and Verheyen, G. (1986). Physiological basis of induced moulting and tissue regeneration in fowls. *World's Poult. Sci. J.* 42 (1): 56–68.

6

Gamebird Housing and Handling

Bill MacFarlane and Casey W. Ritz

Gamebirds have unique characteristics that require special considerations in their housing and handling. In this chapter, the housing management for two of the most common gamebird species will be discussed.

6.1 Pheasants

The commercial pheasant industry is ever-changing and adapting. As new ways of raising pheasants are discovered, protocols change. Currently there are about 6 million pheasants produced in captivity in the US annually. This chapter provides an overview of that industry, and how an individual interested in raising pheasants on a smaller scale could set up their farm.

6.1.1 Breeding Pheasants

When raising pheasants, it is important to know how to manage breeders. Most commercial pheasant breeder operations colony breed pheasants outdoors on the ground. Colony breeding means having hundreds of hens and a much smaller number of males (one male for every 10 or 12 hens) in one single pen. Increasingly, commercial pheasant farms are breeding pheasants indoors in poultry facilities (either new installations or former chicken or turkey sheds). Battery breeding units in Europe consist of 10 hens with one cock bird in a 1 m × 1 m outdoor wire-bottomed cage. Often the cock birds are switched to a new battery unit once a week. There are some large operations in China where hens are housed in cages and are artificially inseminated. Hens are usually artificially inseminated once or twice a week. Generally, the more feral pheasants lay the fewest eggs in cages and the most domesticated hens lay the most. Caged breeding, therefore, genetically selects for more docile or tame birds (Figure 6.1). This may be good in the food market, but not for birds being bred for hunting purposes.

Some metrics to consider for breeders include that pheasants require 0.7 inch linear feeder space and 0.1 inch. linear waterer space per bird. Breeders will eat approximately 1–1.5 pounds of feed per week. Ringneck breeder feed is typically 20% protein feed. Colony-bred pheasants on commercial farms usually are peeped. Peepers are small plastic devices that clip onto the beaks of pheasants, making it difficult for the pheasant to see other birds (Figure 6.2). The purpose of these peepers is to reduce aggression among pen mates.

Gamebird Medicine and Management, First Edition. Edited by Teresa Y. Morishita and Robert E. Porter, Jr.
© 2023 John Wiley & Sons, Inc. Published 2023 by John Wiley & Sons, Inc.

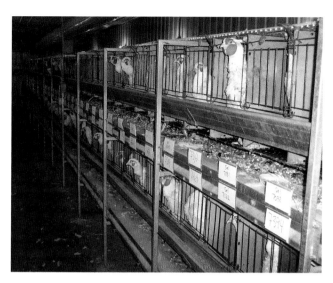

Figure 6.1　Pedigree white pheasant breeder cocks in breeder battery cages.

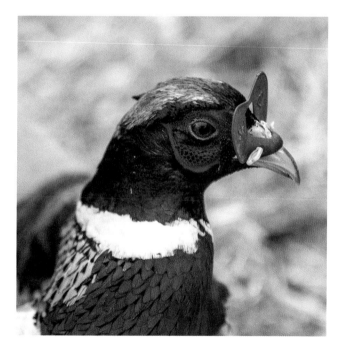

Figure 6.2　This male ringneck pheasant is fitted with peepers (spectacles), which are clip-on plastic flaps that obscure forward vision and reduce aggression among penmates.

Outdoor pheasant density when breeding on the ground is usually in the 20–30 square feet (sq ft) per bird range. Indoor breeder density is in the 5–10 sq ft per bird range. European breeding units are denser, but only hold 10 hens and one cock per unit in a cage a few feet off the ground. Pheasants are also bred in movable pens that sit directly on the ground in Europe. About once every week or two, the pen is moved to fresh grass. Again, outdoor colony breeder ratios are commonly 10–12 hens per cock. Ironically, the higher square footage per hen, the fewer cock birds are needed to keep the hens fertilized. Indoor breeder ratios are commonly 12–18 hens per cock.

All aforementioned systems utilize artificial lighting to induce earlier than natural egg production, which is preferred because commercial farms want to have their first ringneck chicks as early as mid-March. Chicks that hatch earlier than mid-March reach a physiological sexual maturity while the days are still getting longer (before June 20). This can result in young hens laying eggs and cocks attempting to breed other birds. In light of this, hatching ringneck chicks for hunting-type markets before mid-March is not a successful strategy. Breeders induced with artificial light to lay earlier eggs will lay more eggs in total for the season per hen than those raised in natural daylight.

6.1.2 Pheasant Egg Production

Egg production varies by breed, but the most common commercial pheasant breed is the Chinese ringneck pheasant. Chinese ringneck hens weigh about 2.25 pounds at maturity, while Chinese ringneck cocks weigh about 3 pounds at maturity. In some parts of the world, the most common bird is a Mongolian ringneck pheasant but the Chinese ringneck is preferred in the US for its flying ability. The estimated egg production per season from Chinese ringneck breeders would be in the 60–80+ eggs per hen range, while the Mongolian ringneck would lay around 50 eggs per hen. Caged ringneck hens that are artificially inseminated can be expected to lay over 100 eggs through the breeding cycle.

Cull rate percentage indicates what percentage of eggs are not useable for incubation and hatching. Utilizing good management, the cull rate can be held to 4%. One of the biggest influences on curtailing cull rate is the number of daily collections, which can vary from once a day to 10 times a day, depending on the operation. The more often one collects, the lower the cull rate. Other factors affecting cull rate are straw in corners in outdoor pens, the density at which the breeders are kept, and the use of huts in both indoor and outdoor facilities. Huts are plastic or wooden structures that allow the hens to lay in the dark on straw, similar to a "nest" in the chicken industry. Hens will prefer to lay eggs in huts rather than in the open, some could say for privacy.

Placing straw in outdoor pens is necessary because of mud created during seasons of rain. Bacteria such as *Escherichia coli*, a bacterium present in feces, can be found in the soil. Contaminating the outer shell with wet soil will allow this bacterium to penetrate the egg via the shell pores if the egg remains outside for an extended period of time. When a hen lays an egg, the temperature of that egg is close to 100 °F. As the egg remains outside, especially in cooler temperatures, it cools. As the egg cools, any contaminates that are on the shell can be drawn into the egg via the eggshell pores. For this reason and to reduce potential contamination to the eggs, it is critical to collect eggs repeatedly throughout the day, especially during the rainy season.

6.1.3 Incubation and Hatching

Whether it is a small operation or large commercial farm, pheasant eggs are incubated and hatched with machines holding just a few eggs all the way up to incubators holding tens of thousands of eggs. Pheasant eggs can be held in a cool humid environment for up to 10 days before incubation without adversely affecting the percentage of chicks that will eventually hatch (hatchability rate). Pheasant eggs held longer than 10 days tend to not hatch nearly as well. If eggs are held more than 20 days, the hatch rate declines severely. Eggs are usually held with the point of the egg down so the air cell can develop at the wider end of the egg. Some hatcheries turn the eggs during the holding period on a daily basis. Once eggs are placed in the incubator, the eggs need to be turned once every hour throughout incubation (Figure 6.3).

The incubation period for pheasant eggs is halfway between chicken eggs (21 days) and the incubation period for turkeys (27 days). Pheasant eggs are usually incubated 21 days in incubators and

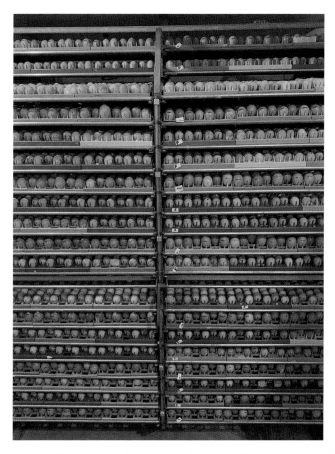

Figure 6.3   Eggs are arranged in racks for a large-volume incubator. The support arm will tilt/rock the eggs every hour throughout incubation.

held in hatchers for 3 days for a total of 24 days from the setting of the egg until the chicks hatch. The process of hatching from the time a pheasant chick starts to break its way out of the egg until it is dry and fluffy is approximately 24 hours. Once chicks are hatched and dry, they are boxed and taken to the brooder house or shed, whether processing a few eggs or thousands of eggs. At this stage, they can also be transported through the United States Postal Service (USPS) without significant chick mortality since the chicks can survive on the yolk for 3 days.

6.1.4   Brooding Pheasant Chicks

In backyard operations, a small number of pheasant chicks can be raised in a facility as small as 10 × 10 ft. One hundred day-old pheasants heated with one or two infrared heat bulbs in an insulated building would be a good place to start, with a goal starting temperature of 98 °F. The birds could stay inside the facility day and night until they are 3 weeks old as long as the temperature is dropped on a regular basis after about 5 days of age. A small run off the brooder could allow the chicks to get fresh air and exercise. The run could open up into the pen where the birds could be placed once they have reached 6 weeks old. The number 1 mistake people who start raising pheasant chicks make is to crowd the birds, so it is important to give the birds adequate space to reduce cannibalism.

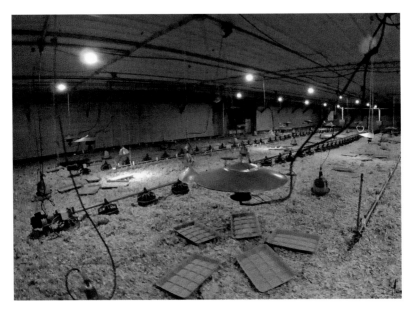

Figure 6.4 This pheasant brooder house with litter floor has been prepared for the chicks. Drinkers, feeders, and extra feeder trays are numerous and widely distributed so that the chicks will easily find them after placement.

Commercial pheasant operations are brooding pheasant chicks in increasingly larger facilities, emulating the commercial chicken poultry industry. Housing often consists of post frame brooder buildings with concrete floors equipped with automatic brooding, feeding, ventilation, and watering (Figure 6.4). Though automation of rearing might seem to result in tamer pheasants, the truth is quite opposite: more feral pheasants occur with less human interaction. Automation reduces the amount of imprinting of humans onto pheasant chicks. Common chick densities are four chicks per square foot from placement at a day old up until 3 weeks of age. Density at 3 weeks is usually increased to two chicks per square foot and kept at that density until the birds are moved into the outdoor pens at 6 or 7 weeks old. Adequate ventilation is critical and air exchange can be as often as one change every few minutes. Since most commercial pheasant farms brood primarily in the summer, it is still economical for those farms to move a lot of air to ensure adequate ventilation.

There are many lighting systems. All involve some sort of dimming capability where the room is bright when the chicks are first placed, and the lights are dimmed down as the birds get older. Most operations use some sort of brooder in the 0–3-week "A" room, but many operations switch to whole-room heating in the 3-week plus "B" room. There are many types of bedding, the most common being woodchips or chopped straw, but other bedding types are utilized depending upon what is available in the region.

Most operations use some sort of valve waterer such as a nipple line or bell drinker. The most common anticannibalism device used in the industry is a peeper, therefore nipple waterers are not used to any great extent because birds with peepers are not effectively able to hit a nipple to get water. Peepers are most commonly attached to pheasants between 31 and 37 days. Other methods used in the industry to control cannibalism and aggression include placing mouth bits (bitting), beak trimming, and hoods, which are a larger form of peeper (Figure 6.5). Day-old chicks are fed a 28% or 30% protein feed similar to turkey feed, and perform best on crumbles, as with mash the chicks can pick out pieces of corn, etc. resulting in an unbalanced diet.

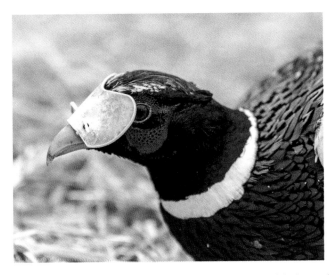

Figure 6.5   A plastic hood, a larger form of the peeper, has been placed on this ringneck pheasant.

Coccidiosis is probably the biggest threat to the health of young pheasant chicks. Keeping the chick room dry is the most effective management tool to ward off coccidiosis outbreaks. Most feeds include a coccidiostat to help prevent coccidiosis in the pheasant flock.

6.1.5   Outdoor Pens

Because the majority of pheasants raised on commercial farms are used for hunting, it is imperative that the birds be raised outside and acclimated to the weather. There are many variations of outdoor pens. An overview of common traits of pens will now be discussed.

Polyethylene or nylon netting is most often used on the tops of the pens. Nets need to be treated during the manufacturing process with ultraviolet protection to prevent them from becoming brittle and able to be ripped open. Netting with a hole size of approximately 2 in. is most commonly used, as the hole size is small enough to keep the pheasants in and big enough to allow wet snow to fall through the net. One of the biggest issues in pheasant pen construction is the ability of the pen to withstand snow. Most farms use wire on the sides of the pens attached to some sort of post every 10 or 12 ft on center. The majority of farms bend the outer fencing wire at ground level for 2 ft out from the pen and under the soil around the pen in order to restrict predators from digging under and into the pen. Overall pen dimensions vary among farms, but the most common dimensions are 60–100 ft width and 150 or more feet length (Figure 6.6). Pens that exceed 100 ft in width often collapse during wet snowfalls.

Commercial farms have developed many systems to avoid pens falling down due to snow. These systems include winching systems to raise and lower the pens, and PVC counter-weighted center prop poles where the netting moves up and down the PVC as the snow accumulates. The most common system uses 2×4 prop posts that can be easily moved or, in the event of a surprise storm, break and allow the netting to rest on the vegetative cover in the pen. Pheasant pens need to be high enough for humans to easily walk inside them. Most producers have lanes or catch pens to facilitate easy catching of pheasants. Most pen systems have a double-entry system to decrease the likelihood of a door being left open and the birds escaping. Many types of vegetative growth are

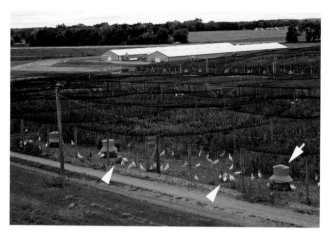

Figure 6.6 An external view of a typical outdoor pheasant flight pen includes support poles with netting and an adequate number of strategically placed feeders (arrow) and drinkers (arrowheads).

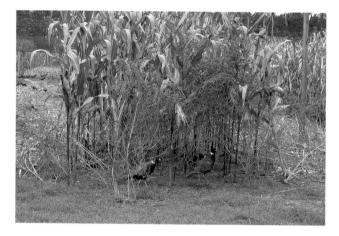

Figure 6.7 Dense vegetation, such as amaranth grasskosha, lamb's quarter, corn or milo, provides excellent shelter and forage areas for the pheasants.

used in pens, with amaranth grasskosha (*Bassia scoparia*) being the most common, followed by lambs' quarter (*Chenopodium album*), corn, or milo (Figure 6.7).

Pens are most effectively located away from ponds, creeks, rivers, trees or woods where predators may live and stage an attack. Sandy, well-drained soil is the best type for pheasant pens. Heavy clay soils cake on the pheasants' tails and create broken or frayed tails. The downside to sandy soil is the pens can become overly dry and the vegetative cover suffers from the drought. Some farms utilize irrigation systems on their pens to eliminate rainfall as a wild card in successful raising of birds.

Feeders and waterers are located in the pen to facilitate filling and monitoring. Feeder and waterer spaces are critically important in successfully raising top-quality pheasants. Each bird requires 0.7 linear in. of feeder space. Waterer space of 0.1 in. per bird is sufficient. Once pheasants reach 6 or 7 weeks old and are moved into the outdoor pens, they should be fed a 20% protein small pelleted feed. Density is one of the most important metrics since raising too many birds per square foot results in loss of vegetative cover in the pen. If this happens, birds' tails can break from

(a) 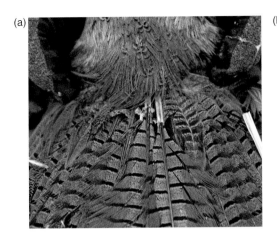 (b)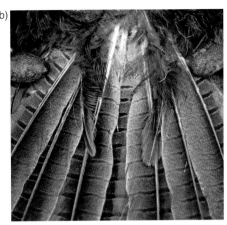

Figure 6.8 Adult pheasants are not suitable for crating and shipping until the feathers are mature with stiff quills and rigid, interlocking feather barbs ("hardened" or "set"). (a) Soft, nonhardened tail feathers with frayed feather barbs; (b) hardened tail feathers.

being dragged through the mud, and birds can also begin to cannibalize each other. Successful commercial pheasant farms usually raise birds at 15–20 sq ft per hen and 20–25 sq ft per cock when using peepers. If peepers are not used, bird density needs to be cut in half in order to have successful, well-feathered birds with undamaged tails.

To be able to ship adult pheasants, their tails need to be matured so they are "hardened" (stiff quill/calamus and firm feather barbs that are interlocked to form a smoother feather contour) or they will fall out during shipment (Figure 6.8). For April and May hatched pheasants, the birds need to be at least 23 weeks old for their tails to be mature and "hardened." June or July hatched pheasants' tails will be mature as young as 20 weeks of age, because the cold nights of October and November speed up hardening of the tails. Pheasants are most commonly shipped in well-ventilated crates in several different configurations. With the topic of biosecurity becoming increasingly important, modern pheasant crates are made of plastic, not wood, so they can be easily disinfected between uses. Pheasant crates are most commonly 9 in. in height and 2 × 3 ft in area (Figure 6.9). Once the birds are shipped, it is important that the recipient of the shipment

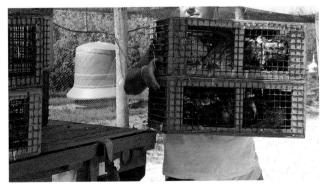

Figure 6.9 Mature pheasants are placed in 9 in. high, stackable crates prior to being placed on the delivery truck. Most pheasant shipping crates are now plastic to facilitate cleaning and disinfection.

knows how to care for the birds. Hence, there are a lot of factors to take into consideration when deciding to raise pheasants.

6.2 Bobwhite Quail

The Bobwhite quail is one of the most widely distributed and hunted gamebirds in the United States. Wild populations have declined steadily over the past several decades which has given rise to confinement rearing of quail for release. Each year, approximately 15 million Bobwhite quail are produced nationwide and marketed for use at public and private shooting preserves and plantations. Most states require that shooting preserves obtain an annual license through the State Department of Natural Resources. Approximately 200 shooting preserves are permitted annually nationwide. The number of preserves and plantations, particularly in the southeastern US, provides an excellent market for Bobwhite quail producers.

  Bobwhite quail production has received attention as an alternative enterprise for many farming operations. Successful quail producers raise breeders with the intent to market the day-old chicks to grow-out producers; grow-out producers specialize in raising of day-old chicks until approximately 16–18 weeks of age for sale as flight-ready birds to shooting preserves. Often, quail operations combine both aspects of quail production. Breeder producers typically sell day-old chicks at $0.35–0.40/bird, whereas flight-ready producers will market birds at approximately $3.75–4.00/bird. The quality of bird produced and the time of year they are available may greatly influence the price received for flight-ready Bobwhite quail.

6.2.1 Breeder and Hatchery Management

6.2.1.1 Lighting

Like all birds, quail are photoreceptive and their growth and reproductive maturity depends on the amount of light stimulus that they receive. While young breeders may begin to lay a few eggs as early as 18 weeks of age, do not expect consistent egg production until about 24–26 weeks of age. Young chicks and immature birds are maintained in a dimly lit environment to reduce cannibalism and allow uniform sexual development. Immature birds can do well on as little as 10 hours of light/day. However, a set 14–16 hours of light per day from day of hatch to sale for release is common with larger operations. In order to reduce cannibalism, light intensity should not exceed 0.5 fc. Interior walls of the house should be light-colored to reflect the light provided and reduce dark areas in the house. It is extremely important to maintain day length once it has been elevated. Any sudden decrease in hours of light per day will cause a decline in egg production.

  The ease of maintaining a lighting program depends on the cost of labor and building construction. For birds receiving natural daylight, add the additional hour(s) of light equally at the beginning and end of the natural daylight. For example, when birds have reached the point that they require 16 hours of light daily, but the natural daylight and time of year produces 12.5 hours of daylight daily, breeders will require an additional 3.5 hours of light per day. Use an automatic timer device to turn lights off and on each day. Turn lights on (or set an automatic timer) about 2.0 hours before the normal daylight begins; set the timer to turn off about 1.5 hours after sunset. Producers who raise birds in total blackout facilities (not exposed to natural day lengths) should have no problem meeting the recommended lighting schedule (Table 6.1) [1].

  Proper light stimulation is extremely important if the birds are to develop sexually. After egg production has begun, do not reduce the hours or intensity of light the birds receive each day. Otherwise, overall production can be severely disrupted.

Table 6.1 Lighting requirements for
Bobwhite quail at different ages.

Bird age, weeks	Hours of light per day
19	11
20	12
21	13
22	14
23	15
24	16
25	17

6.2.1.2 Breeder Housing

Breeders should be maintained in a comfortable, well-ventilated environment and with temperatures between 65 °F and 85 °F to achieve acceptable feed conversion and egg production levels. Ambient temperatures lower than 65 °F will increase the energy requirement, which will lower feed efficiency and, more importantly, reduce egg production. At temperatures greater than 85 °F, feed intake is often reduced, which may also lead to reduced egg production. In contrast to most other domesticated birds, Bobwhite quail often peak in egg production during periods of warmer environmental temperature, possibly suggesting they are more heat tolerant. However, excessively high ambient temperatures often result in reduced fertility in other avian species. A properly designed and operated negative-pressure evaporative cooling system may increase profitability in areas with extended high environmental temperatures. Benefits include a significant increase in egg production, shell quality, and fertility during summer and early fall [1].

Regardless of temperatures, ventilation in the breeder facility must be maintained to remove excess dust, ammonia, and moisture. The ventilation system should not subject the birds to a direct draft, although in the warm summer months this poses less of a problem.

Breeders are typically housed in one of three ways: in large community floor pens, in smaller communal cages designed for 10–20 birds each, or caged as pairs or trios. Each of these house types can have its drawbacks.

Floor pens, in the traditional sense, may be the least desirable type of housing for breeder quail. When birds are housed directly on the floor, collecting eggs is often more difficult and time-consuming, which often leads to less frequent egg gathering. Infrequent collection can cause egg loss due to shell damage and contamination, birds consuming eggs, or preincubation of the developing embryos. These factors will lead to reduced egg harvest, lower hatchability, and poorer chick quality. In addition, there is normally a significant increase in the number of dirty eggs from birds housed on the floor. Dirty eggs cause increased egg contamination, which will also reduce hatchability and chick quality. With floor-laying flocks, producers cannot identify and cull low- or nonproducing birds. Birds raised and maintained on the floor have increased exposure to parasites or other disease-causing pathogens [2].

Housing birds on slatted floors similar to the traditional floor pen setup has been successful. The house design is the same but the problems associated with birds raised directly on bedding are eliminated. There is an added expense to cover the majority of the floor of the house with a removable slatted or wire-type floor, but many producers have benefited from this arrangement.

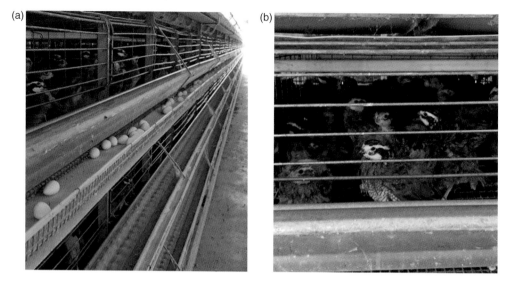

Figure 6.10 (a) Breeder quail cage system with automated egg collection. (b) Closer view of breeder quail hens.

Bird health and eggshell quality is often improved with raised flooring systems. Birds can have a tendency to lay eggs on the slatted floor instead of in nest boxes and this will still result in more direct contact with feces.

Placing breeder birds in wire cages has several advantages over a floor pen design (Figure 6.10). Eggshell quality is improved and the eggs do not come in direct contact with fecal material, as they will roll away from the bird shortly after being laid. Cleaner eggs increase hatchability and chick quality. In some cases, this system enables the use of automated egg collection, which further improves egg quality as the egg-gathering process is faster than by hand and can promote more frequent collection. In addition, when new breeding stock is to be produced from the current flock of breeders, it is possible to select replacement birds based upon genetics and performance. As mentioned earlier, identification and removal of low- or nonproducing birds from the breeding stock is possible with this housing design. Use of nipple or cup waterers and trough feeders is preferred. Flooring should be of quality ½″ welded wire. Eggs from cage breeders will cool more rapidly and be much cleaner than floor-type housing. Pecking and cannibalism will not be a factor if approximately one-third of the upper beak of all birds is removed at placement.

Placing birds in wire cages can have disadvantages that must be considered. Since the birds will spend their entire life on the wire, the bottom of the cages must be smooth and free of sharp points to ensure that the bottom of the feet are not damaged. Injured and sore feet result in reduced fertility as mating frequency is drastically reduced. In addition, any open wounds increase the chance of infection, disease, and premature death of birds. Greater equipment expense is incurred and additional attention to detail is often required as each cage must be equipped with a feeder and drinker. The female-to-male bird ratio should be maintained at 2.5–3.5 females to each male. Having only one or two males per cage can result in reduced flock fertility. Communal cages, or cages designed for 10–20 birds per cage, will often alleviate the suppressed fertility from breeders maintained in cages. Caged birds will require a minimum of 0.5 sq ft per bird. Cannibalism is often a bigger problem with birds housed in smaller cages as they are not able to escape and hide from the more aggressive birds. Lights may be dimmed to 0.5 fc to reduce aggression and pecking. However, lower light levels will result in reduced mating activity.

Fertility of hatching eggs can be linked to management practices in the breeder house. Potential causes of reduced fertility from within the breeder barn include improper ratio of males to females; leg problems in the males, which will reduce mating activity; elevated environmental temperatures that result in reduced mating activity; and improper or inadequate lighting. Each of these problems, if not prevented or corrected, can reduce the fertility of hatching eggs [3].

6.2.1.3 Incubation

Hatching egg sanitation often determines the quality and quantity of chicks hatched. To optimize the number of clean and viable hatching eggs, frequent collection is required. Make the final egg pickup late in the day to minimize the time eggs spend in the breeder house. This is particularly important during the warmer summer months. The most desirable eggs are those that are clean, free of shell defects, and of consistent shape for the breed. The temperature of 68 °F is considered to be "physiological zero." If the temperature of the egg goes above physiological zero, embryonic development will begin. To stop excessive development and weakening of the embryo, cool eggs shortly after they are laid. Repeatedly starting and stopping embryo development due to temperature swings usually causes poor hatchability and increased embryonic mortality.

Store hatching eggs until an appropriate number of eggs are obtained in order to produce the quantity of chicks desired from a single hatch. Store eggs with the large end up in clean egg flats in an egg room or cooler. Maintain the egg storage room at 55–65 °F and 70–80% relative humidity. Egg storage beyond 7 days will reduce hatchability, therefore the date the eggs were laid should be clearly marked on the egg flats. Many producers prewarm hatching eggs for several hours prior to setting. When eggs are prewarmed, they are removed from the cool room and allowed to gradually warm to room temperature. Gradually warming the eggs reduces "sweating" or the condensation of water on the eggshell surface. "Sweating" enables bacteria on the egg shell surface to multiply and allows motile bacteria to penetrate the eggshell. Prewarming, if not properly done, may reduce hatchability and chick quality. The prewarming environment must have good airflow so that condensation moisture is exhausted from the room.

For successful incubation, a number of factors must be controlled: temperature, humidity, egg turning, ventilation, and sanitation. Temperature, humidity, and turning are the three most critical factors with hatching eggs (Table 6.2). Bobwhite quail eggs will hatch 23–24 days from the time they are set in the incubator. The ideal temperature in a forced-air incubator is 99–100 °F with a relative humidity at 80–85%. Temperature fluctuations may prolong or shorten the exact length of incubation. Eggs are generally transferred to a separate hatcher on day 21 of incubation where egg turning is suspended. Using separate setters and hatchers results in cleaner chicks and less

Table 6.2 Incubation time and requirements for Bobwhite quail.

Item	Optimum value
Incubation time, days	23–24
Forced air temperature[a], °F	99.75
Humidity[b], %	84–86
Operating temperature last 3 days of incubation[a], °F	99
Humidity last 3 days of incubation[b], %	90–94

a) All operating temperatures are given in degrees Fahrenheit – dry bulb.
b) Humidity is presented as degrees Fahrenheit – wet bulb.

cross-contamination between the hatching eggs and any newly set eggs. The relative humidity in the hatcher should be a little higher at 90%, with a slightly lower temperature of 97–99 °F. However, the ideal temperature will vary between machine types and hatcher room conditions.

Noticeably prolonged or shortened incubation periods or unusually low hatchability may be caused by warm or cool spots within the incubator. To verify this condition, place several accurate thermometers within the incubator and check them several times daily. If this is the problem, contact the incubator manufacturer for suggestions. Severe or prolonged temperature variability in the incubator room may affect conditions within the incubator itself, especially if the incubator is inadequately insulated. Such variations may adversely affect chick quality [1].

Incubators are of either the still- or forced-air ventilation type. Both types can be successfully used, but forced-air machines provide a more uniform environment for hatching eggs. Developing embryos require oxygen, with an increasing requirement during the latter stages of incubation. Therefore, it is critical to remove carbon dioxide (CO_2) and moisture from the incubator. Forced-air incubators ensure a steady flow of incoming and exhaust air through the machine.

Ventilation in the incubator room is equally important. Be sure to maintain an adequate flow of fresh incoming air into the room. Maintain room temperature and humidity in a way that ensures quality, moist air going into the incubator.

During incubation, eggs require regular turning to prevent the embryo from sticking to the internal shell membrane. Mechanical egg turning devices are recommended and are necessary with large numbers of eggs. If relatively few eggs are being incubated, the eggs can be manually turned and marked with an X on one side of the egg to ensure all eggs are turned each time. Incubating eggs should be turned no less than three times per day and this should continue until they are moved to the hatching machine. Eggs are placed on their sides in enclosed baskets within the hatcher. After hatch, leave the chicks in the hatcher until 90% of the chicks are dry. Then remove them to the brooder.

After 7–10 days of incubation, candling a sample of eggs provides valuable information if hatchability problems are occurring. Remove those eggs lacking a distinct blood vessel network – "clears" – and perform a "breakout" of these eggs to determine the cause of embryonic failure (Table 6.3). Record early embryonic mortality during the egg breakout for trouble-shooting

Table 6.3 Causes of poor hatchability.

Problem	Possible causes
Early embryonic death	Temperature too high or low; preincubation of eggs
Embryos dead, second week of incubation	Improper turning; temperature too high or low
Embryos dead, last week of incubation	Improper positioning of egg with small end up instead of down
Air cell too large	Humidity too low
Air cell too small	Humidity too high
Chicks hatch early	Temperature too high; humidity too low; inaccurate measurements
Chicks hatch late	Temperature too low; humidity too high; inaccurate measurements
Chicks dead after pipping shell	CO_2 content too high; improper turning of eggs
Sticky chicks	Humidity too low; temperature too high

problems in hatchability. Patterns of embryo loss will enable identification and separation of fertility, egg handling, or incubation problems.

To reduce the possibility of exploding eggs within the incubator, be sure to not set cracked or leaking eggs. Eggs explode because of bacterial production of gas within the egg. Exploding eggs potentially shower the incubator's interior with bacteria and mold spores which contaminate the other eggs and may impact the developing embryos within any contaminated egg.

6.2.1.4 Brooding

The brooding period is the first 2 weeks of a chick's life. This critical period is important in getting the chick off to a good start. It is a basic fact of gamebird management that after hatching, chick quality cannot be improved, but it certainly can be impaired. It is imperative that there are preparations made for chick arrival. Cleaning, disinfecting, and quail brooder house setup should be complete several days before the chicks' arrival. Regardless of the season, the brooder stoves should have been running for at least 24 hours before placement and the bedding temperature should be approximately 95 °F.

Chicks have difficulty self-regulating their body temperature for the first 10–12 days of life. They may lose significant quantities of heat through their feet, which emphasizes the need to maintain the bedding surface temperature at 95 °F. Chilling causes the chicks to huddle and makes them more susceptible to disease. Brooder temperatures must be monitored at chick height because temperature can vary as much as 5–8 °F from the ground to 4 or 5 ft above the floor. Reduce brooder temperatures by about 5 °F per week until a temperature of 70 °F is reached.

Brooding is generally accomplished in circular units about 7–8 ft in diameter called "brooder rings." The rings are commonly made of cardboard or $1/4$ mesh screen material. The function of the brooder ring is to keep the chicks in the vicinity of the heat, water, and feed. Brooder rings should be set up so that the chicks can escape the heat of the stove yet not be subject to cold corners or drafts. Chicks will begin to fly over the ring within 10 days of age, so remove the rings at 5–8 days of age and give the birds access to the remainder of the brood chamber. Stocking density within the rings can be as high as 10 birds/ft^2 during brooding.

It is important that the chicks find the water source shortly after arrival to prevent dehydration and death. To assist the chicks in getting a good start, place a vitamin mix in the water. Chicks have sufficient material in their yolk sac when hatched to survive 2–3 days without feed (assuming the incubation temperature is correct), but it is recommended that they have immediate access to feed as well as water upon placement in the brooding rings. Many quail producers now use nipple waterers which significantly reduce the occurrence of wet bedding, sustain better water quality, and are simpler to clean than trough or bell waterers. As a general rule, each nipple will supply water to approximately 40–50 birds. Those producers who continue to use bell type or trough waterers should clean them out at least twice weekly during cooler weather and more frequently in the warmer seasons. Manure should be removed from waterers and feeders before they are disinfected. The water supply may also be chlorinated. Chlorine levels at the point of consumption should approximate 1.0 ppm [3].

6.2.1.5 Grow-out

At 3 weeks of age, chicks are typically given access to the entire grow-out facility or, for flight pen birds, moved at 6 weeks into outside flight pens until the birds are marketed. Birds kept in confinement can be maintained at a density of 0.5 ft^2 per bird. The density of birds placed in a flight pen should equate to 2 ft^2 per bird to accommodate for cover vegetation and sun/weather shelter.

Within flight pens, approximately 20% of the total pen space consists of shelter and dry space for feeder and waterers. Flight pens are relatively inexpensive, typically consisting of wire or netting and wooden support posts. The configuration of flight pens is variable and the actual cost depends on purchased supplies and resources available on the farm. The disadvantage of flight pens can be a higher rate of mortality which can occur due to environmental temperature fluctuation, inclement weather, physical trauma, and predation.

When constructing outdoor pens, pay attention to the drainage. Standing water in flight pens will increase the potential for disease. Conversely, drainage of fecal or toxic material can cause problems from both management and environmental standpoints. Place and maintain feed and water containers so fecal contamination is minimized. For flight pen scenarios, this may include elevated feed platforms constructed of ½–1 in. hardware cloth to allow for dry and manure-free feeding and drinking areas. Wire should be free of any sharp protrusions so birds do not damage themselves. Producers must make a point of checking state or local regulations regarding environmental laws pertaining to their operation. Outdoor environmental conditions create increased potential for disease outbreaks such as quail bronchitis, capillaria, histomoniasis, and ulcerative enteritis (for more information, please see disease chapters).

Conversely, some growers raise Bobwhite quail in scaled-down "broiler houses" (housing used for commercial broiler production) for the entire production period (Figure 6.11). The primary advantage of a quail barn is that the birds are housed within a controlled environment for the entire production period (Figure 6.12). Pine shavings are usually placed in the house at a depth of 4 in. The incidence of mortality is relatively low in this type of facility because of the warm, dry environment it provides. Growers producing quail in an enclosed facility have experienced flock mortality as low as 4–5%. This reduction in mortality can help offset the increased building cost associated with a quail barn.

Additional advantages of quail barns include a lower incidence of cannibalism and reduced feed cost. From 5 to 14 weeks of age, birds are grown in low light conditions to prevent cannibalism. The dim light should be sufficient to still stimulate feed consumption so that birds will have adequate energy reserves for flying when marketed at 16–18 weeks of age. Another advantage with raising quail in barns is that feed consumption may be decreased compared with flight pens. The increased feed consumption with flight pens is a result of temperature variations and feed wastage. Outside temperatures can vary as much as 40 °F when birds are raised in flight pens during a grow-out period. During cold temperatures, birds consume additional feed to compensate for lower

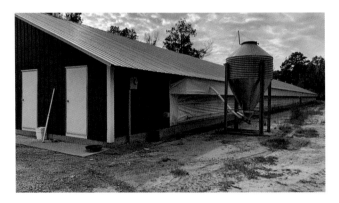

Figure 6.11   An outside view of a quail barn.

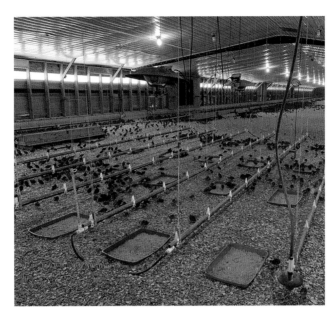

Figure 6.12 An inside view of a quail barn showing both feeders and drinkers. Source: Teresa Morishita.

environmental temperatures. The use of barns provides protection for the young birds and reduces the entry of wild birds and rodents. About 2–3 ft along the border of the brooding barn should be devoid of vegetation in order to reduce rodent traffic.

One of the biggest challenges for Bobwhite quail producers is preventing disease outbreaks which can result in significantly increased mortality and morbidity within a flock. Only a few medications are approved for Bobwhite quail so producers must identify and execute a preventive management plan to minimize disease outbreaks.

The three most common diseases that occur with Bobwhite quail production are quail bronchitis, ulcerative enteritis, and quail pox. However, other diseases (myoplasmosis, botulism, coccidiosis, and *Capillaria* worms) have also been problematic with quail. These diseases are described in other chapters. Prevention of these diseases starts with good management practices such as avoiding the introduction of new birds into existing flocks, thorough sanitation throughout all phases of production, and monitoring flock density.

6.2.2   Key Points for Quail Production

1. Bobwhite quail production can be a viable enterprise if birds are managed properly.
2. It is recommended that quail producers either raise hatching egg chicks or grow out quail from hatching until marketing for flight. Combining both enterprises at the same location can present additional biosecurity challenges.
3. For growers starting out in the business, it is strongly recommended that they learn how to grow birds before producing hatching eggs because of the additional management and investment required with breeder production.
4. Have biosecurity measures in place as you begin farm planning and construction. Good biosecurity measures throughout all phases of the operation will help to alleviate many disease challenges associated with gamebird production.

References

1 Bramwell, K., Dozier, W.A. (eds) (2009). Bobwhite Quail Production and Management Guide. University of Georgia Cooperative Extension, Bulletin 1215. https://extension.uga.edu (accessed 15 March 2022).

2 Merck Veterinary Manual. www.merckvetmanual.com (accessed 15 March 2022).

3 Walker, W. and Smith, T.W. (n.d.). *Raising Bobwhite Quail for Commercial Use*. Mississippi State University Cooperative Extension Publication www.poultry.msstate.edu/pdf/extension/raising_quail.pdf.

7

Gamebird Nutrition
Al Hollister

Gamebird nutrition and feeding is a multistep process that involves not only the determination of the nutrients required for the birds to grow and reproduce, but also the selecting of feed ingredients from those available of adequate quality to meet those requirements, processing as needed and presenting the final feed in a form that will be consumed – all at an acceptable cost. The nutritionist also must consider nonnutritional inclusions in the feed to retain quality, improve palatability, maximize digestibility, and protect the birds from disease and parasites.

Feed is often the most expensive part of any gamebird operation, amounting to 50% or more of the total cost of production. It is made up of many ingredients and processes which must be carefully monitored, since small differences often can contribute to large changes in the performance of the birds. Total variables that the nutritionist needs to be aware of include 13 vitamins, at least nine macro- and microminerals, up to 20 amino acids, and the numerous ingredients that provide protein, carbohydrates, fats, fiber, and water (the most important, but often overlooked nutrient), plus up to 10 nonnutritional ingredients. Even with the use of premixes for vitamins and trace minerals, there can be as many as 25 different ingredients to monitor in a typical feed.

This chapter will briefly describe nutritional and nonnutritional ingredients, processing, presentation, quality control, testing (ingredients and finished feed), feed formulation based on age and species, and the symptoms, diagnosis, and troubleshooting of nutritional problems.

7.1 Feed Type

Although birds in this group (Galliformes) are often considered primarily seed eaters, they are actually omnivorous, especially as young chicks. With limited gut capacity, and in order to get the concentrated high-protein and high-energy diet they need for rapid growth, it is necessary to consume animal protein (insects, worms, small mammals, or reptiles) that are nutrient-dense foods high in protein and fat while low in fiber. The high water content of these creatures also reduces the amount of drinking water needed.

Gamebird Medicine and Management, First Edition. Edited by Teresa Y. Morishita and Robert E. Porter, Jr.
© 2023 John Wiley & Sons, Inc. Published 2023 by John Wiley & Sons, Inc.

Using protein as an example, live common insects are about 20–25% protein and 60–80% water. If we convert that to 10% water like most prepared feed ingredients, crickets, grasshoppers, and earthworms average 50–60% protein. Grains and seeds are on average somewhat less protein dense but contain more energy (starch and oil). Corn (maize), wheat, milo (sorghum), grass seeds, and many plant buds range from about 7% to 18% protein (again dried to 10% water). Whole soybeans (unprocessed) are an exceptional plant protein source in that they are about 30% protein and 20% fat, and after fat extraction they are 46–48% protein. These plant sources have an amino acid balance that is not complete and must be supplemented, whereas the amino acid balance in animal protein is very close to estimated requirements. To mimic the ration of the free-living gamebird, it would be appropriate to include some animal protein in formulated feed to provide the necessary amino acids. However, it is possible to duplicate that amino acid profile with plant-based materials when necessary.

7.1.1 Suggested Nutrient Levels

The nutrient requirements of game birds have not been well researched. Most of the published data is based on chicken and turkey research [1, 2]. The research with chickens and turkeys, as well as the small amount done with gamebirds, was done under the low-stress, nearly ideal conditions in research facilities. Therefore, the information presented in Table 7.1 on suggested nutrient levels is based not on minimal nutrient levels under research conditions, but on the common industry practice of utilizing overages of some nutrients to compensate for unknown requirements and losses of nutrients during processing and storage, plus experience under actual field conditions. Table 7.1 is not meant to be all-inclusive and should be considered only a basis or minimum for formulators or those troubleshooting a suspected nutrition-related problem. Due to limited space, only the amino acids likely to be limiting in a corn-soybean diet are included. Formulas made up of other ingredients will need to consider the other essential amino acids. Nutritionists will find it necessary to make additional adjustments based on species, strain, age, management, the rearing environment, and feed storage conditions. Table 7.1 is designed for birds in three general groups: (i) birds that are to be released; (ii) birds that are of the same species but raised for meat production; and (iii) birds that do not require the higher protein (more nutrient-dense) diet. The sequence of diets for each group is identified with numbers referring to diet crude protein and metabolizable energy (ME); for example, 28 : 1250 is a feed containing 28% protein and ME of 1250 kcal/lb.

Group 1 is gamebirds that would be released and includes ring-necked pheasants, partridge, bobwhite quail or wild turkeys and the sequence would be 28 : 1250 starter >20 : 1250 grower >18 : 1200 flyer >14 : 1150 maintenance >18 : 1273 breeder. Under cold climate conditions, a switch to 1250 ME maintenance may be necessary. Smaller, more active strains could use alternate 24 : 1300 breeder. Group 2 are the same birds as Group 1 but used for meat production and would use the numbers in parentheses in the table as follows: 28 : 1250 starter >22 : 1318 grower >20 : 1350 finisher. Group 3 birds are the coturnix (Japanese) quail, guineafowl, and wild-type mallard ducks and would use 24 : 1250 starter #2 > 20 : 1250 grower >16 : 1250 maintenance >18 or 20 : 1273 breeder. Peafowl or species of pheasants, partridge, and quail not used for release or meat would use the Group 1 sequence to prevent excess body fat and use an alternate breeder diet containing only 1.5% calcium to prevent articular gout. For those preferring metric numbering, remember to multiply the kcal/lb. or mg/lb by 2.2 to get kcal/kg or mg/kg (ppm).

Table 7.1   Suggested nutrients[a] for pheasants, partridge, bobwhite quail, wild turkey (Group 1), meat birds (Group 2) or guineafowl, coturnix quail and mallard ducks (Group 3).

Nutrient[b] – %, IU/lb, mg/lb	Starter	Starter #2	Grower[c] (meat)	Flyer (finisher)	Maint- enance[d]	Breeder[e] (small)
Protein %	26–28	23–24	20 (22)	18 (20)	14–16	18–20 (23–24)
ME kcal/lb	1250	1250 (1318)	1250 (1318)	1200 (1350)	1150 (1250)	1273 (1300)
Calcium %	1.25	1	1	0.75	0.7	2.5 (2.6)[f]
Phosphorus (avail.) %	0.65	0.5	0.5	0.4	0.4	0.55
Sodium %	0.16	0.16	0.16	0.16	0.16	0.16
Chloride %	0.15	0.15	0.15	0.15	0.15	0.15
Met + Cys %	1.1	0.95	0.8 (0.85)	0.6 (0.75)	0.6	0.75
Lysine %	1.65	1.4	0.95 (1)	0.8 (1.0)	0.75	0.95
Threonine %	1.1	1.05	1	1	0.7	0.75
Tryptophan %	0.26	0.25	0.25	0.25	0.18	0.2
Vitamin A (IU)	6000	6000	5100	4800	4200	6500
Vitamin D (IU)	2500	2500	2125	2000	1750	3000
Vitamin E (IU)	40	30	20	20	10	50
Vitamin K (mg)	2.2	2	1.8	1.7	1.5	2.2
Thiamine (mg)	3	3	3	2	2	3
Riboflavin (mg)	7	5	4	4	3	7
Pantothenic acid (mg)	15	15	12	12	10	15
Niacin (mg)	70	60	40	40	30	75
Folic acid (mg)	3	3	2.55	2.4	2.1	2
Pyridoxine (mg)	5	5	4.25	4	3.5	5
Choline (mg)	900	900	765	720	630	900
Vitamin B12 (mg)	0.03	0.03	0.03	0.024	0.02	0.03
Biotin (mg)	0.3	0.3	0.255	0.24	0.2	0.3
Iodine (mg)	1.5	1.4	1.3	1.2	1.05	0.5
Manganese (mg)	70	60	60	50	40	60
Copper (mg)	15	10	10	10	10	15
Iron (mg)	60	50	50	50	40	50
Zinc (mg)	100	80	80	80	40	100
Selenium (mg)	0.13	0.13	0.13	0.13	0.13	0.13

a) The amounts represent as-fed. Assume 90% dry matter. See the text for diet selection procedure for Groups 1, 2, or 3.
b) Amino acids: only those most likely to be limiting in corn-soy diet are included.
c) Grower or finisher refers to strains raised for meat or flying (strains for release).
d) Maintenance range: higher energy may be required in colder climate conditions.
e) Breeder (small) refers to smaller, more active strains.
f) Breeder calcium: use 1.5% for breeds with small clutches (peafowl, etc.).

7.2 Feed Ingredients

Most basic poultry and gamebird diets can be formulated with the relatively small numbers of ingredient types. This would include carbohydrate from grains like corn (maize), wheat, or milo (sorghum), protein from soybean meal, canola or corn gluten meal, animal (meat meal, fish), plus calcium carbonate, dicalcium phosphate, salt, vitamin-mineral premix, methionine, lysine, and fat. For birds that need to be kept lean and athletic for release, additional low-energy ingredients (wheat middlings or alfalfa) may be necessary to provide less nutrient-dense formulations and will be discussed later in this chapter. Finally, nonnutritional feed additives like pellet binders, mold inhibitors, mycotoxin binders, antibiotics, coccidiostats, probiotics, enzymes, and wormers may be required.

7.2.1 Ingredient Quality

To accurately formulate a diet, the nutritionist must know the specifications of each ingredient. For grains and protein sources, this would include crude protein, fat, ME, moisture, amino acid profile, crude fiber, calcium and phosphorus – at the very minimum. Averages of these numbers are often obtained from research with ingredients that are assumed to be of uniform quality (i.e., most corn is US #2), and are reported in publications like NRC Poultry (1994) or the Feedstuffs Reference Issue and Nutrition Guide. However, these specifications should be considered only a guide because crops change from year to year and by region grown, and should be verified with test results. Due to space limitations, only the more common ingredients will be covered in this presentation.

7.2.2 Corn (Maize)

Corn is the most widely used energy source for all kinds of livestock. It is highly digestible for gamebirds and does not contain antinutritive factors. Although the amino acid profile is not ideal, this can be easily resolved through the use of a good protein source like soybean meal and small additions of amino acids, like methionine and lysine.

Standards for grading corn and other grains are provided for and defined in the Official United States Standards for Grain, US Department of Agriculture (USDA) Agricultural Marketing Service, Grain Division. This includes information on minimum pounds per bushel (one bushel = 2150.42 cu in.), maximum percentages of moisture, broken kernels, foreign materials, and damaged kernels. US grade #2 corn must be a minimum of 54 pounds per bushel, 15.5% or less moisture, 3% or less broken kernels and foreign material, and less than 5% damaged kernels. Similar guides are provided for wheat and other grains (includes soybeans). The disadvantages to the use of corn (high levels) include poor pellet quality and the potential for mold or mycotoxin contamination in some locations (weather-related stress) or if it is not stored properly.

7.2.3 Soybeans and Soybean Meal

Soybeans are an excellent source of vegetable protein and have an amino acid profile that works well in combination with corn. Usually, only methionine is needed to complete the amino acid profile (and sometimes lysine). Soybeans are normally available in a whole, roasted form averaging 38% protein and 18% fat, or as dehulled and solvent processed soybean meal which is usually 46–47% protein and 2% fat. Like corn, detailed standards for grading soybeans are provided by the Official

United States Standards for Grain. Disadvantages can result from poor processing; if not enough heat is used, antinutrients (like trypsin inhibitors) are not destroyed, while overheating may result in reduced availability of the important amino acid lysine. Soybean meal also contains nonstarch polysaccharides (NSP) which are hard for young birds to digest. It is recommended that an enzyme be used in high-protein starter diets, especially those without other nonsoybean protein sources (meat meal, fish meal, corn gluten meal, etc.); this will be discussed later with enzymes.

7.2.4 Wheat and Wheat Middlings

Wheat is commonly used primarily for flour production for human consumption, but if wheat is available at a reasonable price and corn is unavailable or too costly, it can replace corn in gamebird diets. To prevent problems with excessive viscosity that causes poor digestibility and wet manure, the addition of an enzyme (xylanase) is necessary when using high levels of wheat. The byproducts of flour production, like wheat middlings, retain small amounts of starch, making them excellent pellet binders. In addition, the low energy resulting from starch removal makes middlings an excellent low-energy addition to diets for gamebirds for release.

7.2.5 Meat Products (i.e., Meat and Bone Meal, Fish Meal)

Although the (estimated) amino acid needs of gamebirds can be met with the use of vegetable proteins and pure amino acids, most nutritionists include animal protein products like meat and bone meal or fish meal to achieve a better amino acid balance, and to reduce the amount of soy NSP (especially in starter diets). Although good-quality fish meal has become expensive and hard to source, and bovine meat and bone meal is avoided due to the threat of bovine spongiform encephalopathy (BSE), porcine meat and bone meal are still readily available. In addition to the protein, meat and bone meals are a good source of phosphorus that often provide an economic advantage. Disadvantages include inconsistent levels of calcium and phosphorus and the potential presence of pathogens if not processed properly.

7.2.6 Fat, Oil

Fats and oils can be a major source of energy in feed, due to their content of an average of 2.5 times as much energy as that in grains. However, the extra energy is only needed in high-energy meat bird diets (and some breeder diets), while birds for release should be provided lower energy levels to perform well. Although added fat is helpful for controlling dustiness and improving palatability in mash diets, its use in pelleted diets must be limited to a maximum of approximately 2% because of the negative effect it has on pellet quality.

Fats and oils are made up of a glycerol molecule with three attached side chains of fatty acids usually containing 8–24 carbon atoms. The carbons are linked by single or double bonds indicating saturation or unsaturation. Fat is solid at ambient temperatures (more single bonds, or saturation), whereas oils are liquid (more double bonds).

Evaluation of quality is based on features such as color, fatty acid profile and saturation or unsaturation, the percentage of free fatty acids, and MIU (moisture, insolubles, unsaponifiables). For feed fat, color is not as important as it is in human or pet food, but it may be an indicator of abuse in processing. Fatty acid profile depends on the source, with animal fats trending toward more saturation while vegetable oils usually contain more unsaturated fatty acids, which are more digestible for poultry. Free fatty acids are those that have separated from the glycerol molecule, and high percentages may indicate oxidative damage. The higher quality feed fats contain no more than 10% free fatty acids. Feed fat should contain no more than 1.5% moisture, 0.5% insolubles (like fiber, hair, minerals) and a maximum of 1% unsaponifiables (like sterols, pigments) if from animal fat, or 4% if from vegetable oil. The ideal MIU maximum would be 2–2.5%. A standard fat testing protocol (especially fat from a new supplier) should also include scanning for PCBs and pesticides. Finally, antioxidants like ethoxiquine, BHT (butylated hydroxytoluene) or BHA (butylated hydroxyanisole) should be added to all fats to prevent oxidation and rancidity.

7.2.7 Minerals, Vitamins, Amino Acids, and Nonnutritional Ingredients

Definitions of all approved nutritional and nonnutritional products are listed in the Association of American Feed Control Officials (AAFCO) (2021) [3] but only minimal additional information is included.

The American Feed Industry Association (AFIA) Feed Ingredient Guide (1995) [4], although out of print, contains information that is hard to find elsewhere, including factors that influence quality, availability, physical properties, and major feed applications. Manufacturers or distributors of ingredients provide specification sheets detailing the composition of their product. This information is essential for accurate formulation. As with grains, proteins, and fats, all ingredients from an unproven supplier should be tested independently to confirm that they meet specifications.

7.3 Mold Control

Molds are always present, averaging 500 000 cfu/g while levels above 1 million cfu/g are considered of concern. Mold itself is usually not dangerous. In high-moisture conditions, it grows, digests feed, and reduces the feed's value to the bird. However, under suitable conditions, molds produce mycotoxins which can be very dangerous to gamebirds. At times when feed may be stored for too long (more than 3–4 weeks) or there is the increased possibility of water condensation due to temperature fluctuations (spring or fall seasons), a mold inhibitor is highly recommended.

Pheasants, ducks, and turkey poults are quite sensitive to the effects of mycotoxins. Aflatoxins can cause reduced performance when present in the 10–20 parts per billion (ppb) range. Many other common mycotoxins like T-2 or fumonisins are dangerous in the parts per million (ppm) range, cause liver and kidney damage, and are to be avoided when possible. The most common symptoms reported are lesions in the mouth and throat; poor eggshell quality in layers and breeders; and stunting, poor growth, and rickets in growing birds as a result of liver, kidney, and intestinal damage. In other livestock, feed refusal, poor growth performance, and poor reproductive performance are observed.

Almost every year, weather conditions cause stress on the corn and other crops. That stress increases the potential for mold growth before harvest. Inadequate storage of the previous year's crop also leads to after-harvest mold growth during storage. It is common to see more than one type of mold or mycotoxin in a sample and toxicity may be from multiple sources.

Areas where feed manufacturers can reduce problems include ingredient storage and preparation, feed manufacturing changes, use of additives and nutrition-related changes to reduce or overcome symptoms. These measures will prevent or reduce mold growth, but will not affect mycotoxins that are already present.

7.3.1 Controlling Mold Growth in Ingredients

Ingredient storage and handling measures to reduce mold growth include: (i) evaluating all incoming corn with a black light (UV, although it only detects aflatoxin) and rejecting any corn that appears moldy; (ii) monitoring for moisture level; 12% or less will prevent mold growth; (iii) controlling insects that damage grain; (iv) ensuring bins are cleaned and leak proof; (v) utilizing only the best corn for young animals or substituting other grains (wheat, milo); (vi) using caution with grain byproducts like screenings and DDGs which are more likely to contain higher levels of mycotoxins; (vii) reducing handling damage to grain as much as possible to minimize broken kernels and fines; (viii) grinding grain only as needed and keeping storage time of ground grain to a minimum; and (ix) adding mold inhibitors to stored ingredients.

7.3.2 Controlling Mold in Feed

In finished feed, steps can be taken to prevent mold growth (as with ingredients) as well as to control mycotoxins and their symptoms. (i) Select, add or subtract ingredients based on quality, risk, species to be fed or age (wheat and milo may be safer during a bad corn year); (ii) adjust deliveries so that feed storage time is minimized; (iii) use pelleted feed; (iv) as with ingredients, make sure bins are clean and dry; (v) increase crude protein, and add animal sources and pure amino acids to provide a better amino acid balance; (vi) increase digestibility by adding enzymes; (vii) increase vitamin/trace mineral levels (especially D3), in feed and water; (viii) add mold inhibitor; (ix) add antioxidants (in premix or separately); and (x) add a mycotoxin binder.

Nutritionally, the most common mycotoxins cause damage to the gut, liver, kidneys or immune system. Damage to the gut, liver, and kidney results in malabsorption or interference with nutrient utilization or distribution. Hence, if extra, more digestible nutrients are added, more of these nutrients get absorbed. Similarly, the gut damage prevents absorption of vitamin D (and other vitamins) and/or the liver-kidney damage interferes with vitamin D metabolism. Therefore, increasing vitamin levels will be beneficial.

7.3.3 Mycotoxin Testing

Because there is usually more than one mycotoxin present and they are difficult and expensive to test for, it may be quicker and easier to first treat the symptoms using several methods at once. Then, especially if there are distinctive symptoms, testing using mycotoxin screens may be helpful for selecting more specific treatments.

7.4 Water and Water Quality

Although not an ingredient, water is often considered the most important nutrient. At the same time, it is also the most often overlooked. Water makes up 65–85% of the body, depending on age. It is involved in all metabolic functions, including temperature regulation, digestion, transport of nutrients, and elimination of waste. As the "universal solvent," water is the carrier of nutrients, even fats and fat-soluble vitamins which it carries as "micelles" that are formed by surfactants (i.e., bile) that make them soluble.

7.4.1 Water Temperature

The ideal drinking water temperature is between 60 and 75 °F. During hot weather, care must be taken that water does not reach too high a temperature as rejection may occur. Water rejection and dehydration are especially critical if the birds are being fed an ionophore coccidiostat, as ionophore toxicity (often referred to as "knockdown") can occur in birds that are dehydrated.

7.4.2 Consumption

Water consumption/bird by weight averages twice the weight of feed (water is 8.3 lb/gal). During hot weather, water consumption may increase to three or four times the average. Hence, in growing birds, water consumption can be a valuable diagnostic tool. Any fluctuation in consumption may be an indication of how the flock is doing.

7.4.3 Water Supplements

All manner of supplements or treatments may be delivered in the water: vitamins, electrolytes, probiotics, antibiotics, vaccines, coccidiostats, and wormers. The advantage of water treatment is that it can be started and stopped at very short notice, unlike the feed, which oftentimes must be ordered in large quantities. In situations where birds are stressed or sick, they will often go off feed, but they will almost always drink water.

7.4.4 Water Quality

The quality of water is evaluated based on the level of bacteria and minerals present (Tables 7.2 and 7.3).

Coliforms are a good indicator of water contaminated by livestock (runoff from concentrated animal production areas) or human waste (failed septic system). More than 50 cfu/mL coliforms suggests it is definitely a good idea to treat the water supply, possibly with shock chlorination. The following guidelines should be used to determine when water supplies should be tested for bacteria: noticeable change in color, odor or taste; flooding has occurred near the well; person or animal becomes sick from waterborne disease; recent maintenance on water supply system; persistent poor performance; or loss of pressure in the water system.

Table 7.2 Water quality standards for poultry: bacteria.

Contaminant	Levels considered average	Maximum acceptable level	Comments
Bacteria Total bacteria (TPC) cfu/mL	0 cfu/mL	1000 cfu/mL	Total bacteria is an indicator of system cleanliness; high numbers do not necessarily mean the bacteria present are harmful but it does mean that the system can potentially harbor pathogenic organisms. High bacteria levels can impact taste of water resulting in reduced consumption by birds.
Total coliforms	0 cfu/mL	50 cfu/mL	
Fecal coliforms	0 cfu/mL	0 cfu/mL	
			Presence of any fecal coliforms means water is unfit for consumption by poultry or humans

Source: Adapted and edited from Dr Susan Watkins, University of Arkansas (pers. comm.).

Table 7.3   Water quality standards for poultry: minerals.

Contaminant	Levels considered average	Maximum acceptable level	Comments/treatments
pH	6.5–7.8	8	A pH below 5 can be harmful to drinker equipment, causing corrosion to metal components. A pH above 8 impacts effectiveness of water sanitizers. High pH is also associated with high alkalinity which may result in reduced water consumption in poultry due to "bitter" taste
Total hardness	60–180 mg/L	110 mg/L	Hardness can also be determined by adding the calcium and magnesium content. Hardness causes scale which can reduce pipe volume and cause drinkers to leak or be hard to trigger
Calcium (Ca)	60 mg/L	No known level considered unacceptable	No upper limit for calcium; birds are very tolerant of calcium but values above 110 mg/L may require water softener, polyphosphates or acidifier to prevent scaling
Magnesium (Mg)	14 mg/L	125 mg/L	Higher levels of Mg may cause flushing due to laxative effect, particularly if high sulfate is present
Iron (Fe)	0.2 mg/L	0.3 mg/L	Birds are tolerant of iron metallic taste but high iron causes leaking drinkers and promotes the growth of *E. coli* and *Pseudomonas*. Treatment includes oxidation with chlorine, chlorine dioxide or ozone followed by filtration
Manganese (Mn)	0.01 mg/L	0.05 mg/L	Mn can result in black grainy residue on filters and in drinkers. Also, manganese is a food for pathogens. Manganese may interfere with copper uptake and utilization. Treatment includes oxidation with chlorine, chlorine dioxide or ozone at a pH of 8 followed by filtration. Green sand filtration is an option
Chloride (Cl)	50 mg/L	150–200 mg/L	When combined with high sodium levels, Cl creates salty water that can act as a laxative (causing flushing). Salty water can promote the growth of enteroccoci organisms that can lead to enteric issues and can damage reproductive tract in breeder birds, causing shell quality issues. Treatment with reverse osmosis, lower dietary salt level or blend with nonsaline water. Keep water clean and use daily sanitizers such as hydrogen peroxide or iodine to prevent microbial growth

(Continued)

Table 7.3 (Continued)

Contaminant	Levels considered average	Maximum acceptable level	Comments/treatments
Sodium (Na)	50 mg/L	150–200 mg/L	When combined with high chloride levels causes salty water: see comments and treatments for Cl above
Sulfates	15–40 mg/L	200 mg/L	Sulfates can cause flushing in birds. Rotten egg odor (hydrogen sulfide) indicates the presence of bacteria. The system will require shock chlorination. Sulfates can be removed by aerating water into a holding tank or treatment with hydrogen peroxide, chlorine or chlorine dioxide and then filtration. With elevated sulfate levels, hydrogen peroxide is preferred (stronger oxidizer) since it requires an almost 2 to 1 ratio of sanitizer to sulfate for oxidation
Nitrates (NO_3)	1–5 mg/L	25 mg/L	If nitrates convert to nitrites, this can result in poor growth and feed conversions due to the nitrites tying up blood hemoglobin. Plus presence of nitrates may indicate fecal contamination so also test for bacteria. Can be removed with reverse osmosis
Nitrites (NO_2) More nitrate>nitrite	0.4 mg/L	4 mg/L	
Lead	0 mg/L	0.014 mg/L	Long-term exposure can cause weak bones in growing birds and fertility problems in breeders
Copper	0.002 mg/L	0.6 mg/L	Continuous exposure to elevated levels of copper can result in proventriculitis
Zinc		1.5 mg/L	No known issues

Source: Adapted and edited from Dr Susan Watkins, University of Arkansas (pers. comm).

Moreover, all drinking water has some amount of dissolved minerals (Table 7.3). Most of the time, these dissolved minerals are well within acceptable ranges. However, if contaminants are not within desired levels, the result may be poor performance; equipment failure or damage; or the increased presence of harmful bacteria or fungal slime (some minerals can act as a food supply for these).

7.4.5 Potential Water Treatments

For water treatment, a target level of chlorine that should be achieved is 3–5 ppm. A target level of chlorine dioxide is 0.8–2 ppm while a target level of hydrogen peroxide is 50–100 ppm

7.5 Feed Ingredients – Nonnutritional

7.5.1 Pellet Binders

Once birds get used to eating crumbles or pellets, they tend to ignore any fines in the feeders, so maximum pellet quality is desirable to prevent waste. To achieve pellets with minimal fines, a pellet binder may be needed. Some ingredients (wheat and wheat middlings) are natural binders due to the binding ability of the gluten when it is gelatinized by the heat, moisture, and pressure present during the conditioning and pelleting process. When wheat products are not available or not needed in the formula, other products like bentonite, molasses, lignin, gelatin, and urea formaldehyde-based binders may be used.

7.5.2 Mold Inhibitors

As mentioned above, molds can reduce ingredient quality and produce mycotoxins. Mold inhibitors, usually based on propionic acid or other organic acid, are highly recommended for feed that will be stored for extended periods or that will be exposed to fluctuating temperatures and high moisture. Metal bins are especially prone to condensation in the spring and fall seasons.

7.5.3 Mycotoxin Binders

Binders (often sold as "flow agents") are selected for their ability to tie up and carry toxins out of the digestive tract in the feces, or to change the toxin structure to a less toxic form. Binders may contain refined clay portions (sodium-aluminosilicates), yeast cell wall fractions, enzymes, or a combination. The enzymes digest the toxin to a less harmful form. Most clay-based products bind aflatoxins but binding of other mycotoxins is variable depending on the product and its ingredients. Some toxins can be deleterious if present in ppb (parts per billion), and many have detrimental effects at ppm (parts per million), so it recommended to use a toxin binder in all feeds, especially starter and breeder feeds, as a precaution.

7.5.4 Enzymes

Enzyme mixtures include the addition of xylanase, beta-glucanase, pectinase, and phytase and are commonly used in meat- or egg-producing poultry to improve digestibility and feed conversion. This practice is also true for *some* gamebird feeds. In very young birds, endogenous enzyme production is not yet fully functional. Since starter feeds commonly have 27–28% crude protein, the high percentages of NSP in soybean meal can result in poor digestion and pasty vents (fecal staining of the vent region) unless an enzyme is added. The demands of egg production also make enzymes helpful for breeders. But in growing gamebirds for flight, the increased digestibility can be counterproductive. Because it is desirable to keep these birds lean and athletic, it is better to provide a low-energy, high-fiber diet without added enzymes. In addition to reducing fat deposition and preventing birds from becoming overweight poor performers, bulking agents induce satiety and take more time to consume. Thus, these gamebirds are less likely to have the time or inclination to peck at their penmates.

7.5.5 Antibiotics and Coccidiostats

Only one antibiotic and five coccidiostats are approved for gamebirds in the US, so extra-label use under the direction of a veterinarian is required for others. The one approved antibiotic, bacitracin methylenedisalicylate (BMD®), is used routinely in bobwhite quail feed because of their frequent problems with ulcerative enteritis due to *Clostridium colinum*. The coccidiostats monensin (Coban®) and salinomycin (Bio-Cox®) are approved for quail; amprolium for pheasants; and lasalocid (Avatec®) or sulfadimethoxine-ormetoprin 5 : 3 (RofenAid®) for partridges. Because resistance has developed to some of these products, it is often necessary to rotate to other products with a different mode of action. Moreover, the ionophores (monensin and lasalocid) can cause ionophore toxicity (knockdown) and mortality during times of hot weather or reduced water consumption and should be avoided in those situations.

7.5.6 Probiotics (Direct Fed Microbials – DFM)

While antibiotics are used as a treatment, probiotics are most effective when used as a preventive. For maximum effect, these beneficial bacteria need to reach the gut and be allowed to colonize and provide normal healthy gut flora before any potential pathogens that might arrive in the feed, water, litter or air. Delivery can be in the drinking water; in hatchling supplements (like GroGel Plus®); by spray in chick boxes; or mixed in the feed. Many suppliers offer probiotics for feed delivery that contain one or a few species (usually *Bacillus*), primarily because these spore-formers are relatively stable in storage and during feed processing. Although some of these cultures have been demonstrated to provide performance or health benefits, it is unrealistic to expect that they could consistently work under the multitude of conditions found in the field and/or replace the hundreds (or thousands) of species present in normal, healthy bird intestines.

A major disadvantage is that *Bacillus* species do not colonize the gut, so must be fed continuously. Thus, the most consistently effective probiotic cultures contain many additional species performing different functions. For example, while *Bacillus* sp. function mainly in the lumen as they pass through, others like *Lactobacillus* sp. and *Bifidobacteria* sp. attach to the cells of the gut wall and colonize. By covering the surface, these bacteria can provide competitive exclusion of pathogens by physically occupying attachment sites. Additionally, different species competitively inhibit potential pathogens by competing for nutrients, producing inhibitory substances (i.e., organic acids), or assisting the bird with digestion (enzyme production). Many of the more effective species are not spore-formers and thus require protective coatings to provide stability in the feed or must be delivered in the drinking water or in a hatchling supplement.

7.5.7 Wormers

Floor-reared and pen-reared poultry have always been, and will always be, troubled by parasites that are carried into the pens where they can be consumed by the birds. Parasites like worms not only cause damage to the lining of the digestive tract and internal organs, but also may lead to secondary invasion from bacteria. Mortality is not always high, but even a minor infestation costs money in feed, bird performance, and health. No wormers are approved for gamebirds in the USA. While fenbendazole (Safe-Guard®) is likely the most widely used and effective wormer available, and has been researched for many years in gamebirds, it is yet to be approved. It is broad spectrum, acting against roundworms, cecal worms, and some capillary and gapeworms. It is usually provided in the feed for 5–7 days and repeated after 3–4 weeks. Water-soluble fenbendazole (Aquasol®) was recently introduced to provide some convenience for those not able to use it in the feed. Plus, it eliminates problems with feed delivery time, ordering amount, bin space, etc. This newer version does not have the problems with settling out seen in the earlier water-delivered product.

Piperazine (Wazine®) is another old water-delivered wormer that is effective for intestinal roundworms. Depending on the size of the operation and availability of veterinary assistance, it may be an easier option. It is not considered effective for other worms.

Hygromycin B (Hygromix®) is an approved wormer for chickens and is said to be effective for control of roundworms, cecal worms, and capillary worms. Hygromycin B is slower acting than fenbendazole and is recommended to be fed continuously. This may be an advantage for some growers who do not have bin space for segregation of fenbendazole-treated feed or do not buy enough quantity to meet their feed mill's minimum order.

Diatomaceous earth (DE) is a "natural" mined product that is popular in the organic portion of the poultry industry. The sharp spines on the skeletons of tiny organisms can puncture or damage the soft skin of worms. It does not kill all worms but damages many, and only while they are in the digestive tract. It has no effect on those that have penetrated the gut lining and moved elsewhere, so it is better at prevention. Advantages are that it is inexpensive and can be included in any feed.

7.5.8   Plant Extracts

Plant extracts like saponins (yucca, quillaia) have long been known to increase membrane permeability and cause damage to some parasites and microorganisms. They are not usually sold for that purpose but might be worth consideration as a dual-purpose additive (along with ammonia control). Similarly, with increased interest in reducing the use of antibiotics, other plant extracts like oregano oil (carvacrol), thyme oil (thymol), and many others are currently being evaluated. There is some indication that they also affect membrane permeability in worms.

7.5.9   Grit

For breeders, large particle size calcium carbonate or oyster shells may be included in a mash diet or fed free choice. Insoluble grit (granite grit) is usually not required for feed that is processed, but in the case of birds that are free ranging, given whole grains or vegetable matter, it is advisable to provide insoluble grit free choice. When introducing grit, it must be done gradually to prevent overconsumption and impactions.

7.5.10   Treatments for External Parasites

For mites, sulfur-based products can be included in the feed or provided in a dust bath. Diatomaceous earth can also be provided via feed or dustbath.

7.5.11   Nutritional Considerations Regarding Worms

Because most worms migrate into or through the gut lining and other organs, they may cause extensive damage and blood loss to those tissues and allow penetration by pathogenic bacteria. Therefore, it is essential that a quality vitamin-mineral premix is used in the feed. Because absorptive tissues of the digestive tract may be compromised, it is especially important to add extra vitamins in the feed. In addition to the feed, it can be beneficial to supplement the water with a "stress pack" vitamin product to reduce stress, support the immune system, and promote healing of tissues. These vitamins include A, D, E, and K. Minerals like zinc are also important for healing and tissue repair.

7.6   Feed Form

Upland gamebirds, like chickens and turkeys, prefer bite-sized particles of food like pellets or crumbles. But because they have a relatively dry mouth, they can do well on ground feed (mash). This is in contrast to ducks and other waterfowl which have a "wet mouth" and will waste mash feed while trying to wash it down with water. Ground feed must be treated with care, but can be used successfully if the ingredients are ground to a uniform particle size. This is necessary to prevent sorting by the birds and settling and separation of finer particles, like vitamins and trace minerals. Particle sizes of about 0.5–1 mm (quail and Hungarian partridge) and 1–2 mm (pheasants) for a starter and 3–4 mm for older birds are good targets. The inclusion of slightly "sticky" ingredients like meat and bone meal or fat (0.5%) is also necessary to reduce separation and dustiness.

Pelleted feed, although more costly, has advantages: uniform distribution of nutrients; reduced waste; no sorting; less bulk; and better flowability. In addition, the heat and pressure of conditioning and pelleting result in reduced bacteria and molds and increased digestibility due to cooking and inactivation of growth inhibitors (trypsin inhibitors). For starter feeds (as with mash), the pellets must be crumbled to decrease particle size (1–2 mm for pheasants), and for some species very fine (or even reground) crumbles are necessary (about 0.5–1 mm for quail and Hungarian partridge). For all other feeds, a mini-pellet size of 3/32 to 1/8 in. (2.4–3.2 mm) is ideal, or a larger pellet cut very short.

Disadvantages of pellets include higher cost; also, the heat created during processing not only kills some beneficial bacteria along with pathogens but denatures some enzymes and some vitamins. Hence, suppliers must compensate by providing specially selected or protected probiotic bacteria and enzymes and add vitamin overages.

7.6.1 Feed Testing

A simple series of tests can determine if feed is mixed as formulated: tests for crude protein, crude fat, crude fiber, calcium, phosphorus, sodium, and a trace mineral (i.e., zinc) will often tell if the feed has been mixed correctly. This type of test is usually inexpensive, and most labs can perform it without problems. Since vitamin testing is quite expensive, testing for a mineral will help to indicate if the premix is at the correct level. Of course, this is only for vitamin trace mineral premixes that are a combination product. If the feed mill is using separate vitamin and mineral premixes, then it becomes necessary to test a vitamin as well. Additional tests, like mold count, bacterial counts or mycotoxin screens, may be needed.

7.7 Formulation of Gamebird Feed

Formulation is the process whereby nutritional ingredients are assembled in the correct ratio to meet specific nutrient requirements based on age or stage of bird at the best cost, at the same time incorporating nonnutritional ingredients based on their need in the formula (feed form, disease prevention, etc.). Protein and energy ingredients occupy approximately 85% of formula, while minerals, vitamins, and nonnutritional ingredients form the remainder of the formula.

After the nutritionist or formulator provides the restrictions (minimums and maximums for each nutrient or ingredient), modern computer programs designed for "best fit" or "least cost" formulation can perform the thousands of simultaneous calculations necessary to provide the required amounts of each of those components. In actual practice, modern manufacturers provide vitamin and mineral premixes that are precalculated to provide the correct amount of each nutrient. This combination of some 20+ ingredients into one reduces the total number of calculations necessary to provide a formula from the remaining 10–20 ingredients. In a standard corn-soybean diet, restrictions are usually reduced to protein, calcium, phosphorus, ME, salt, methionine, and lysine. Additional restrictions may be needed for fat or fiber to adjust nutrient density or pellet quality.

Most gamebird feed programs include a starter, grower, finisher (meat birds) or flight conditioner (birds for release), maintenance and breeder. Table 7.1 provides suggested nutrient levels and Table 7.4 provides examples of formulas. The feeds required for pheasants, partridges, quail, and wild turkey are very similar, using a high protein starter (26–28%), a grower (20%), or several growers from 20% to 24% protein, a finisher for meat birds or a flight conditioner for release birds (18–20%), and a maintenance diet (12–15%; flight birds or breeders). Guineafowl, coturnix quail, and mallard ducks need only 23–24% protein in the starter (starter #2), while other diets are similar to those used for the other species. Breeder diets may also require some adjustments to allow for strain differences; smaller, more active strains often perform better with a slightly more nutrient-dense feed (breeder #2) and for species that are not heavy layers (like peafowl), a lower calcium level (1.5%) is sufficient (and also reduces the chance of experiencing gout). If there is not access to gamebird-specific formulations, a turkey starter feed will work well for most gamebirds; however, turkey grower and finisher diets are usually too high in energy for birds that are to be released (see Tables 7.1 and 7.4).

7.7.1 Possible Hand Calculations

In situations where the formulator or producer does not have access to formulation software or changes must be made quickly "by hand," it is worth mentioning Pearson's square. This is a simple method of calculating the amounts of two ingredients. A very practical example would be a producer who keeps multiple ages or several species of birds but only has two feed bins, one for 28% protein starter and one for 20% protein grower feeds. Ideally, it would be better to have an intermediate grower of approximately 23–24% protein instead of making a potentially stressful switch from the 28 to the 20. Or the grower may have another species that requires only a 23% protein starter (guineafowl or coturnix quail). The correct protein level can be found by a mix of the 28% and 20% feeds. But, how much of each is needed?

As an example, if we have a 28% protein starter diet and a 20% protein grower diet and we wish to feed an intermediate starter diet of 23% protein, they are set up on the left two corners of a square with the desired amount in the center of the square (see diagram below). Ignoring negatives, subtracting across diagonally from corner to corner, we get 28–23 = 5 and 23–20 = 3. Adding the total parts, 3 + 5 = 8. Then divide each by the total, 3/8 = 0.375 and 5/8 = 0.675. Multiply each by 100 (to get %) and the result is that the 28% formula will be 37.5% of the mix and the 20% formula will be 62.5% of the mix.

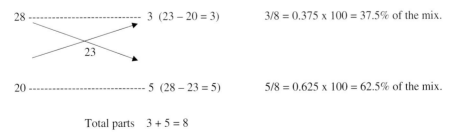

This procedure can be used with more than two ingredients if they are first blended into one.

Table 7.4 Examples of gamebird formulas (in pounds per 2000 pounds).

Ingredients	28% Starter[j]	24% Starter[k]	20% Grower	Meat finisher	Flight finisher	Maint-enance	Breeder #1	Breeder #2[l]
Corn[a]	830	1030	1090	1260	995	940	1160	1050
Soybean meal	850	670	545	450	385	177	470	575
Meat and bone[b]	150	150	50	150	50	50	150	150
Wheat middlings[c]	100	100	225	100	505	769	100	100
Salt	5.15	5.15	6.8	5.15	6.85	6.85	5.15	5.2
Calcium carbonate	19.5	27	42	14.2	27	28	98	93
Dicalcium phosphate	16	3	20	–	13	12.5		
Fat	5	–	–	–				10
Vitamin/mineral[d]	8	7	7	7	7	6	9	9
dl-methionine	5	4.2	4.2	4.25	3.9	4.25	2.3	3.3
Lysine	2.6	–	–	–		4.15		
Mycotoxin binder[e]	2	2	2	2	2	2	2	2
Mold inhibitor[f]	1	1					1	1
Enzyme[g]	1	1		1				1
Coccidiostat[h]	1	1						
Antibiotic[i]	1	1	1					
Probiotic	1	1	1	1	1	1	1	1
Analysis								
Protein (%)	28	24	20	20	18	15	20	22
Met Energy (kcal/lb)	1250	1250	1250	1350	1200	1150[m]	1250	1280
Calcium (%)	1.3	1.1	0.95	0.95	0.85	0.85	2.6	2.5
Phos (avail) (%)	0.65	0.5	0.45	0.45	0.4	0.4	0.45	0.45
Salt (%)	0.37	0.37	0.37	0.37	0.37	0.37	0.37	0.37
Meth + Cyst (%)	1.1	0.95	0.85	0.85	0.75	0.65	0.75	0.85
Lysine (%)	1.75	1.3	0.95	0.95	0.85	0.85	0.85	0.95

a) Corn: can be replaced with wheat or milo with adjustments for protein, etc.
b) Meat meal (or fish): some markets for meat birds may request all-vegetable formulas.
c) Wheat midds: minimum of 100 lb/ton for pellet quality or use a pellet binder.
d) Vitamin/mineral pack: this example uses combined vitamin/mineral/choline – some suppliers may add them separately to increase stability in storage.
e) Mycotoxin binder: amount will change with product and challenges.
f) Mold inhibitor: may not be necessary if feed is used within 2 weeks.
g) Enzyme: beta-glucanase for high-soy or xylanase for high-wheat formulas.
h) Coccidiostat: usually needed in starter and grower.
i) Antibiotic: may not be needed; quail usually require BMD to prevent enteritis.
j) Use 28% starter for pheasants, partridge, bobwhite quail, wild turkey.
k) Use 24% as starter #2 for above or as the first starter for guineafowl, coturnix quail or ducks.
l) Use breeder #2 for smaller, more active strains of each species.
m) ME of maintenance may need to be increased in cold weather.

7.7.2   Nonfeed Supplements

7.7.2.1   Water

Fresh clean water and properly formulated feeds *usually* provide all the nutrients that gamebirds need. But under conditions of stress when feed consumption is not adequate, extra supplements in the water may be necessary, and occasionally there is a need to get vitamins or other supplements into the bird quickly without waiting to reorder feed. Water delivery can be started and ended much more quickly than the feed. As an example, say the grower notices a few "wing walkers" (weak legs) in the flock of growing birds. Is it a feed deficiency problem or an absorption problem? The diagnosis of rickets will be the same in either case. Vitamin D is usually the first to show symptoms of deficiency (sometimes B vitamins), and is often diagnosed as rickets caused by calcium, phosphorus or vitamin D deficiency or imbalance in the feed. Actually, it is often a result of poor absorption due to enteritis caused by coccidia, bacteria, virus or mycotoxins. Analysis takes time. It is quicker to add vitamins in the water, and that supplementation will often get them through until the problem resolves or is diagnosed more accurately.

7.7.2.2   Electrolytes

Feed should contain all necessary electrolytes for normal circumstances. During hot weather, birds are often off feed due to a reduced appetite. Electrolytes in the water replace lost electrolytes, stimulate water consumption, and help reduce shrink during long road trips.

7.7.2.3   Combination Products

When birds are off feed for any reason, they do not receive the necessary vitamins, minerals, and electrolytes present in the feed. Stressed birds may not eat but will almost always drink. For any stress situation, including heat or cold, just-placed chicks, crowding and before and after moving, the addition of a multivitamin plus electrolytes product is recommended.

7.7.2.4   Probiotics

As is the case with electrolytes and vitamins, probiotics are often included in the feed. For maximum effect, the beneficial bacteria need to reach the gut before any potential pathogens that might arrive in the feed, water, litter or air. While we are familiar with antibiotics being used as a treatment, probiotics are most effective when used as a preventive. Delivery can be in the drinking water, hatchling supplements (GroGel Plus) or by spray in the hatch trays if feed is not convenient.

7.7.2.5   Wormers

Although wormers are usually delivered in feed, there may be times when water delivery is more convenient. One of the most effective products for most worms (fenbendazole) is now available in water delivery form (Safe-Guard, AquaSol®).

7.7.3   Other Supplements

7.7.3.1   Hatchling Supplements

Excessive dehydration can occur after hatch if there is an extended hatching window, or when chicks are in transit for long periods of time. Hatchling supplements (i.e., GroGel Plus) are green in color to attract the chick, semi-solid (like gelatin) and contain 90% or more water, plus nutrition. When provided at the hatchery or upon arrival at the grow-out farm, they provide much-needed

Table 7.5 Nutrition-related disease, diagnosis, troubleshooting I.

Nutrient	Symptoms of deficiency (D) or excess (E)	Comments
Protein, amino acids	D: Slow growth, poor feathering and egg production. E: Wet manure and high ammonia, articular gout	Test feed for correct protein and amino acids for the age or stage
Calcium, phosphorus	D: Rickets, weak bones, reduced eggshell quality and egg production. E: Gout, rickets (excess Ca > P deficit)	Check Ca/P ratio, vitamin D, malabsorption of D due to enteritis caused by bacteria, virus or mycotoxin. Limit saturated fat in starter diets
Sodium, chloride, potassium	D: Weakness, poor growth, ataxia, soft bones, reduced egg production, cannibalism. In growing ducks – high mortality. E: Ascites, increased water consumption, wet litter	Test feed for proper mix. Test water for excess minerals. Ideal electrolyte balance (Na + K-Cl) is 250–300 mEq/kg
Fiber	D: Feather picking. E: Slow growth, impaction (litter eating)	Fiber (wheat mids, alfalfa) is a good low-energy diluent to prevent overweight birds
Fat	D: Linoleic acid deficiency occurs in no-corn diets. Reduced growth, hatchability, and egg production. E: Above 1–2% added fat > poor pellet quality	Poor quality or rancid fat > destruction of fat-soluble vitamins
Water	D: Dehydration, increased 1st week mortality, reduced feed consumption, renal failure > death. E: Wet feces and litter	D: Look for tight skin on legs. Stimulate 1st day consumption with hatchling supplement, attractants in waterers, adjust nipples to drip, etc. Consider water temperature, taste, ionophore toxicity. E: Excess undigested protein, excess salt or magnesium in feed or water. Add enzymes in high-wheat diets and starter diets with high-soybean meal
Vitamin A	D: Weakness, ataxia, ruffled feathers, eye and membrane disorders, infections, enlarged hocks, poor egg production	Keep premix and feed storage time as short as possible. Add antioxidants
Vitamin D	D: Rickets, weakness (wing walkers), weak bones, poor eggshell quality, and egg production. E: Gout, rickets (excess Ca > P deficit)	Check Ca/P ratio and amounts, vitamin D level. Consider malabsorption of D due to enteritis caused by bacteria, virus or mycotoxin. Add water-soluble vitamin D3
Vitamin E	D: Encephalomalacia (incoordination), muscular dystrophy, reproductive disorders	Check for lack of antioxidant or rancid fat in feed. Selenium can replace in some cases
Vitamin K	D: Poor blood clotting, hemorrhages	Check for cocci or other internal parasites, mycotoxins

Table 7.6   Nutrition-related disease, diagnosis, troubleshooting II.

Nutrient	Symptoms of deficiency (D) or excess (E)	Comments
Thiamine (B1)	D: Loss of coordination, poor feathering, polyneuritis	Amprolium can be antagonistic
Riboflavin (B2)	D: Poor growth, diarrhea, curled toes, poor hatchability	Ducklings have higher requirements. Consider genetics
Pantothenic acid (B3)	D: Ragged feathers, poor growth, dermatitis around mouth, poor hatchability	Consider mycotoxins
Niacin	D: Perosis, slow growth, poor feathering, mouth lesions, enlarged hocks	Requirements in gamebirds and ducks are higher than other poultry
Folic acid	D: Poor growth and feathering, perosis, reduced hatchability and egg production	Depigmentation can occur. Check also copper, iron, and lysine levels
Pyridoxine (B6)	D: Poor growth, feathering, and coordination, reduced hatchability and egg production	
Biotin	D: Foot dermatitis, perosis, broken feathers, poor hatchability	Wheat or barley diets may need extra. Rancid fat, enteritis, and excess litter ammonia increase requirement
B12	D: Anemia, poor growth, perosis, hatchability	Consider also iron, copper
Choline	D: Slow growth, perosis, reduced egg production, feathers, egg size, hatchability	
Manganese	D: Perosis, abnormal bone growth, egg production	Limit excess Ca and P. See also choline & folic acid
Iron, copper	D: Anemia, poor feather color, cartilage and bone disorders. E: Fat destruction	Consider aflatoxins
Iodine	D: Reduced hatchability, delayed yolk sac absorption, poor feathering	
Zinc	D: Retarded growth, dermatitis, poor feathering and egg production. E: Anorexia	
Selenium	D: Exudative diathesis, ruffled feathers, poor egg production and hatchability	Vitamin E can replace some selenium. High Cu or Zn may interfere with uptake

hydration until the chicks find and use the normal sources, thus reducing starve-outs and early mortality. When placed on top of starter feed, hatchling supplements act as an attractant to train the chicks what to eat. These supplements can also serve as a vehicle for delivery of other products such as vaccines or probiotics.

7.7.3.2   Dust Bath

For mites, sulfur-based products can be included in the feed or provided in a dust bath. Likewise, DE can be included in feed or a dust bath.

7.8 Nutritional Diseases, Diagnosis, and Troubleshooting

Although it is possible to encounter nutritional disease symptoms as a result of errors in mixing of vitamin-mineral premix or feed, poor storage, formulation, selection of ingredients, appropriate feed for age or delivery errors, it is necessary to separate these problems from bacteria, viruses, parasites or toxins that can affect digestion and absorption. In other words, is it a deficiency or imbalance of some kind, or malabsorption due to gut damage or disease that results in the same symptoms? Testing of the feed, as described earlier, should tell if the problem is in the feed. Then, an examination of management, feed storage, handling, and disease state can proceed.

Modern prepared feeds usually contain a premix of both vitamins and microminerals, so it is rare to find a situation where an individual vitamin or trace mineral nutrient is responsible for deficiency disease symptoms; it is usually a combination. Still, it is possible under specific circumstances, such as the presence of a particular antivitamin (amprolium and thiamine) or the destruction of some vitamins which are less stable. Vitamins that are less stable in processing and more likely to be damaged by heat or oxidation include thiamine and vitamins A, D, and E. Tables 7.5 and 7.6 list the nutrients, common symptoms of deficiency or excess, and comments that may be helpful in diagnosis. Note that many nutrients have similar symptoms of deficiency, making diagnosis due to a particular nutrient difficult. This data is further complicated by the fact that most symptoms described result from studies with chickens or turkeys, so they are not always seen in gamebirds. Diagnosis often involves a detailed study of management, disease, presence of toxins, feed manufacturing, and nutrition to find the cause of a particular problem.

References

1 Leeson, S. and Summers, J.D. (2005). Feeding programs for gamebirds, ratites and pet birds. In: *Commercial Poultry Nutrition*, 3e (ed. S. Leeson and J.D. Summers), 381–395. UK: Nottingham University Press, Nottingham.

2 National Research Council (1994). Nutrient requirements of ring-necked pheasants, Japanese quail and bobwhite quail. In: *Nutrient Requirements of Poultry*, 9e. Washington, DC.: National Academy Press.

3 Association of American Feed Control Officials (2021). Feed terms and ingredient definitions. In: AAFCO, Official Publication. In: (ed. R.T. Eyck), 331–520. IL: AAFCO. Champaign.

4 American Feed Industry Association (1990). *AFIA Feed Ingredients Guide II*. Arlington, VA: AFIA.

8

Biosecurity for Gamebirds

Rodrigo A. Gallardo and Eva Wallner-Pendleton

The term *gamebird* describes any species of bird that may be used for hunting, including upland gamebirds, waterfowl, and woodland birds. Upland gamebirds include pheasants, chukar partridges, red-legged partridges, Hungarian partridges, bobwhite quail, and wild turkeys. Mallard ducks are the most common waterfowl raised commercially for release (Figure 8.1).

An important program which includes biosecurity in these groups of birds is the National Poultry Improvement Plan (NPIP). The NPIP was established in the early 1930s as a cooperative industry, state, and federal program to reduce and/or eradicate several vertically transmitted diseases and diseases of important economic and regulatory significance in poultry in the USA. This program is discussed at length in Chapter 2. Participation in the NPIP is a very important component of a biosecurity program. Currently exhibition poultry, ornamental and hobby upland gamebirds (such as golden pheasants, impeyans, and Lady Amherst breeds) and backyard waterfowl participate in Subpart E of this program. In 2019 subpart J was added to the NPIP for the large, commercial gamebird industry including raised-for-release gamebirds, gamebird breeding flocks, and gamebirds raised for meat and eggs.

It is important not to confuse the terms *gamebirds*, which are birds raised for hunting purposes, and *game fowl*, which are chickens raised for hobby purposes, breeding, and exhibition. Within this second category there are breeds known as old English game chickens which some have used for illegal cockfighting. Small hobby flock owners often raise multiple bird species including gamebirds, chickens, turkeys, and waterfowl. Large commercial gamebird operations usually have one or two gamebird breeds on their farms but, as the name implies, have thousands of birds on their premises. Because commercial flocks and hobby flocks have different management, flock size, purpose, and biosecurity risks, they will be covered separately in this chapter.

8.1 Commercial Gamebird Production

As hunting opportunities for wild gamebirds declined in the US due to reduced habitat and urbanization, commercial production of gamebirds developed to meet the needs of hunters. Both gamebird production and hunting preserves increase productivity of existing agricultural land and allow farmers to derive income from the land year round, including the winter months.

The gamebird industry is made up of breeding operations, hatcheries, brooding, rearing to release, and hunting preserves. These activities often coexist within one operation with little

Gamebird Medicine and Management, First Edition. Edited by Teresa Y. Morishita and Robert E. Porter, Jr.
© 2023 John Wiley & Sons, Inc. Published 2023 by John Wiley & Sons, Inc.

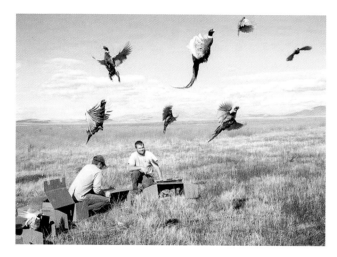

Figure 8.1 Gamebird production and hunting preserves increase the productivity of agricultural land and allow farmers to derive income from the land year round, including in the winter months.

geographical separation. Some gamebird producers also raise multiple gamebird species on the same farm. This consolidation of activities is done for optimization of labor and a hedge against possible fluctuating markets for the various products sold. However, biosecurity measures and confining disease outbreaks to a limited number of animals/pens can be challenging under this type of management.

Gamebirds are usually started indoors in brooder houses similar to those used in commercial poultry. At approximately 5 weeks of age (this age can vary considerable between farms), game chicks are allowed outside access. This can create a biosecurity challenge as exposure to wild birds is possible. In the case of quail chicks, while they can also be moved out to flight pens, many growers, especially in the southern US, keep them indoors until maturity. When birds reach maturity, around 17–21 weeks of age, they can be released onto hunting preserves or sold to outside preserve operators.

Commercial gamebird producers may market several products including hatching eggs, day-old chicks, started birds of various ages, flight-ready birds, and adult breeders. Eggs are usually sold from March to July, chicks are typically marketed from April through August, started birds are sold from June through September, and raised-for-release birds from September through mid-April coinciding with the hunting season. Birds and/or eggs can be sold and transported regionally or in many cases shipped long distances to customers. Most large commercial producers transport birds on their own in specially designed vehicles (Figure 8.2). Smaller flocks of chicks or ducks are often shipped via the United States Postal System (USPS) or other carriers.

(a)

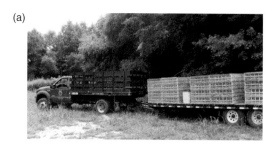

(b)

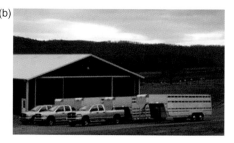

Figure 8.2 Transportation of gamebirds can be tricky and is certainly more specialized than transporting commercial poultry. Several specially designed vehicles are used for this task.

8.2   Biosecurity Recommendations

Biosecurity is a term used to describe a group of measures taken to keep pathogens and disease out or contained in the event of disease occurrence. They consist of measures to prevent the spread of that disease to other units in the same business or to neighbors [1]. These measures are often focused on keeping foreign animal diseases (FADs) out of flocks but also help to prevent the introduction of multiple infectious diseases in gamebirds such as fowl cholera, mycoplasma, erysipelas, botulism, salmonellosis, avian pox, marble spleen disease, Newcastle disease, avian influenza, and histomoniasis. For example, low-pathogenicity avian influenza viruses regularly infect North American waterfowl and shore birds and present a risk to gamebirds. In addition, the NPIP Subpart J (Biosecurity principles for operations with 25 000 raised for release gamebirds or more) states in 9 CFR 53.10 that a written biosecurity plan is mandatory in order to receive 100% indemnity if a FAD infects a premises [2]. There are 13 components that need to be addressed in the written biosecurity plan.

1. The farm must possess a biosecurity coordinator.
2. Regular employee trainings on biosecurity must be held.
3. Lines of separation (demarcate the areas where the birds can roam) must be established.
4. Establishment of a perimeter buffer area (area that separates the barns or pens and other buildings or structures related with the enterprise from areas unrelated to the enterprise) must occur. Upon entrance to the facility, clothes changing stations or protective equipment use should be required. The Danish entry system is an option to physically separate clean and dirty areas and maintain biosecurity inside the premises (Figure 8.3).
5. Clear biosecurity requirements for personnel must be in place, including but not limited to use of protective equipment, not having domestic or pet birds at home, traffic and movement specifications in the farm, etc.
6. Rodent and vermin control plans should be written and in place for flies, rodents, predators, wild birds, waterfowl, etc. (Figure 8.4).
7. A biosecurity plan for equipment and vehicles should be in place. Measures need to be taken to minimize disease introduction and spread due to use of equipment and vehicles, including use of washable crates, off-farm bird transfers, cleaning and disinfection of vehicles and crates before returning to the farm, protective equipment use, tire wash stations, designated parking of vehicles away from bird pens, visitor log sign-in, etc.
8. A mortality disposal plan should be in place and include items such as daily bird pick-up and use of on-site biosecure disposal rather than rendering trucks. For example, carcasses should be stored in closed, vermin-proof containers.
9. The farm should have a litter and manure disposal plan that limits insect, rodents, and wild bird attraction such as properly performed composting.
10. A biosecure replacement bird plan should be in place, such as obtaining birds from NPIP-certified hatcheries.
11. A clean water supply should be available, ideally from a municipal source or well as opposed to surface water sources that might attract wild waterfowl, and the water should be tested for microbial contamination and treated if necessary.
12. Feed and replacement litter should be stored in a biosecure manner, limiting exposure to wild animals or vermin. Spilled feed should be disposed of promptly.
13. Unexplained elevated mortality should be investigated to rule out any reportable disease. Submission of a sample of the mortality to an animal diagnostic laboratory for testing is recommended.

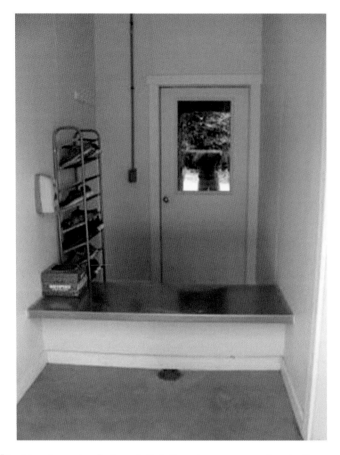

Figure 8.3 The "Danish entry system" allows full clothes change or use of protective equipment upon entry to a commercial or noncommercial facility. The physical barrier between dirty and clean sites helps organization and cleanliness.

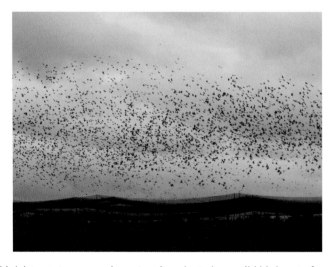

Figure 8.4 Wild bird deterrents are very important in order to keep wild birds out of commercial premises. These birds can carry pathogens that might affect gamebirds in captivity.

This biosecurity plan is audited by each state NPIP coordinator. The NPIP has added avian influenza surveillance and testing for upland gamebirds and raised-for-release waterfowl. Testing requirements and intervals can be viewed at www.poultryimprovement.org/documents/Biosecurity-Principles-and-Audit-Guidelines-2017-2020.pdf.

Because of the way in which gamebirds are managed, unique aspects need to be addressed as they affect biosecurity. Since the different productive units may be a part of the same premise, disease containment is one of the biggest challenges in these flocks. Biosecurity measures related to physical separation of breeding facilities and hatcheries from commercial birds and hunting preserves are mandatory. In addition, personnel should not be shared between these units. Breeding facilities and hatcheries should be highly biosecure since they are composed of expensive birds that are difficult to replace. Hatching eggs need to be aseptically processed in hatcheries, avoiding infections that might affect the chicks.

Most raised-for-release gamebirds are kept outdoors in flight pens. This can pose additional challenges to biosecurity. Perimeter fences and overhead netting are key to preventing predators gaining access to the birds (Figure 8.5). While overhead netting prevents the entrance of starlings, raptors, shore birds, and wild waterfowl, it does not prevent the access of small songbirds. Sometimes blackbirds and starlings roost on the netting, allowing their droppings to enter the gamebird pens. Noise cannons and other scare devices can be used to discourage roosting on the nets. Predators such as birds of prey attempt to capture birds near the netting, causing severe trauma to some of them (Figure 8.6). In addition, dogs, coyotes, foxes, mink, weasels, skunks, and racoons will try to dig underneath the fence. Sturdy fencing with underground and perimetral gravel is effective in deterring digging. Plastic sight barriers and electric fencing are also helpful. For rodent control, a holistic approach should be taken, including gravel surrounding the pens, bait stations in two perimeters outside the bird area, mowing weeds, and avoiding clutter. Bait stations need to be monitored for bait consumption and that information recorded to understand rodent activity. Finally, dead birds need to be collected immediately and properly disposed of to prevent scavengers and household pets from inadvertent poisoning.

Flight-ready birds are often sold and delivered within a wide geographical area. In order to minimize disease risk to the seller, it is recommended to unload birds in a mutually agreed location away from the buyer's farm. Transfer of birds to the buyer's crates and transportation in the buyer's

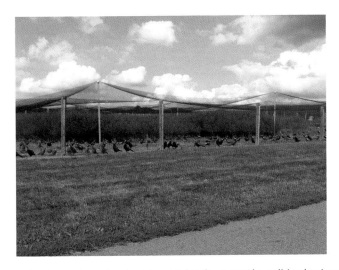

Figure 8.5   Perimeter fencing and overhead netting are key in preventing wild animal access to the birds.

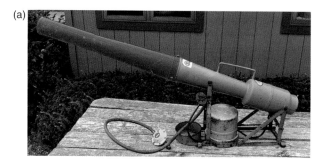 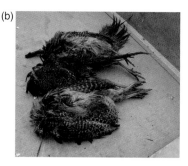

Figure 8.6 (a) Noise cannons are used to deter nuisance birds and predators from commercial premises. (b) One of the consequences of wildlife interaction is headless birds due to predation between perimetral fencing.

vehicle to their premises help avoid contaminated equipment from bringing disease back to the seller's farm. In some instances, multiple bird deliveries to different customers may be made in the course of one trip. Unloading off site helps to prevent the vehicle from becoming contaminated between farms. When all birds have been offloaded, the delivery truck and crates should be cleaned and disinfected thoroughly, preferably before reentering the home farm.

Mixing mallard duck production and upland gamebird production is a potentially risky practice for introduction of diseases such as avian influenza and fowl cholera [1]. If there are enough direct or close indirect interactions between these species, cross-infection may occur. Raised-for-release waterfowl and upland gamebirds should ideally be kept on separate farms, with different personnel and separate equipment. Furthermore, gamebird producers should be discouraged from rearing poultry such as chickens and turkeys for disease prevention purposes [1]. Several diseases such as *Mycoplasma gallisepticum* and histomoniasis can be passed from poultry to gamebirds. A disease such as *M. gallisepticum* is also vertically transmitted from breeder to offspring via the hatching egg. This could potentially infect valuable gamebird breeding stock and is very difficult to eradicate. The disease can then be transferred to birds sold to customers, creating a serious problem for them and bad customer relations. In hunting preserves, the idea is to minimize comingling of birds from different suppliers, and to keep the birds for only a short time for the sake of flock health, so it is suggested to obtain only the number of birds needed for 1–2 weeks.

Mild forms of avian influenza are considered endemic in waterfowl and shore birds in North America. The genotypes affecting these birds are variable and most produce little or no clinical disease in their hosts however, highly pathogenic strains may cause increased mortality. Low pathogenic avian influenza (LPAI) and highly pathogenic avian influenza (HPAI) infections in upland gamebirds are uncommon. If they occur, they are usually the consequence of close or indirect contact with wild or domestic waterfowl. Waterfowl do not need to come into direct contact with gamebirds to transmit infection. The virus is excreted in large numbers in droppings. Fecal matter can be carried on shoes, farm equipment, and surface water. There have been instances of avian influenza infecting pheasants after the same equipment used for mowing vegetation around a pond was used near a pheasant pen. In another instance, gamebirds and waterfowl were separately penned but after heavy rain, virus-infected temporary streams were formed and those carried the virus from the waterfowl into the pheasant pens.

Preventing avian influenza in upland gamebirds is of crucial importance for many reasons. Avian influenza is a reportable disease in poultry and gamebirds in all states. A positive avian influenza test will result in quarantine of those premises while state and USDA officials investigate the type of avian influenza present, including the serotype and pathogenicity. This may take several weeks and prevent inter- and intra-state transport of birds during the investigation. In cases of low-pathogenicity H5 and H7 subtypes of avian influenza, controlled marketing (allowing the flock to develop immunity, stop virus shedding and go to processing) is not a business-viable option to producers growing raised-for-release gamebirds. There are extremely few gamebird meat-processing facilities and holding birds for several weeks would result in a huge economic loss. The disease would also be very difficult to contain on a large multistage, multiage premises to one pen. Prevention through biosecurity and monitoring for the disease is therefore especially important for gamebird producers.

One practical suggestion is that if caretakers go out hunting waterfowl or fishing near waterways used by ducks or other wild birds, they should clean and disinfect their vehicle, shower, and launder clothing before going back to the farm to care for birds. Contaminated footwear is especially dangerous, as it can hide viruses and bacteria in crevices and is extremely difficult to disinfect. Therefore, dedicated footwear should be supplied that is used only on the farm. A minimum of 48 hours of downtime (period before coming back to premises) is also suggested, in addition to the recommendations explained above.

If an H5 or H7 avian influenza virus is detected on a gamebird operation, especially if a high-pathogenicity form of the virus is found, depopulation will be necessary. Depopulation methods are challenging, especially because breeders and raised-for-release birds are housed outdoors. Herding them together and moving them into an enclosed space would be necessary to achieve euthanasia via CO_2 gas or foam methods. Small groups of gamebirds could be euthanized by trained teams using cervical dislocation [3]. After depopulation, disinfecting outdoor pens involves cleaning and disinfection of feeders, drinkers, and nest boxes. Netting material might need to be destroyed if it cannot be properly disinfected. Vegetation such as cover crops should be mowed down and the soil tilled and composted. Brooder houses can be cleaned and disinfected similar to commercial poultry buildings. Placement of sentinel birds and environmental sampling on the premises should be used to verify that the virus has been effectively destroyed in the environment [3].

Even though some strains of avian influenza have zoonotic potential, those strains are not known to be present in the Americas at this time. However, it is important to follow certain guidelines to prevent zoonotic infections for hunters and people who process gamebird meat.

1. Avoid close contact with birds that appear sick.
2. Do not butcher gamebirds or waterfowl that have been found dead or sick.
3. Do not eat, drink, or smoke while handling or butchering gamebirds.
4. Wear rubber gloves when processing birds.
5. Wash tools and countertop surfaces with a detergent and water followed by disinfecting the area with a 10% bleach solution.
6. Wash hands thoroughly after cleaning and disinfection are complete.
7. Cook gamebirds to an inside temperature of 165 °F.

8.3 Small Gamebird Flocks

Many people raise small numbers of gamebird species as a hobby or to release on their own property. These hobby growers frequently have other species of birds such as fancy chickens, waterfowl and turkeys. Since these flocks vary in size, equipment and management conditions, biosecurity recommendations can be drastically different and case-by-case recommendations are needed.

Attempts to characterize small flocks have occurred but mainly focused on poultry species. The USDA has three comprehensive reports to date, known as Poultry 04′, Poultry 07′, and Poultry 10′. In these reports, the USDA attempts to define numbers, types of birds, bird health, movement and biosecurity practices in four major cities in the US [4–6]. While not directly mentioning gamebirds, studies such as this generate useful information that can be extrapolated to small gamebird flocks or flocks that have gamebirds as part of a small flock. For example, while more than 90% of backyard hobby flocks have less than 100 birds, approximately 58% have less than 20 birds. The exception are game fowl flocks in which 57% have between 100 and 499 birds.

The categorization used by diagnostic laboratories considers small flocks as flocks consisting of 1000 birds or less [7]. This is important since small flock diagnostic testing is available in most states in the US. Many states charge a reduced fee for necropsy and diagnostic work for backyard flocks. Some states even offer free diagnostic testing for small flocks. Animal diagnostic laboratories are usually managed by the State Department of Agriculture and Animal Health and/or by the universities imparting veterinary medicine which are present in most states. To find animal diagnostic laboratories in your state, contact the National Animal Health Laboratory Network (NAHLN). In addition, you can contact the State Veterinarian's office in your state. See links below.

- www.aphis.usda.gov/animal_health/nahln/downloads/all_nahln_lab_list.pdf
- www.usaha.org/upload/Federal%20and%20State%20Health/STATE_ANIMAL_HEALTH_OFFICIALS%20-%20Copy%205.pdf

The characteristics and composition of small flocks are extremely variable. Small flocks exist in a wide range of rural, suburban, and urban settings. The housing and management of these birds also vary considerably from complete confinement to semi-confinement to free range. Common problems affecting small flocks may occur because of lax standards in predator control, cannibalism, inadequate understanding of nutritional needs, breed-related characteristics, and basic bird behavior.

8.4 Biosecurity Considerations

Noncommercial poultry raising has numerous challenges in terms of biosecurity. However, there are numerous simple strategies that can be taken to reduce disease risks.

8.4.1 Do Not Mix Multiple Bird Species Together in One Flock

Keeping multiple species of birds penned together is a risky practice. For instance, waterfowl can carry and spread avian influenza to gamebirds and other poultry. Chickens are often infested with cecal worms (*Heterakis* sp.) that can transmit histomonads (blackhead organisms) in the worm eggs. Chickens are fairly resistant to blackhead, but quail, partridges, and peafowl often get quite sick from this disease. Currently, other than regular deworming and biosecurity, there are no legal preventive or treatment medications available in the US. Other pathogens such as *Pasteurella multocida*, *M. gallisepticum*, and *Mycoplasma synoviae* can also be transferred by bird-to-bird contact in mixed flocks.

8.4.2 Biosecurity Measures for Visitors

It is extremely difficult to control where people have been, especially when premises are small and urban. One way of avoiding the introduction of pathogens to small flocks is preventing the entrance of anybody who has no business visiting your poultry flock. Special care is needed when visitors are fellow breeders since there is a big chance of disease spread. Some pathogens can persist for hours or even days in shoe crevices, even after cleaning and disinfection [8]. Shoes and clothes can also act as fomites carrying pathogens. Humans are very important disease carriers, even if they do not become infected. They can carry poultry pathogens not only on their clothes and shoes but also in their nostrils, hair, and skin. The NAHMS Poultry 04′ survey states that more than 50% of small flock breeders never allow entrance of visitors [4]. It is common in outbreak situations to have a neighbor or fellow breeder come and examine sick birds. This practice should not be allowed as it can spread disease to other flocks

8.4.3 Avoid Comingling with Other Birds or Mammals

The openness of these flocks in terms of contact with animal species poses risks to the health of the birds. Rodents, wild birds, cats, dogs, etc. can carry *Salmonella* sp., *P. multocida*, mycoplasmas and other avian pathogens. Mycoplasmosis is unfortunately very common in small flocks. Once *M. gallisepticum* (MG) or *M. synoviae* (MS) are introduced into a flock and the infection is established, the agent persists indefinitely in a continuously stocked premises. Several diseases in domestic birds have been associated with comingling with pets, i.e., dogs and cats, poultry, etc. Mechanical transmission through sharing of cages and other equipment between farms can also spread disease. Humans can act as fomites as well. For instance, if a person visits a bird auction or exhibition (Figure 8.7) and then returns to the home flock without changing clothes, shoes, and showering, they can unwittingly introduce disease into their flock. Birds that are free ranging are also more likely to encounter wildlife such as predators and rodents which may introduce disease into the flock.

8.4.4 Use of Available Resources

Small flock owners are encouraged to use their regional animal diagnostic laboratories as an important source of information to craft prevention strategies in small flocks. State laboratories across the US have programs that reduce and sometimes eliminate costs incurred in diagnostics and testing for flocks below 1000 birds. The appropriate use of a diagnostic laboratory as a source of information and the use of this information to craft prevention strategies is key in disease prevention and bird-keeping success. Studies in small flocks in central California have shown that these flocks

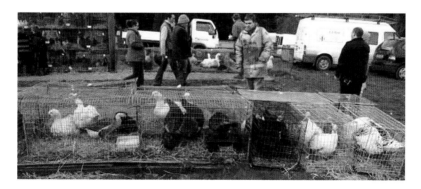

Figure 8.7 At bird auctions, many birds are grouped together and their source is not fully known. Avoid visiting bird auctions but if you do, complete clothes changing and shower are needed to prevent the introduction of diseases into your flock.

are exposed to respiratory pathogens and develop immune responses from this interaction [8]. Knowing which pathogens are present allows the design of better prevention strategies that are specific to each flock. Additional resources exist in almost all states through university poultry extension services. Disease, management, behavior, and nutrition information is readily accessible through websites, factsheets, videos, and podcasts. Becoming familiar and working with your state extension office or poultry extension specialist is recommended for all gamebird producers. In a quick search on a web browser using the words "poultry extension resources," at least 10 different poultry extension services in different states and universities were found. These web pages catered for poultry information specifically for small flocks.

8.4.5 Informed Vaccination

The availability of a vaccine does not mean that the vaccine needs to be used. An informed vaccination strategy is crucial for the well-being of poultry. Unfortunately, there are no approved vaccines for gamebirds. However, some poultry vaccines have been used in gamebirds under the supervision of a veterinarian if needed to control a specific disease. It must be remembered, however, that some vaccines may be risky to use since they can revert to virulence after improper vaccination. Others may introduce live organisms into an environment that did not have that organism present before, exposing nonvaccinated neighbors to the pathogen and potential disease.

Finally, vaccination does not make up for poor management. Most diseases in birds are caused by poor management, which is why revisiting management and health programs and elaborating preventive strategies, including necessary vaccinations, is key for a healthy flock.

8.4.6 Use of Dedicated Shoes and Clothing

The simplest way of avoiding the introduction of pathogens to a flock and taking pathogens from one flock to the other is using dedicated shoes and clothes in poultry premises. Even though this is a simple measure, it is not frequently used in small or backyard gamebird flocks. Showering and changing clothes between flocks is also very helpful to prevent disease spread. Many bacteria and viruses can be transported on shoes, clothing, hair, and nostrils of people visiting other facilities or even feed stores. The use of dedicated shoes and clothes when working or visiting small flocks minimizes risks particularly of introduction and dissemination of pathogens. For example, avian influenza virus can be carried in boot crevices protected in fecal droppings from infected birds even after treatment of these boots in disinfectant footbaths [9]. It is recommended to also use rubber mats inside vehicles that can be removed, washed, and disinfected between flock visits.

8.4.7 Handwashing

As with changing clothes or using protective equipment, handwashing prevents the entrance of pathogens to a poultry flock, particularly if feed, water, and/or birds are handled. Numerous commercial poultry facilities have changed from handwashing stations to using alcohol-based hand sanitizers. For small flock owners, this would be important before entering and after leaving the farm to prevent introduction of outside pathogens and spread of any potential pathogen that might be inside the premises. The NAHMS Poultry 04′ report reflected that handwashing was practiced more frequently after than before handling birds – 58.1 vs 71.8%, respectively [4]. This reflects the need for additional outreach to explain the basis of biosecurity measures in order to protect poultry flocks.

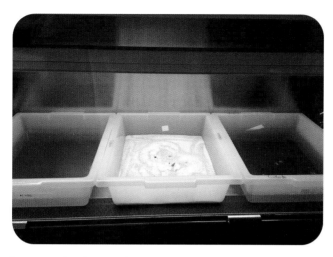

Figure 8.8 Footbaths prepared under experimental conditions and used for a period of 1 week. From left to right: quaternary ammonia, bleach powder, and phenol. Most of the organic material gets dissolved in the liquid footbaths. In contrast, the cleanliness of the bleach powder is striking compared with the liquid footbaths.

8.4.8   Adequate Cleaning and Disinfection

While in most instances, facilities and the environment where small gamebird flocks are located are difficult to clean and disinfect, maintaining premises organization and avoiding clutter allow good air and sunlight circulation that naturally helps with disinfection and dryness of bedding material. In addition, periodical cleaning and disinfection of equipment such as feeders, drinkers, nest boxes, and scratch areas help to reduce pathogen load to a minimum.

When you select cleaning and disinfection products, keep in mind not only price but also effectiveness and practicality of use in your facilities. If you are thinking of having footbaths, keep in mind that these need to be periodically maintained otherwise their effectiveness is null (Figure 8.8). In addition, studies have shown that bleach powder is more effective at killing low and highly pathogenic avian influenza in dedicated boots [9].

8.4.9   Mortality and Disposal

While mortality in birds after hatch can be higher (between 1% and 3%) during the first 7–10 days, it should decrease to less than 0.1% during the pullet/cockerel period. In adults mortality should be very low (less than 0.01%). This is important to keep in mind since unexplained and elevated death loss should be investigated, and the information obtained should be used to establish preventtive measures for the flock. This concept is called "preventtive medicine" and is the way in which poultry and gamebird flocks should base their management and health programs.

Disease investigation is usually handled by diagnostic laboratories. Almost every state in the US has poultry or animal diagnostic laboratories that receive birds or carcasses for diagnostic work. There are even poultry programs for which there is a reduced fee or free diagnostics. In addition to ruling out FADs such as Newcastle disease and avian influenza, these laboratories investigate causes of death and are able to detect and sometimes culture most of the pathogens that affect poultry. In addition, diagnosticians are also trained to detect toxic, accidental or management-related death causes. The results of these investigations should be used to improve management, nutrition, and disease prevention. In case this information is not understood by the farmer-owner, universities across the US have poultry extension agents who are trained in disease diagnostics and should be able to help you in the results interpretation process.

Disposal of dead birds in the trash and/or leaving carcasses in the floor adjacent to the rest of the flock are not suitable methods of disposal, since vermin will be attracted and infectious diseases could be transferred from the dead bird to the rest of the flock. Another disposal method is to bury birds in the ground, covering them with abundant lye before the dirt cover. A good option before deciding on bird disposal is to spray them with a 10% bleach solution or commercial Lysol®, which would help reduce pathogen load on the surface of the birds while decisions on how to dispose of them are taken.

8.4.10 Litter Disposal

Litter is a great way of reducing moisture buildup and increasing comfort for the birds. At the same time, it is a material that needs to be changed and maintained. Manure also needs to be kept dry and heavy buildup can increase ammonia and negatively affect bird health. Composting manure or bedding material is a great way of reducing the infectious load of the byproducts generated by poultry keeping. When composting, the temperature of the composted pile should increase over 50 °C (122 °F). This temperature is able to inactivate pathogens such as *Salmonella*, *E. coli,* and avian influenza [10, 11]. Contact the poultry extension specialist at your local university for more information about composting.

8.4.11 Introduction of New Birds into a Flock

A significant number of disease introductions may occur when new birds are added to an existing flock. If possible, day-old chicks purchased from a NPIP participating hatchery or breeders should be used. Ideally, the hatchery and the breeders are screened for pullorum disease, MG, MS, and *Salmonella enteritidis*. This information is available on the NPIP website (www .poultryimprovement.org). Purchasing birds from a livestock auction, swap meet or even from neighbors or bird clubs can be very risky (Figure 8.7). If obtaining birds from these sources is unavoidable, it is recommended to keep the new birds isolated in a separate area for ~3 weeks. During that time, they can be checked for external and internal parasites by your veterinarian and treated if necessary. They should also be blood-tested for exposure to diseases (your diagnostic laboratory can advise). During the 3 weeks, the birds are watched for any signs of disease. This procedure reduces disease introduction but is not foolproof as some illness in birds result in asymptomatic carrier state and the birds may still transmit infections to the existing flock. The best way to prevent diseases is to keep a closed flock and use all the biosecurity tools mentioned in the previous paragraphs.

Focusing on the above-mentioned points will allow owners and veterinarians to formulate disease prevention strategies and incorporate crucial information that is unique for each flock. This should be the gold standard for disease prevention and, from a practical perspective, is the cheapest way of keeping disease out of your flock. Proper biosecurity practices have been correlated with lower Newcastle disease antibody titers in small flocks [8]. The same correlation is true for *Salmonella* prevalence [12] and most- ikely the same happens with MG and MS. These two pathogens are transmitted vertically to the progeny, perpetuating the infection if birds are not obtained from reputable sources and no eradication efforts are in place in breeders. MG- and MS-positive birds can suffer more intense and prolonged respiratory diseases if infected with common pathogens such as the virus that causes infectious bronchitis, *P. multocida* (fowl cholera), *Avibacterium paragallinarum* (infectious coryza), infectious laryngotracheitis virus (ILT), and many others.

8.5 Flock Concept

Health management in poultry and gamebird flocks is not a task that should focus on birds as individuals. Even though we care about individual birds, the approach is flock based even if you have one bird in your flock. As a manager or owner, the emphasis should be not only on the birds but also on their environment. Temperature, humidity, access to feed and water, sanitation and disinfection strategies, nutrition and supplementation, hatching, breeding, raising, maintenance, and conditioning are all activities and topics that need to be considered. The information we gather from them and from services such as diagnostic laboratories should help us come up with management and health programs which can be followed and corrected if failure is noticed. In veterinary medicine, this is called "preventative veterinary medicine, herd or flock medicine." A big portion of these plans is biosecurity, and incorporating the above-mentioned biosecurity strategies will make management programs strong and will help to keep disease and other problems out of your flock.

References

1 Wallner-Pendleton, E.A. (2011). Biosecurity considerations for gamebird operations. In: *A Practical Guide for Managing Risk in Poultry Production.* (ed. R.L. Owen), 261–266. Jacksonville, FL: American Association of Avian Pathologists.

2 Wallner-Pendleton, E.A. (2011). Biosecurity for the gamebird industry. North American Gamebird Association Meeting.

3 Wallner-Pendleton, E.A. and Hulet, M. (2013). Gamebird industry. In: *Poultry Industry Manual FAD PReP* (ed. USDA-APHIS), 132–149. Ames, IA: Center for Food Security and Public Health, Iowa State University.

4 USDA-APHIS (2004). *Poultry 04' Part IV: Reference of Health and Management of Backyard/Small Production Flocks and Gamefowl Breeder Flocks in the United States.* Fort Collins, CO: USDA-APHIS-VS, CEAH, National Animal Health Monitoring System.

5 USDA-APHIS (2008). *Reference of Management Practices on Small Enterprise Chicken Operations in the United States, 2007.* Fort Collins, CO: USDA-APHIS-VS, CEAH, National Animal Health Monitoring System.

6 USDA-APHIS (2011). Poultry 2010, Reference of the Health and Management of Chicken Flocks in Urban Settings in Four U.S. Cities. Fort Collins, CO: USDA-APHIS-VS, CEAH, National Animal Health Monitoring System.

7 Dunn, P.A. (2011). Special considerations for backyard flocks and the urban live bird marketing system. In: *A Practical Guide for Managing Risk in Poultry Production* (ed. AAAP), 267–275. Jacksonville, FL: AAAP.

8 Derksen, T., Lampron, R., Hauck, R. et al. (2018). Biosecurity assessment and seroprevalence of respiratory diseases in backyard poultry flocks located close to and far from commercial premises. *Avian Dis.* 62: 1–5.

9 Hauck, R., Crossley, B., Rejmanek, D. et al. (2017). Persistence of highly pathogenic and low pathogenic avian influenza viruses in footbaths and poultry manure. *Avian Dis.* 61: 64–69.

10 Biswas, S., Nazmi, A., Pitesky, M. et al. (2019). Thermal inactivation of *Escherichia coli* and *Salmonella typhimurium* in poultry carcass and litter at thermophilic temperatures. *J. Appl. Poultry Res.* 28: 307–317.

11 Figueroa, A., Derksen, T., Biswas, S. et al. (2021). Persistence of low and highly pathogenic avian influenza virus in reused poultry litter, effects of litter amendment use and composting temperatures. *J. Appl. Poultry Res.* 30: 100096.

12 Derksen, T, Lampron, R., Gallardo, R.A. (2018). Backyard poultry flocks Salmonella sp. seroprevalence. In: *Proceedings of the 67th Western Poultry Disease Conference*, April 16–18, Salt Lake City, UT. https://aaap.memberclicks.net/assets/WPDC/wpdc_2018_proceedings_final.pdf (accessed February 2022).

9

Field Investigation, Medication, Vaccination, and Diagnostics for Gamebirds

David D. Frame, Douglas Anderson, and Mark C. Bland

This chapter will address multiple issues and on-farm decisions that a veterinarian must address when working with gamebirds in the field, including how to conduct a field investigation; how to appropriately medicate and vaccinate gamebirds; and, finally, how to use the diagnostic services that are available for medical practice with gamebirds.

9.1 Field Investigation

It is important to keep in mind that field investigations deal with a flock problem; therefore, the investigation by definition becomes an exercise in population health management.

There are a number of components that can make a field investigation challenging. These consist of management practices, environmental factors, feeding and watering issues, and presence or absence of disease agents. The interaction among these variables can be complex. For this reason, it is important to ask relevant questions and make keen observations in order to get a clear understanding of the situation. Note taking during the farm visit may later prove to be invaluable.

9.1.1 Case History

Typically, a request for an on-site visit is initiated by the flock owner. During the initial visit, interacting with the owner and asking relevant questions will help increase perspective. An accurate and complete case history will go a long way in gaining an understanding of the problem. Although not exhaustive, Table 9.1 provides a checklist that may be a reasonable starting point.

9.1.2 Management and Environmental Evaluation

A good way to look at management and environment is to use a mental checklist such as FLAWS. This is an acronym that represents **F** for flock and feed, **L** for lights and litter, **A** for air (ventilation), **W** for water, and **S** for sanitation and [bio]security. See Table 9.1 for a fundamental checklist based on FLAWS.

Gamebird Medicine and Management, First Edition. Edited by Teresa Y. Morishita and Robert E. Porter, Jr.
© 2023 John Wiley & Sons, Inc. Published 2023 by John Wiley & Sons, Inc.

Table 9.1   Checklist for field visit observations.

Item	Notes
☐ Clinical signs	
☐ Morbidity and mortality	
☐ Contiguous flocks or cohabitation with other avian species	
☐ Feeders and feed: condition and types	
☐ Lighting	
☐ Litter and bedding condition	
☐ Ventilation	
☐ Types of waterers and water quality	
☐ Sanitation: cleaning and disinfecting protocol	
☐ Biosecurity practices	

9.1.3   Diseases and Clinical Signs

Although diseases and abnormalities of gamebirds are discussed in other chapters, the presence or absence of typical clinical signs will help in identifying potential cause(s). Field observations may reveal depression typified by ruffled feathers, inappetence, and reluctance to move. Respiratory signs of snicking or labored breathing may be present. Ambulatory issues, such as limping, paralysis, or abnormal joints, might be observed.

9.1.4   Equipment for Farm Visit

The following describes basic equipment to have with you so that you can adequately examine birds while on the farm. Personal protective equipment (PPE) should include clean reusable or disposable coveralls, disposable bouffant (head covering), plastic disposable boots or rubber pull-over boots, disposable gloves, heavy-duty plastic garbage bags, hand sanitizer, and aerosol disinfectant.

Necropsy tools consist of a sharp boning knife, scalpel blade (#10 BP), necropsy shears, several small and large scissors (sharp/dull tip), and mouse-tooth forceps. It is highly recommended that a microscope with slides and coverslips be brought along to examine intestinal scrapings.

For sample collection, bring a transportation crate (for transporting live/dead birds to the diagnostic laboratory), 3 cc syringes, with 20- and 22-gauge × 1 in. needles, 1.5 mL microcentrifuge tubes or 5 mL red-top blood tubes, several sizes of whirl packs, small specimen containers with and without formalin, and sterile swabs

9.1.5   Postmortem Examination

The objective of the field necropsy is to provide information that can be combined with flock history and field observations that will help to determine causes of performance problems, morbidity, and/or mortality. When necessary, euthanasia methods should follow AVMA guidelines [1]. The preferable protocol is to use CO_2 gas using a small chamber or garbage can. Cervical dislocation can be employed as an alternative if no other recourse is available. The disadvantage of cervical dislocation is that the tissues in the neck are disrupted, thereby potentially hindering accurate assessment for potential upper respiratory or alimentary tract abnormalities.

The necropsy technique of gamebirds in the field can vary, but it is imperative that one proceeds in an orderly fashion. This will reduce the chance of overlooking something. The necropsy procedure is described in detail in Chapter 15. Field necropsy should be backed up with appropriate laboratory diagnostic investigations on whole birds, tissue samples, serology, feed, and environment samples.

9.2 Medication Administration

Years ago, things were easier for the gamebird grower. Treatment of a mortality issue could be quickly solved with an antibiotic in the feed or water. Minimum tonnage requirements made it quick to change. There were numerous antibiotic options available and if these were not suitable, water-soluble therapies were also readily available. Drugs might be used in combination or in off-label levels. Drugs not intended for poultry could find their way into the feed system or drainage system as runoff to nearby water sources. Attention might be given to medication withdrawal times, or these withdrawal times might be ignored or interpreted incorrectly.

In more recent times, some of the issues are the same. For example, feed versus water, drug resistance/sensitivity, and off-label drugs/usages are important considerations when treating a flock. Although still considered poultry, gamebirds are often fed and watered in different manners. Netted outdoor flight pens might have a water system that will not permit the use of a proportioner, stock barrel/bulk tank, or water line, so there would be no way to get medicated water to them. Increasing ambient temperature may result in overconsumption and toxicity of certain sulfa drugs. Brooding rooms and dark houses should have a system that can supply medicated feed or water.

Newer methods of administering medication include selecting an appropriate feed antibiotic with a VFD (Veterinary Feed Directive) or a water-soluble antibiotic prescription (Rx) label as well as a source [2]. For example, salinomycin has a legal level, but some mills will refuse to carry the product because of its toxicity to horses. Farm stores used to carry many of the water-soluble antibiotics over the counter (OTC), but since the 2017 deadline for VFDs and Rx, they now require veterinary oversight (Table 9.2).

It is important to select the right product to provide the most judicious use of medication in order to prevent drug resistance [3]. Federal directives that provide oversight over the use of drugs by veterinarians are described below.

9.2.1 Extra-label Drug Use (ELDU)

Extra-label drug use is any alteration of the drug label in dose, frequency, concentration, species, etc. No ELDU is permitted in the feed. The VFD must follow the label.

9.2.2 Animal Medicinal Drug Use Clarification Act (AMDUCA)

This Act, instituted in 1994, addresses ELDU by veterinarians. It allows veterinarians to prescribe ELDU when the health and welfare of an animal are threatened or when suffering or death may result. It requires a valid VCPR (veterinarian–client–patient relationship). The veterinarian determines if a script is necessary. Only FDA-approved drugs are permitted and must be intended for prevention, treatment, or control. They are not permitted if the drug results in an illegal food residue and cannot be used for ELDU in medicated feed.

Table 9.2   Gamebird approved drug list [2].

Active ingredients	Route	Withdrawal time (days)	Dose	SPP
Bacitracin-MD	Feed	0	200 g/ton	Quail
Amprolium	Feed	0	159 g/ton	Pheasant
Lasalocid	Feed	0	113 g/ton	Chukar
Monensin	Feed	0	73 g/ton	Quail
Salinomycin	Feed	0	50 g/ton	Quail
SDM/Ormetoprim	Feed	0	113.5–68.1 g/ton	Chukar

9.2.3   Veterinary Feed Directive

In an attempt by the FDA to eliminate the use of low-dose antibiotics with medically important antibiotic usages (critical in human medicine) for the purpose of growth promotion and feed efficiency, the VFD was developed. Further, the goal was to place the remaining drug use under the supervision of a licensed veterinarian. A VFD can only be issued by a licensed veterinarian with a valid VCPR. In discussion with the client, examination of the patient/environment, and if available for followup care, the veterinarian accepts responsibility. Antibiotics can be used for prevention, control, and therapeutic purposes but not asgrowth promotants or for feed efficiency. Coccidiostats are not affected by the VFD. See the VFD form (Figure 9.1) for the required information.

The VFD is written by the veterinarian and a copy is given to the feed mill and to the client. The Directive must be maintained for two years.

9.2.4   Minor Use/Minor Species (MUMS)

This Act was instituted in 2004 to give veterinarians access to drugs that are not otherwise available. Minor use is for limited usage (infrequent, small numbers) in major species (horses, cattle, dogs, cats, pigs, turkeys, chickens). Minor species treatment is for all other species. Gamebirds are considered minor species. This declaration allows the veterinarian to use poultry dosages in gamebirds. It still cannot change the feed labels, but it can allow the use of nonlabeled gamebird antibiotics.

Despite the special allowances, there are certain drugs that are prohibited under any circumstances for use in food animals. They include the following: chloramphenicol, clenbuterol, diethylstilbestrol, dimetridazole, ipronidazole, nitroimidazoles, furazolidone, nitrofurazone, fluoroquinolones, and glycopeptides. The two drugs most abused are fluoroquinolone and dimetridazole; the use of enrofloxacins or metronidazoles is not permitted. Withdrawal establishment and supervision is the responsibility of the veterinarian.

9.2.5   Compliance Policy Guide (CPG) for Extra-label Use of Medicated Feeds for Minor Species

CPG 615.115 directs FDA inspectors to make medicated gamebird feed a low enforcement priority. It does not make medicated feed legal, just low priority. A declaration of this statement can be added to the VFD or Rx. See the VFD form.

Veterinary Feed Directive

All parties must retain a copy of this VFD for 2 years after the date of issuance.

Veterinarian: _____   Client: _____

Address: _____   Address: _____
                                         (business or home)
_____   _____

Phone: _____   Phone: _____

Fax or email (optional): _____   Fax or email (optional): _____

Drug(s) Name: _____   Drug(s) Level: _____ g/ton   Duration of use: _____

Species and Production Class: _____   Number of reorders (refills) authorized: _____
                                                        (If permitted by the drug approval)

Indication for use (as approved): _____

Caution (related to this medicated feed, if any): N/A _____

USE OF FEED CONTAINING THIS VETERINARY FEED DIRECTIVE (VFD) DRUG IN A MANNER OTHER THAN AS DIRECTED ON THE LABELING (EXTRA LABEL USE) IS NOT PERMITTED.

Approximate Number of Animals: _____

Premises: _____

Other Identification (e.g., age, weight) (optional): _____

Special Instructions (if any): This VFD is being issued in accordance with CPG 615.115. _____

Affirmation of intent (for combination VFD Drugs) (check box)*:

☐ This VFD only authorizes the use of the VFD drug(s) cited in this order and is not intended to authorize the use of such drug(s) in combination with any other animal drugs.

☐ This VFD authorizes the use of the VFD drug(s) cited in this order in the following FDA-approved, conditionally approved or indexed combinations(s) in medicated feed that contains the VFD drug(s) as a component.

Drug(s)	Drug Level(s) and any Special Instructions

☑ This VFD only authorizes the use of the VFD drug(s) cited in this order any FDA-approved, conditionally approved or indexed combinations(s) in medicated feed that contains the VFD drug(s) as a component.

▶ Withdrawal Time (if any): This VFD Feed must be withdrawn __7__ days prior to slaughter. ◀

VFD Date of Issuance: _____ (Month/Day/Year)

VFD Expiration Date: _____ (Month/Day/Year)
                                                       (As specified in the approval; cannot
Veterinarian's Signature: _____   exceed 6 months after issuance.)

Figure 9.1   Veterinary Feed Directive. The VFD form provides veterinarians in all states with a framework for authorizing the use of medically important antimicrobials in feed when needed for specific animal health purposes.

9.3   Vaccines and Vaccine Administration

Vaccination is the practice of exposure of a flock to a pathogen to produce antibodies which will protect the vaccinated flock from the effects of the pathogen in the future. Since the vaccines are not designed for gamebirds, there is some risk in the response. Until the bird's reaction is known, vaccinate with great care and use the mildest vaccine available. A small trial is not a bad idea to protect against creating a greater problem.

As with most atypical species, there are usually very few or no vaccines marketed for the gamebird industry. This creates the situation where commercially produced poultry vaccines created for other species (chickens and turkeys) are used for vaccination of gamebirds. Considerations for selecting poultry vaccines for use in gamebirds would include a nearly identical strain of the infective organism; ease of application; type of application; killed vaccine; safety of a modified-live vaccine (mlv); and availability of vaccine. Vaccines that have been considered or used in gamebird production include those for quail pox, fowl pox, pigeon pox, cholera (*P. multocida*), hemorrhagic enteritis (HE)/marble spleen disease (MSD), erysipelas (*Erysipelothrix rhusiopathiae*), and infectious coryza (*Avibacterium paragallinarium*). Rarer vaccines include those for Newcastle disease (NDV or APMV-1), *Ornithobacterium rhinotracheale* (ORT), and avian encephalomyelitis (AE). Coccidia vaccines are one of the latest considerations.

At the time of writing, there are no longer vaccines labeled for gamebirds. The last available product was for quail pox in bobwhite quail. Unfortunately, quail pox vaccination is ineffective against fowl pox of pheasants or partridges. The reverse also holds true: fowl pox vaccination is ineffective against quail pox in bobwhite quail. Currently, the license and rights to quail pox vaccine are pending investment for production.

Cholera vaccine (*P. multocida*) is variable in effectiveness, based on serotype isolated. Commercial poultry vaccines are typically composed as a combination of serotypes 1, 3, and 4. Gamebird isolates range from serotypes 1 to 17 and often are nontypable. The less the similarity, the less the cross-protection. Use of the least reactive strains or a vaccination method like wing web inoculation should be considered to reduce exposure. Make sure the birds are examined for vaccine "take" to ensure vaccine exposure was completed.

Hemorrhagic enteritis of turkeys is the same virus as MSD of pheasants. Be aware that vaccination may still create an unacceptable reaction. Confer with a veterinarian, vaccine producer or technical service personnel to evaluate the threat in your situation. In minimal cleanout programs of the brooder area, preexposure from the previous flock might result in a reaction from a vaccine exposure.

Erysipelas and infectious coryza (IC) are bacterial diseases that are commonly observed in gamebirds. These vaccines would only be used if the threat of disease was imminent or nearby commercial flocks were undergoing a serious epizootic. *O. rhinotracheale* has the potential to reoccur and create havoc just as gamebirds begin to reach release age.

Coccidiosis vaccine usually depends on a shortened precocious period or consumption of low numbers of sporulated oocysts. The biggest dilemma lies in the species-specific nature of coccidia. Pheasant coccidia will not infect quail, chukar, or partridges, etc. The reverse is true. Since the strains differ, infection will not occur and immunity will not follow. Some gamebirds, such as chukar partridges, are more sensitive to infection. While pheasants can develop immunity on a wire floor or ground, chukars will develop a serious infection if raised on the floor without a coccidiostat.

If vaccination is needed and an appropriate product is not available, a couple of alternatives might be considered. One is an autogenous vaccine. This includes the use of isolates from the farm to create a vaccine made specifically for the problem strain. Drawbacks include safety issues that may arise from autogenous vaccine use, strains may need to be collected yearly, and the volume of vaccine needed (minimum volume purchase) may be excessive for the farm size. As another option, under the specific requirements of 9CFR.107.1 (Veterinary Practitioners and Animal Owners) and 9CFR.107.2 (Products under State License), an owner may be allowed to create a product needed for immunization. Interested individuals should contact their State Department of Agriculture for more information and to determine whether the owner is qualified.

Proper vaccine administration is the key to effectively immunizing a flock. Failure to follow directions will result in insufficient protection or even a disease outbreak. Among the vaccines available, there are five common vaccination methods: water, spray, eye drop, wing web, and injection [4].

Water vaccination is usually based on a short period of thirst followed by return of the water with vaccine, with the goal of allowing all the birds a chance to drink at least one dose [5]. The time required to create thirst and result in vaccine coverage will vary depending on the climate and rate of consumption. Do not over-thirst the birds to the point of dehydration. In warm weather, do not deprive the birds of water for more than one hour. Vaccine materials should be restricted to vaccine use only because residual disinfectant will destroy any vaccine. One should inspect and prepare the drinker system for vaccine delivery several days before the procedure. The water delivery system should be fully flushed with dilute powdered skim milk (1 cup/25 gal). The same buffering solution can be used to perform the vaccination. If the skim milk does not go into solution easily, use distilled water for dilution, then further dilute as needed. Water vaccination usually occurs in the brooder barns.

Spray vaccination is not a frequent practice in gamebird operations but could be utilized if needed. The procedures have been well described in commercial poultry [6]. Most often, the

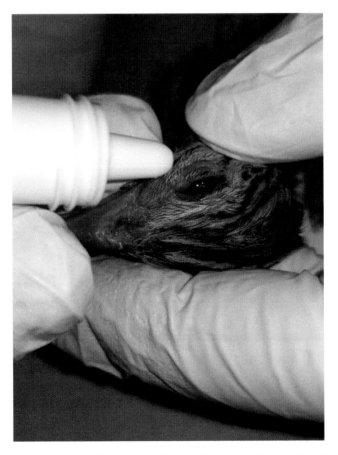

Figure 9.2   Fluid vaccine drops placed into the eye through the open eyelids (eyedrop administration) can serve as a substitute for spray vaccine in some instances. Source: Photo courtesy of Elisa Castaneda.

vaccination will be done in closed flight pens or dark houses. A sprayer capable of producing a coarse spray of 100–150 μm will be needed (sprayer volume at 5 gal per 20 000 birds). If possible, the spray vaccination should occur early in the morning depending on the climate and with the ventilation fans turned off and lighting as dark as possible. During the process, the vaccinator can watch and evaluate the coarseness and output of the sprayer. After vaccination, leave the ventilation fans off for another 15–30 minutes if climate permits.

Eye drop vaccination (Figure 9.2) may be used in place of spray vaccination or the reverse. It would require some bird handling but could be done during specs, blinders, and bits. Optimize your handling to prevent getting the wrong vaccines or contaminant in the eyes.

Wing web vaccination is probably the most common of gamebird vaccination methods. It does require a large amount of bird handling which could be combined with specs, blinders, and bits, if the timing is right. The vaccine comes with a two-pronged applicator. Once the pellet is hydrated, the applicator is dipped in the vaccine and from the underside of the wing, pushed clear through the wing web without injuring the bones or muscles (Figure 9.3). Do not remove one of the prongs to make the applicator a little easier to manipulate (cuts vaccine dose in half). In a week's time, the birds can be checked for a scab or a "take" at the injection site [7]. A couple of the vaccines can be given at once (one per side). Cholera, fowl pox, and AE would be the most likely wing web vaccines.

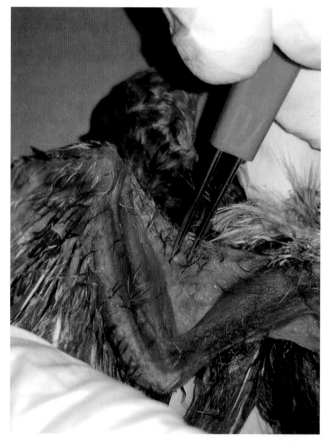

Figure 9.3 To perform wing web vaccination, the double-pronged needle carrying vaccine fluid is inserted through the thin skin of the web (patagium). Source: Photo courtesy of Elisa Castaneda.

Vaccination by injection rarely occurs except for the possibility of an autogenous vaccine and maybe more often injecting antibiotics. Subcutaneous (SQ) injection is vaccine placement just under the skin, often in the midneck or inguinal area. Lift a pinch of skin away from the neck and place the needle in the tented area. For the inguinal SQ injection, lifting the leg will open the area from the lower breast to the medial thigh area. Intramuscular injection (IM) is vaccine placement in the muscle of the breast or lateral thigh. Needle placement and direction at any site should be away from the liver to prevent an accidental injection.

9.4 Diagnostic Services

Because of the potentially complex nature of many gamebird diseases, coupled with the lack of extensive microbiologic and serologic tools available in most general veterinary practices, the clinician often has to submit samples to a diagnostic laboratory for a definitive or confirmatory diagnosis. There may also be opportunities for practicing veterinarians to assist clients in flock monitoring for disease prevalence or to help them evaluate general health maintenance and vaccination programs. Diagnostic laboratories have the tools to help in these endeavors.

It is recommended that a veterinarian involved with gamebird clients who require ongoing assistance develop a relationship with a trusted diagnostic laboratory that can help accomplish the requisite diagnostic and health-monitoring objectives. Contact the State Department of Agriculture or closest land-grant university for the location of veterinary diagnostic laboratories that accept poultry and gamebirds. The NAHLN maintains a list of qualified laboratories [8].

9.4.1 When and How to Use the Veterinary Diagnostic Laboratory

Before submitting birds or tissues, call the laboratory, introduce yourself, and explain the situation. You may wish to speak to a diagnostician who specializes in poultry and gamebirds if one is available. Find out what samples they would suggest sending, and if there is a submission form online that can be filled out beforehand to accompany the specimens. Explanatory background information and case history are especially important and could help the diagnostician to determine what tests need to be run to arrive at a quick and accurate diagnosis. The case history should include species, age, number of birds on the premises or in the flock, clinical signs, daily mortality, type of feed, style of waterers and feeders, and any unusual circumstances, such as a recent water leak, rain or snow storm, predation, etc.

9.4.2 Sample Collection

When collecting and packaging samples, always use appropriate PPE if you suspect possible zoonotic diseases. Veterinarians will generally have three reasons to submit gamebird specimens to diagnostic laboratories.

1. Obtain a diagnosis of an apparent disease outbreak.
2. Do surveillance testing for presence/absence of specific diseases in order to comply with government regulations.
3. Monitor vaccination programs.

The kind of sample to be collected is dependent on the objective.

9.4.2.1 Whole Birds

In a suspected disease outbreak, the submission of intact birds is often the most successful way of obtaining an accurate diagnosis. The diagnostician will then have all tissues, lesions, and carcass conformation at their disposal. It is important to submit a number of birds showing typical clinical signs and lesions. Carcasses should be submitted refrigerated but not frozen. The addition of artificial coolant or refrigerant during transit to the laboratory will prolong preservation.

9.4.2.2 Oropharyngeal (Tracheal Opening and Choanal Cleft) or Cloacal Swabs

Collection of oropharyngeal swabs is often recommended when respiratory disease is suspected. They are routinely used for monitoring avian influenza and Newcastle disease. Oropharyngeal sampling is preferred on live birds; on dead birds, tracheal swabs are best obtained from fresh carcasses (Figure 9.4). Avoid swabbing into the esophagus. Use synthetic or semisynthetic swabs (polyester, rayon, nylon, etc.) with plastic handles. Do not use cotton or calcium alginate swabs or swabs with wooden handles, as these may interfere with test results.

After swabbing the pharynx or trachea, swirl each swab in a tube containing at least 3 mL of brain heart infusion broth or other prescribed transport medium and then squeeze out the excess liquid from the swab against the side of the tube. Withdraw the swab and discard in a zip-lock bag for later aseptic disposal. If birds are very small (e.g., quail), the use of flocked pediatric nasopharyngeal swabs may be necessary to obtain proper oropharyngeal samples. A maximum of five swabs (i.e., birds) are pooled into each tube of 3 mL of transport medium if submitting samples for avian influenza or Newcastle disease antigen detection. In some cases, the only feasible way to obtain samples is by swabbing the cloaca. Do not mix oropharyngeal and cloacal swabs in the same tube(s). Although a pool of 11 oropharyngeal swabs *is* allowable in 5.5 mL of transport medium with antibiotics, this procedure is *not* indicated for cloacal swab collection [9, 10].

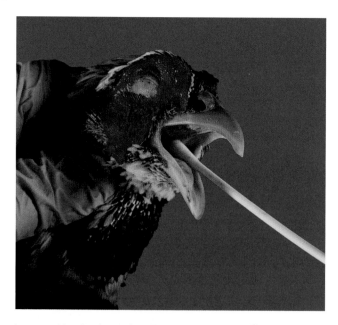

Figure 9.4 An oropharyngeal/tracheal sample collected with a Dacron® or polyester tip swab is suitable for a variety of molecular analyses (e.g., PCR) as well as bacteriology.

Each composite tube must be clearly identified as to flock origin, building, and collection date. This same information must be accurately recorded on a hard-copy list or accession sheet that will accompany the tubes to the laboratory.

9.4.2.3 Blood Samples

Blood sampling of multiple birds in a flock is a convenient method for antibody detection when assessing a potential disease outbreak or for evaluating vaccination programs. In order to achieve statistical and practical relevance, it is generally recommended that a minimum of 20–30 birds are tested per flock. Blood samples are routinely submitted for flock surveillance for presence of antibodies to certain potential pathogens, such as avian influenza or Newcastle disease. Because most laboratory tests require serum, receptacles free of anticoagulants are indicated; however, check with the laboratory to make sure plasma is not necessary. The use of round or conical bottom 1.5 mL microcentrifuge tubes is preferred because of convenient size and ease of handling and shipping. Polypropylene tubes are preferred because there is less chance of breakage than with glass or polystyrene.

Proper collection and storage of avian blood are very important in order to render high-quality serum. In general, the following procedure will yield satisfactory results. Use a 20 gauge needle for larger birds and a 20–22 gauge for medium or smaller birds. Use the largest needle feasible to reduce turbulence during collection and dispensing of the blood sample. Turbulence and delay in time needed to extract the sample may increase the probability of hemolysis and premature clotting. Slowly fill the syringe with approximately 1.25 mL of blood. *Slowly* dispense enough blood into a 1.5 mL microcentrifuge tube until the tube is two-thirds to three-quarters full. Do not overfill or cause bubbling or excessive turbulence during ejection into the tube. Place each filled tube in a rack or other holder that will permit the blood-filled tubes to clot while tilted at about a 30° angle. Do not disturb until *all* blood samples have coagulated. This takes patience and time but is extremely important for optimal serum quality and yield. Allow blood to clot at room temperature (about 75 °F).

Once all samples are firmly clotted, gently shift the tubes to vertical and let them rest in that position overnight at room temperature. The serum can then be easily poured or pipetted off into clean, appropriately labeled tubes. All tubes containing serum should be stored at refrigerator temperature (about 45 °F) until shipment to the laboratory. If samples are sent to the laboratory with serum still on the clot, keep samples cool but not frozen during storage and transit.

9.4.2.4 Environmental Sampling

It may be necessary to submit other sorts of samples besides blood or whole birds to the laboratory. Samples such as litter, water, and feed are useful for monitoring the environment for presence or prevalence of potential pathogens. Check with the laboratory for specific ways in which these materials should be gathered and submitted. Specimens should be collected in sterile containers and kept cool until shipment. Environmental samples will most often be collected for detection of bacterial or protozoal pathogens; therefore, it is important that a representative sample be collected.

Litter might be collected in order to determine general nematode or coccidial load in a pen or enclosure. A good way to do this is to collect several hand grabs or scrapings of litter from various locales in the house or pen. Samples should be collected near waterers and feeders as well as from other areas where the birds tend to congregate. These individual grab samples are combined into a larger bag and thoroughly mixed. A representative homogenous sample from the combined collection is then extracted as a composite sample, placed in a separate bag, and sent to the diagnostic laboratory for subsequent culture or microscopic evaluation.

Water samples for bacterial culture or PCR should be collected in sterile 15–50 mL capacity tubes. They should be drawn from various areas of the drinking system. The filled tubes could be homogenously combined into one composite, or submitted as separate samples, depending on the diagnostic objectives of the clinician.

Other than for the analysis of nutrient content, feed samples would most likely be sent to a diagnostic laboratory for evaluation for the presence of *Salmonella*, or perhaps to look at other bacterial loads, such as *Escherichia coli*. Samples should be taken from various areas of the feedline, discharge chute, or truck load. Depending on the objective, the individual samples could be sent to the diagnostic laboratory as a pooled composite or as separate samples.

For *Salmonella* monitoring of bird-occupied premises, the use of drag swabs is the generally accepted method. A drag swab is a sterile gauze pad or small sponge moistened in sterile skim milk attached to a pole or string. Absorbable shoe cover swabs may also be used. The principle is to wipe or drag the swab through the litter, equipment, and environment in a methodical pattern. The swab acts as a wick by picking up bacteria as it moves along the substrate. These swabs are then put into properly labeled, sterile sealable bags and transported to the laboratory on ice packs. For detailed procedures, refer to US FDA [11] and National Poultry Improvement Plan (NPIP) [12] protocols.

9.4.3 Sample Packaging and Submission

Proper packaging of samples is essential to minimize breakage and prevent leakage and contamination during transit. Be especially careful to make sure caps on microcentrifuge tubes are securely attached, bags are properly sealed, and everything is accurately labeled using waterproof pens or markers.

The packaging must consist of three components: a primary receptacle, secondary packaging, and a rigid outer packaging shell. The primary receptacle contains the sample itself. Examples of primary receptacles are the grab bags of litter, tubes of blood, serum or water, and bagged carcasses. All carcasses and specimens should be double-bagged in sealable laboratory or freezer bags. These are to be placed in a convenient-sized Styrofoam® container. If the surrounding Styrofoam is not leak proof, it is recommended to place all specimens collectively inside an additional large leak-proof sealable bag or container (Figure 9.5). This serves as the secondary packaging. The refrigerant is added and then the contents packed with enough absorbable material, such as shredded newspaper or a commercial absorbent, to wick and hold the maximum conceivable quantity of

(a)

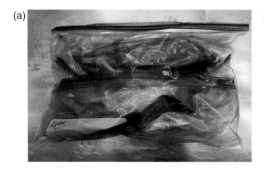

(b)

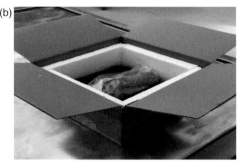

Figure 9.5 Proper packaging of carcasses for shipment to the diagnostic laboratory. (a) Two carcasses are double-bagged in sealable bags. (b) The double-bagged carcasses are then placed between coolant surrounded by Styrofoam within a cardboard shipping box.

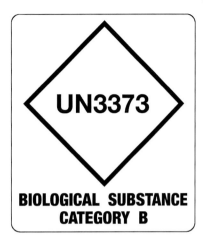

Figure 9.6 A "biological substance, category B" label should be applied to the outside of shipping boxes containing biological specimens or samples.

potential moisture leakage. This container is sealed shut with tape. The submission form is placed in a sealable plastic bag and attached to the top of the secondary container.

The sealed secondary container is then placed in an appropriately sized cardboard mailing box, which serves as the outer final shipping packaging. Additional cushioning material may be needed between the secondary and outer packaging to eliminate looseness and motion during transit. The cardboard box is then sealed and labeled with the mailing information. For "Biological Substance, Category B," this label must be present in letters at least 6 mm high and must be marked on the outer package adjacent to a diamond-shaped UN3373 label (Figure 9.6). These labels can be found online. Send by a reliable carrier for overnight or next-day delivery to the laboratory [10, 13].

9.5 Diagnostic Services Commonly Requested for Gamebird Field Investigations

Listed below are common tests that a veterinarian working with gamebirds would most likely request. Ability of diagnostic and testing services will vary between laboratories, so it is important to contact the laboratory and explain specifically what is being requested before submitting samples.

9.5.1 Full Necropsy

Laboratories will vary as to what additional services are included in a necropsy request in addition to a gross examination. It is recommended that the clinician submit enough carcasses to insure that predominant necropsy findings reflect the true significant problem observed in the field. About 5–10 carcasses, depending on age, size, and suspected field problem, are sufficient to get a reasonable diagnosis. Submit only fresh carcasses and keep them cool during storage and transit.

9.5.2 Histopathology

The histologic examination of tissues may or may not be included in the base price of a full necropsy. If special staining procedures are needed, such as periodic acid–Schiff (PAS) for visualization of fungal hyphae, additional costs may be incurred.

9.5.3 Direct Smear and Fecal Flotation

These are basic techniques that most laboratories can perform. They are commonly employed to detect internal parasitic infections, such as *Ascaridia* spp., *Heterakis* spp., *Syngamus trachea*, or *Capillaria* spp.

Direct smears of tissues are sometimes made to get a quick idea of a suspected problem. A specific dye or staining procedure might be applied, such as the Kinyoun-modified Ziehl–Neelsen acid-fast procedure for detection of *Mycobacteria* spp. A Giemsa-stained blood smear might be prepared to help in detection of blood-borne parasites.

9.5.4 Immunohistochemistry

This technique uses the principle of an in situ antigen–antibody reaction using a visible marker, such as a fluorescein dye or enzyme-attaching technique. The advantage of this process is that it can be performed on formalin-fixed tissues, thereby allowing both conventional histologic techniques, such as H&E staining, and specialized immunohistochemistry methods to be employed on the same tissue block.

There are direct and indirect immunohistochemistry methods. The indirect technique, using a secondary antibody labeled with an indicator such as fluorescein dye, is more often employed because of greater flexibility of conjugate applications.

Immunohistochemistry techniques have been successfully used for detection of antigens within tissues or cells for a number of pathogens potentially affecting gamebird health, such as adenovirus, Newcastle disease, fowl pox virus, AE virus, and *Mycoplasma* spp. [14]

9.5.5 Bacteriology

Time-tested basic culture techniques must still be regarded as indispensable in the search for many bacterial diseases. Standard aerobic culture is employed when suspecting typical avian disease-causing bacteria, such as *P. multocida*, *Bordetella avium*, *E. coli*, *Pseudomonas* spp., *Staphylococcus* spp., *E. rhusiopathiae*, or other aerobic pathogens. Tissues or samples suspected of harboring *Salmonella* spp. are preenriched and subsequently placed in selective enrichment broth before being plated on *Salmonella*-selective agars. There are also commercially available rapid detection systems for *Salmonella* spp. Techniques using specialized media may be necessary for more fastidious organisms, such as *Mycoplasma* spp. or *Avibacterium paragallinarum*. Anaerobic culture methods are used for isolation of clostridial species, such as *Clostridium perfringens* (necrotic enteritis) or *Clostridium colinum* (ulcerative enteritis).

Additional tools have been developed to assist in rapid identification of bacteria. For example, automated biochemical-based identification systems that compare an isolate's biochemical results with a database library of standard profiles are becoming more common in diagnostic laboratories. Matrix-assisted laser desorption/ionization-time of flight mass spectrometry (MALDI-TOF) is also a very useful tool that is available in many laboratories. The process uses laser ionization of large molecular fragments that are distinctive for identification of specific microbes. The technique is useful for either primary identification or as a supplementary confirmatory tool to conventional biochemical or other methods. MALDI-TOF also offers additional uses, such as strain identification of microbes in epidemiologic studies.

9.5.6 Rapid Plate Agglutination (RPA) Test

The rapid plate agglutination test is frequently used as a flock screening test. There are variations of RPA tests, using either whole blood or sera.

Briefly, the blood or serum sample is collected and a small amount is placed on a glass slide or in a shallow concave depression in a ceramic plate. A predetermined quantity of antigen reagent is dropped into the blood/serum. The combined mixture is lightly blended together and then gently rocked or rotated for a prescribed period. Any appreciable amount of antibody in the blood will agglutinate with the antigen (usually dyed for easy visualization) and form visible clumps.

In order to comply with basic NPIP certification, breeder flocks must be tested for antibodies against *Salmonella Pullorum* and *S. typhi*. This requires whole blood, so the test is typically performed bird-side. Each bird is accurately identified and secured until the test is completed.

Other useful gamebird flock RPA screening tests using sera are performed for the detection of antibodies against *Mycoplasma gallisepticum* or *M. synoviae*. Monitoring for these potential pathogens is important if NPIP certification is sought for MG/MS-Clean or MG/MS-Monitored status [15, 16].

9.5.7 Agar Gel Immunodiffusion (AGID) Test

This test, also known as the agar gel precipitin (AGP) test, is based on an antigen–antibody reaction taking place in a semisolid medium, most typically in agar. It is commonly available in diagnostic laboratories and has the advantage of being relatively inexpensive, easy to set up, and fairly straightforward in interpretation of results. The test is done by pouring liquid agar into a Petri dish or onto a clear glass slide and allowing it to cool. Once hardened, circular holes of equal diameter are punched in the agar, positioned so there is one center hole surrounded by six others equally spaced around its perimeter. The plugs in the holes are removed by aspiration. Depending on the test being performed, the size of holes and distance between them may vary slightly. A punch may be purchased or made in-house with the necessary dimensions for the test being performed. Typically, for serologic testing, the antigen is placed in the center well and the individual serum samples and controls are placed in the outer wells. The antigen and antibodies in serum (if present) diffuse toward each other and form a visible precipitate line. Results are reported qualitatively as "detected" (visible precipitate line) or "not detected" (no line).

A common use for the AGID test in gamebird diagnostics is for determining flock status to avian influenza exposure in compliance with avian influenza surveillance programs [15, 17]; however, other uses could also be applied, such as looking for antibodies to AE virus.

9.5.8 Enzyme-linked Immunoassay (ELISA) Test

The ELISA test is the prevalent screening test used in most poultry laboratories. The test is based on the principle of reaction rate. The amount of enzyme-driven visible color change of a substrate is dependent on the quantity of antigen present in the serum sample. Each sample is compared to the positive and negative controls to yield a sample-to-positive ratio, which is then transformed into a titer value by a double regression calculation. The ELISA test is generally performed using 96-well plates and computer-assisted functions. This makes it especially useful for flock screening by processing many samples quickly and simultaneously. The ELISA test is an excellent tool for assessing vaccination response in a flock.

Most of the companies producing commercial kits have accompanying software packages that allow clear visualization of results in graphic format. There are commercial kits available for many common poultry diseases, but not all are necessarily approved for gamebirds. Nonetheless, ELISA testing can be a valuable tool for evaluating flock prevalence of antibodies to avian influenza, Newcastle disease, MG, MS, and AE.

9.5.9 Polymerase Chain Reaction (PCR)

This technique amplifies DNA directly or, in the case of RNA viruse,s by amplification of synthesized DNA from RNA using reverse transcriptase in the first step of the reaction. Real-time PCR uses a thermocycler to amplify DNA. A fluorescent dye is incorporated that is read by the computer at the end of each cycle. The degree of fluorescence is correlated to the amount of DNA present. These data are plotted and displayed graphically. Depending on the PCR method used, it can detect if a sample passes a cycle threshold (i.e., positive or negative) or it can be quantitative, specifying amount of antigen in the sample.

These PCR techniques are very versatile and can be used for the detection of many antigens associated with gamebird diseases.

9.5.10 Antigen-capture Immunoassay (ACIA) Test

The ACIA test is commonly used as a screening test for detection of avian influenza (type A influenza virus) antigen. Commercial kits are available for rapid detection from tracheal or cloacal swabs. These are based on vertical wicking immunomigration on test sticks that are placed in a small quantity of media containing the pooled swab samples. The test is rapid and can yield results in 15 minutes. It is employed as a screening test only, and any positive results must be verified using confirmatory procedures, such as virus isolation (VI) or PCR [18].

9.5.11 Hemagglutination Inhibition (HI) Test

This test can be used to determine serum antibody titer to a variety of disease agents that agglutinate red blood cells, such as *M. gallisepticum*, *M. synoviae*, avian influenza virus, Newcastle disease virus, and some adenoviruses. The HI test is based on the ability to inhibit the antigen from agglutinating red blood cells through neutralization by serum antibodies. The greater the quantity of specific antibody in the serum, the greater the ability to inhibit the antigen's innate propensity for hemagglutination. The serum is mixed in serial dilutions of either $\log_2$ or $\log_{10}$, depending on procedure, with the antigen in a 96-well round-bottomed microtiter plate. Results are reported as the reciprocal of the highest serum dilution that causes complete inhibition of agglutination [14].

Although still very useful, the HI test is not as commonly employed as in the past. Quicker and less labor-intensive antibody-quantifying methods, such as commercial ELISA kits, are now readily available and extensively used.

9.6 Tests That Might Be Required in Special Situations or May Not Be Widely Available

9.6.1 Virus Isolation (VI)

This is a diagnostic procedure that from a clinical standpoint would only be employed if a viral pathogen was suspected and could not be readily identified by other available means. VI requires the propagation of specific substrates and strict biosecurity procedures. The techniques vary depending on type of virus to be isolated. It is not a service offered in all diagnostic laboratories, so consultation with the laboratory is important before submitting samples for VI.

9.6.2 Virus Neutralization (VN) Test

This labor-intensive and expensive test is generally done in research settings and would seldom be feasible in a clinical situation. The technique is useful for identifying unknown viruses or differentiating between viruses [14].

9.6.3 Embryo Susceptibility Test

In the past, the embryo susceptibility test was used to determine the immune status of chicken breeder flocks for AE [19]. Although theoretically useful, it requires inoculating eggs and is time-consuming compared to currently available serologic methods of flock monitoring.

9.7 Conclusion

In summary, the characteristics of many gamebird diseases require diagnostic tools that are often not available in most veterinary practices. Developing a trusted and responsible relationship with a diagnostic laboratory will pay huge dividends in servicing gamebird clients.

References

1 American Veterinary Medical Association (2020). *AVMA Guidelines for the Euthanasia of Animals*. www.avma.org/sites/default/files/2020-02/Guidelines-on-Euthanasia-2020.pdf (accessed February 2022).

2 Lundeen, T. (ed.) (1999). *Feed Additive Compendium*. Minnetonka, MN: Miller Publishing Co.

3 Newman, L.J. and Sander, J.E. (2021). Poultry drug use guide. In: *AAAP Avian Disease Manual*, 7e (ed. M. Boulianne, M. Brash, B. Charlton, et al.). Jacksonville, FL: AAAP.

4 Baxendale, W. (1996). Current methods of delivery of poultry vaccines. In: *Poultry Immunology* (ed. T.F. Davison, T.R. Morris and L.N. Payne), 375–387. Abingdon: Carfax.

5 Sander, J. (1991). Principles of vaccination programs for poultry health. *Poult. Dig* 10: 14–24.

6 Stewart-Brown, B. (1995). Applying poultry vaccines via the aerosol route on the farm: technique and critique. In: *Proceedings, Poultry Vaccination Techniques and Evaluation Workshop*, St Paul, MN, September 16, 1995. American College of Poultry Veterinarians, pp. 30–39.

7 Howell, L.M. (1995). Farm vaccination – wing web method. In: *Proceedings, Poultry Vaccination Techniques and Evaluation Workshop*, St Paul, MN, September 16, 1995. American College of Poultry Veterinarians, pp. 40–45.

8 US Animal and Plant Health and Inspection Service, US Department of Agriculture, National Animal Health Laboratory Network: Laboratories (last modified 2 Jun 2020). www.aphis.usda .gov/aphis/ourfocus/animalhealth/lab-info-services/nahln/sa_labs/panels/ct_labs (accessed February 2022).

9 US Department of Agriculture (2016). FY 2016 HPAI Response: Avian Sample Collection for Influenza A and Newcastle Disease. www.aphis.usda.gov/animal_health/lab_info_services/ downloads/WIAV0020.pdf (accessed February 2022).

10 National Poultry Improvement Plan. Recommendations for Collecting Specimens from Poultry for Viral Diagnostic Testing. WI-AV-0020.07. http://poultryimprovement.org/documents/ WIAV0020.pdf (accessed February 2022).

11 US Food and Drug Administration (2018). Detection of Salmonella in Environmental Samples from Poultry Houses. www.fda.gov/food/laboratory-methods-food/detection-salmonella-environmental-samples-poultry-houses (accessed February 2022).

12 National Poultry Improvement Plan (2014) Program Standards. pp. 26–28. www.poultryimprovement.org/documents/NPIPProgramStandards.pdf (accessed February 2022).

13 Frame, D.D. and A. Van Wettere (2015). Collection Procedure for Submitting PCR Samples to Utah Veterinary Diagnostic Laboratory for Avian Influenza Testing in Turkeys, Chickens, and Game Birds. https://digitalcommons.usu.edu/cgi/viewcontent.cgi?article=1770&context=extension_curall&_ga=2.106336771.143294984.1600187328-102730920.1600187328 (accessed February 2022).

14 Williams, S.M., Dufour-Zavala, L., Jackwood, M.W. et al. (2016). *A Laboratory Manual for Isolation, Identification, and Characterization of Avian Pathogens*, 6e. Athens, GA: American Association of Avian Pathologists.

15 National Archives Code of Federal Regulations (2022). Part 145 Subpart E—Special Provisions for Hobbyist and Exhibition Waterfowl, Exhibition Poultry, and Game Bird Breeding Flocks and Products. www.ecfr.gov/current/title-9/chapter-I/subchapter-G/part-145 (accessed February 2022).

16 National Archives Code of Federal Regulations (2022). Part 146 Subpart E—Special Provisions for Commercial Upland Game Birds, Commercial Waterfowl, Raised-for-Release Upland Game Birds, and Raised-for-Release Waterfowl. www.ecfr.gov/current/title-9/chapter-I/subchapter-G/part-146 (accessed February 2022).

17 USDA-APHIS (2021). Avian Influenza Guidance Documents. www.aphis.usda.gov/aphis/ourfocus/animalhealth/animal-disease-information/avian/avian-influenza/ai-guidance-documents (accessed February 2022).

18 United States Department of Agriculture (2015). HPAI Outbreak 2014–2015. Use of the Antigen Capture Immunoassay. www.aphis.usda.gov/animal_health/emergency_management/downloads/hpai/acia_testpolicy.pdf (accessed February 2022).

19 Taylor, J.R.E. and Schelling, E.P. (1960). The distribution of avian encephalomyelitis in North America as indicated by an immunity test. *Avian Dis.* 4 (2): 122–132.

10

Gamebird Respiratory Diseases
Richard M. Fulton

10.1 Introduction

Respiratory diseases of gamebirds are similar to respiratory diseases of other avian species, more specifically chickens and turkeys. As a general rule, pheasants, quail, and partridges respond similarly to chickens. Peafowl respond similarly to turkeys. Due to how they are raised, in contrast to commercial poultry, gamebirds are at higher risk of respiratory disease from migratory waterfowl, wildlife, and other pests. Causes of respiratory disease include viruses, bacteria, fungi, and parasites.

10.2 Viral Respiratory Diseases

Viral respiratory diseases include avian influenza (AI), Newcastle disease, infectious laryngotracheitis (ILT), coronavirus infection in pheasants, and quail bronchitis viruses (QBVs).

Avian influenza is caused by an enveloped RNA virus in the orthomyxovirus family. The AI virus is considered to be a type A influenza which also infects human beings. Humans may also be infected with type B and C influenza viruses. Type A influenza viruses may infect other animals such as swine, horses, dogs, cats, mink, seals, and whales and is named for the respective species that it infects, such as swine influenza when it infects swine and AI when it infects birds. Wild waterfowl, namely ducks, geese, and swans, appear to be the reservoir for all type A influenza viruses where they cycle as low pathogenic strains (LPAI) and mutate to highly pathogenic avian influenza (HPAI). LPAI causes little disease and death while HPAI causes dramatic disease and death loss. LPAI H5 and H7 viruses circulate for a time in gallinaceous birds and develop into HPAI viruses [1].

Influenza viruses are further classified by the surface antigens on their envelope which are known as H for the hemagglutinin antigen and N for the neuraminidase antigen. Hemagglutinin is responsible for helping the virus attach to the cell membrane. Since viral envelopes consist of lipid, derived from the host cell, soap and water, cooking temperatures, ultraviolet light, and almost any disinfectant can disrupt the membrane, preventing the virus from attaching to the host cell and thus preventing infection. Neuraminidase antigen, also on the virus envelope, allows the newly assembled viruses to escape from host cells. In humans, drugs developed to combat flu viruses are antineuraminidase compounds. There are currently 18 H types and 11 N types recognized [2]. Therefore, AI viruses can be any combination of H type and N type with a total of 198 different possibilities. In the avian species, only H5 and H7 types are of major concern since they have, in the past, been responsible for catastrophic influenza outbreaks, also known as HPAI [1].

Although thought of as primarily a respiratory infection, common AI viruses may also produce gastrointestinal infections. Yet under the right conditions, the H antigen may have the correct amino acid sequence (multiple basic amino acids at the cleavage site) which allows those viruses to be cleaved by enzymes found throughout the body, thus producing general systemic disease. It is through this mechanism that low LPAI viruses become HPAI [3, 4]. In the USA, there have been multiple outbreaks of HPAI [5]. They have cycled between domestic flocks as LPAI and yet seem to change overnight to HPAI. Diagnosis requires laboratory testing, and no treatment or vaccination is used in the USA.

Newcastle disease is caused by an enveloped RNA Avulavirus in the paramyxovirus family and is commonly referred to as avian paramyxovirus 1. It too is considered to be a respiratory disease yet is often mixed with neurologic disease as well. The type and severity of disease caused by Newcastle disease virus (NDV) vary with the type of infecting virus. There are NDV viruses that cause little or no disease, called lentogenic strains, those that cause moderate disease, called mesogenic strains, and those that cause catastrophic disease, called velogenic strains. The milder strains are thought to be endemic in poultry while velogenic strains thought to be endemic in feral pigeons, some domestic poultry, coastal seabirds, and cormorants [1]. Velogenic strains can cause lesions within the body organs and are referred to as viscerotropic velogenic (vvNDV) or neurologic disease alone and as neurotropic velogenic (nvNDV). Although vvNDV is found throughout the world, it rarely occurs in the USA. It is therefore often referred to in the USA as exotic NDV. Over the years, California has had repeated outbreaks of vvNDV due to smuggling of fighting chickens [6, 7]. Diagnosis requires laboratory tests and no treatment is available. Vaccination, with primarily lentogenic strains and some mesogenic strains, is commonly used in commercial poultry flocks in the USA.

Unfortunately, in either HPAI or vvNDV outbreak scenarios, it is very hard to determine which virus is causing the problem without laboratory tests. Both viruses cause large death losses, with or without clinical illness, within flocks and similar, if not equivalent, clinical signs and gross lesions, making it difficult to tell which virus is the source of the outbreak. Gross lesions in both HPAI and vvNDV consist of hemorrhage in multiple internal organs including proventriculus and intestines, hemorrhage and ulceration within the esophagus and hemorrhage in the trachea. Other lesions of vasculitis may include swelling of the face and cyanosis of skin, shanks, and feet. The reproductive system may also be affected.

Diagnosis in either AI and NDV is by polymerase chain reaction (PCR), virus isolation, and other virus identifying techniques. PCR tests are available to first identify the causative virus as either AI or NDV virus and then to differentiate AI as H5 or H7 and NDV as velogenic.

For information concerning HPAI and vNDV, please access the web pages of the United States Department of Agriculture at www.aphis.usda.gov/aphis.

Infectious laryngotracheitis is a herpesvirus that normally infects chickens. In gamebirds, the disease has been reported in pheasants and in a peafowl [8]. The classic lesion of ILT is hemorrhage with or without fibrin in the larynx and proximal trachea (Figure 10.1). Other organs are not generally affected but in some cases, the virus infection may extend to the lungs. ILT may be suspected upon necropsy and confirmed with histopathology (Figure 10.2) and other laboratory tests such as PCR and/or virus isolation. There is no treatment available for ILT yet reportedly

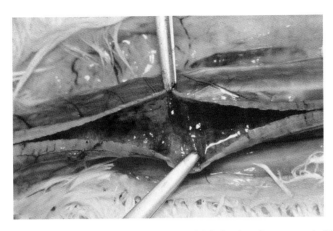

Figure 10.1 Blood and fibrin in the trachea of a chicken with infectious laryngotracheitis.

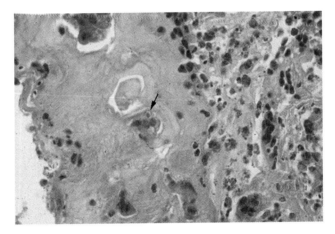

Figure 10.2 Chicken trachea: fibrin, hemorrhage, and syncytial cells with intranuclear herpes viral inclusion in one of the grouped cells (arrow).

increasing the house temperature a few degrees may shorten and lessen the disease effects. Vaccination is used in commercial chickens. Extreme care should be used when deciding to vaccinate for ILT since the chicken embryo-origin and tissue culture-derived ILT vaccine can cause outbreaks in nonvaccinated birds when it spreads from bird to bird [9]. Only genetically modified ILT vaccines should be used since they do not contain the entire virus and thus will not spread and cause disease.

Coronavirus is closely related to infectious bronchitis virus, a respiratory disease in chickens, with some strains causing kidney damage and gout. Coronaviruses, which are enveloped RNA viruses, have been recovered from pheasants with respiratory disease and kidney damage [10]. Mortality has been recorded as 15%, and possibly up to 45%. Although not standard, diagnosis would be a combination of lesions (renal disease), virus isolation with identification. Of course, there is no treatment and no known vaccine is available.

Quail bronchitis is a respiratory adenovirus disease of young bobwhite quail (*Colinus virginianus*) yet may occur in Japanese quail (*Coturnix japonica*). The quail bronchitis virus (QBV) is a nonenveloped DNA adenovirus. Since this is a nonenveloped virus, it persists in the environment for long periods of time and is difficult to inactivate (kill). The disease occurs most commonly in

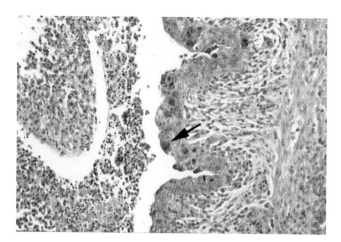

Figure 10.3 Quail trachea with inflammatory exudate in the lumen and numerous epithelial cells with karyomegaly and filling of the nucleus with amphophilic adenoviral inclusions (arrow).

young quail (less than 3 weeks of age). Infection is characterized by high morbidity and mortality, up to 80% death loss, and respiratory disease. Gross lesions in dead birds consist of mucus plugs in the trachea. Diagnosis is by the presence of intranuclear inclusions in the cells lining the trachea, seen with histopathology (Figure 10.3), and/or egg inoculation. There is no treatment or vaccine available [11].

10.3 Bacterial Respiratory Diseases

Bacterial respiratory diseases of gamebirds include mycoplasmosis, pasteurellosis, hemophilosis and ornithobacteriosis. Although some of these bacteria are capable of causing systemic disease, their primary focus is the respiratory system.

Mycoplasmosis in pheasants, quail, and partridges may be caused by *Mycoplasma gallisepticum* (MG) [12]. MG infection in pheasants can cause conjunctivitis, distended infraorbital sinuses, nasal exudates as well as other respiratory sounds with gross lesions of polyserositis and airsacculitis [13]. Similar ocular and air sac lesions were seen in partridges that were infected with *Mycoplasma iowae* [14]. Diagnosis is by necropsy, culture, and identification. Many laboratories are not able to culture mycoplasma and rely heavily on PCR. Unfortunately, the gold standard remains culture and identification since the author has been involved in cases where PCR was positive while multiple attempts to culture the mycoplasma were negative. Treatment only helps to suppress clinical signs yet does not rid the animal of infection and consists of long courses of tetracycline and/or tylosin. Mycoplasma organisms are transmitted through the egg to offspring of infected females (transovarial transmission). The only true method of control is depopulation of all gamebirds and poultry on the premises, cleanup and no restocking for a period of 3 weeks. Since mycoplasma is often a hidden disease, testing of replacement stock would be encouraged.

Pasteurella multocida, a Gram-negative bacterium, is the cause of pasteurellosis, commonly known as fowl cholera. *P. multocida* is capable of causing systemic disease yet causes predominantly respiratory disease in turkeys and is thus considered in this chapter. In chickens and possibly gamebirds, this bacterium causes not only an acute disease but also a chronic disease

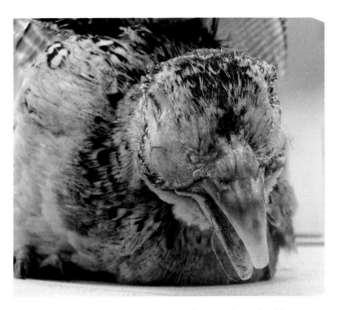

Figure 10.4   Pheasant: sinusitis and conjunctivitis due to *Pasteurella multocida.*

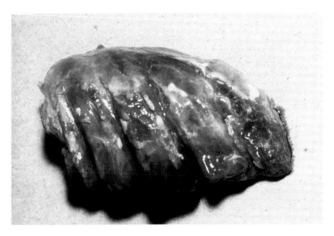

Figure 10.5   Turkey lung: fibrinous pleuritis and bronchopneumonia due to *Pasteurella multocida.*

with swelling of sinuses, eyes, wattles, joints, and feet (Figure 10.4) [15]. Acute disease often consists of mucous discharge from the mouth, diarrhea, and increased respiratory rate. Lesions of acute infection include fibrin within the coelomic cavity and swollen liver with multiple small white areas of necrosis. The ova may be flaccid with fibrin near the ovary. The lungs may contain fibrin within the body of the lung and on the surface (Figure 10.5). Daily mortality is drastically increased with acute infection. Diagnosis is made by bacterial culture and antibiotic sensitivity along with clinical signs and gross lesions.

Treatment consists of use of antibiotics which are shown to inhibit the bacteria, most often sulfonamide or tetracycline. *P. multocida* is transmitted by wild flying birds and is carried in the mouth of asymptomatic racoons, rodents and cats [16]. Thus prevention requires the exclusion of wildlife, rodents, and cats from gamebirds. Turkey farmers have commented about increased incidence of fowl cholera in buildings close to wood lots. Frequent, once every 2–4 hours, removal of sick and dead birds can help control the spread of the disease within the flock. Vaccines are available but must match the infecting serotype to provide protection [17].

Hemophilosis is caused by the bacteria *Avibacterium* (*Hemophilus*) *paragallinarum* which is a Gram-negative bacterium. Hemophilosis is the disease commonly known as infectious coryza. It was identified in a flock of Japanese quail and has been reported to occur in pheasants and guineafowl. The infection consisted of a nasal discharge, sinusitis, and conjunctivitis, and the authors reported a 90% morbidity rate [18]. Diagnosis would be made by bacteriologic culture but the submitter must warn the laboratory that they suspect this bacterium since it requires special culture techniques. Treatment would be via antibiotic, most likely sulfonamide antibiotics. Vaccines are available, yet it is important to match the serotype of the infecting bacterium with that of the vaccine.

Ornithobacteriosis is caused by *Ornithobacterium rhinotracheale* (ORT). ORT is a Gram-negative bacterium which is difficult to culture, and cultures should be kept for at least 72 hours [19]. This disease has also been reported in chickens and turkeys. In pheasants, clinical signs are open mouth breathing and cough that can be heard for a long distance. Gross and microscopic lesions are those of pneumonia and airsacculitis. Diagnosis consists of bacterial culture with associated lesions. Treatment would be tetracyclines, penicillin, and sulfonamides [17].

10.4 Parasitic Respiratory Diseases

Parasitic respiratory diseases of gamebirds include syngamosis (gapeworm) and cryptosporidiosis.

Syngamosis is caused by infection with the nematode parasite *Syngamus trachea*. The infection is known as gapeworm or redworms based upon the clinical signs they cause or their appearance. These parasites live permanently in the trachea. They form a "Y" appearance with the male attached to the tracheal lining and the female surrounding the male (Figures 10.6 and 10.7). Infection may be directly from bird to bird, oral consumption of eggs, or through an intermediate host. The parasite has been reported in pheasants, quail, peafowl, and other domestic poultry [20]. Young pheasants whose tracheal diameter is small may become blocked by the parasites and they die.

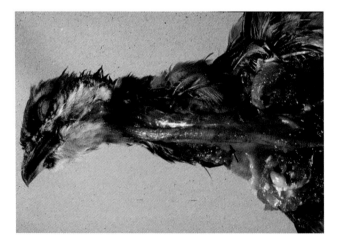

Figure 10.6 Partridge: *Syngamus trachea* in unopened trachea (arrow).

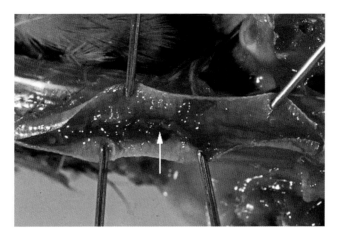

Figure 10.7   Partridge: *Syngamus trachea* in opened trachea (arrow).

Older pheasants suffer from breathing difficulties and increased susceptibility to other infections. Treatment is with fenbendazole or levamisole although caution is suggested since these treatments would be considered off-label usage.

Cryptosporidiosis is caused by a protozoan parasite with a life cycle similar to *Eimeria* sp., the intestinal coccidian parasite of the avian species. Cryptosporidia that have been reported include *Cryptosporidium baileyi* and *C. meleagridis* in red-legged partridges [21], *C. baileyi* in red grouse [22], and *C. baileyi* in Japanese quail [23]. The parasite cycles immediately below the cell membrane of epithelium in conjunctiva and trachea as well as enterocytes. Clinical disease would include eye discharge, respiratory signs, and diarrhea. Diagnosis can be made by direct staining of smears of the surface of the organ and/or histopathology (Figure 10.8). There currently are no known treatments and control is only accomplished by eradication, cleanup and sanitation. Unfortunately, cryptosporidia are extremely resistant to common chemicals used for disinfection.

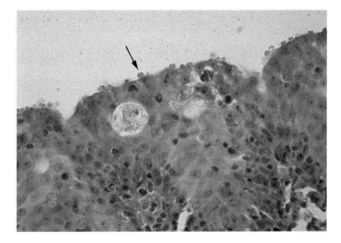

Figure 10.8   Quail: photomicrograph of trachea; note *Cryptosporidium* sp. (arrow).

10.5 Fungal Respiratory Diseases

Aspergillosis is a fungal disease typically caused by the fungi *Aspergillus fumigatus* and *A. flavus* [24]. Aspergillosis had been reported in partridges and pheasants and may occur in any bird species [25]. Gross lesions consist of white to tan nodules within the lung and air sacs but may affect other tissues as well. Where the oxygen tension is high, such as in air sacs, fruiting bodies may be present where the white plaques have a gray felt-like covering. Aspergillosis is typically found in animals debilitated by chronic stresses, including immunosuppressive diseases. Fungal spores are typically found in the litter and are inhaled. In young birds, a respiratory syndrome known as brooder pneumonia occurs when there are granulomas of the lungs. Brooders are typically warm, moist, and dark, a perfect environment for growing fungi. The spores in young birds may be inhaled in the housing (brooder) or from eggs that explode in the incubator and spew fungal spores in the hatching environment. In young and older birds, aspergillosis is fatal. Treatment in large populations is not feasible.

Diagnosis is made based on gross lesions with histopathology. Culture alone, without lesions, is not diagnostic since fungal spores can be found in normal atmospheric air.

References

1 Lee, D.-H., Bertran, K., Kwon, J.-H. et al. (2017). Evolution, global spread, and pathogenicity of highly pathogenic avian influenza H5NX clade 2.3.4.4. *J. Vet. Sci.* 18 (S1): 269–280.

2 CDC (2021). Types of Influenza Viruses. www.cdc.gov/flu/about/viruses/types.htm (accessed February 2022).

3 Stieneke-Gröber, A., Vey, M., Angliker, H. et al. (1992). Influenza virus hemagglutinin with multibasic cleavage site is activated by furin, a subtilisin-like endoprotease. *EMBO J.* 11 (7): 2407–2414.

4 Decha, P., Rungrotmongkol, T., Intharathep, P. et al. (2008). Source of high pathogenicity of an avian influenza virus H5N1: why H5 is better cleaved by furin. *Biophys. J.* 95 (1): 128–134.

5 Animal Plant and Health Inspection Service (2022). Highly Pathogenic Avian Influenza (HPAI). www.aphis.usda.gov/aphis/ourfocus/animalhealth/animal-disease-information/avian/avian-influenza/defend-the-flock-hpai (accessed February 2022).

6 Carvallo, F.R., Moore, J.D., Nyaoke, A.C. et al. (2018). Letter to the editor: Diagnosis of virulent Newcastle disease in southern California, May 2018. *J. Vet. Diagn. Invest.* 30 (4): 493–494.

7 Dimitrov, K.M., Ferreira, H.L., Pantin-Jackwood, M.J. et al. (2019). Pathogenicity and transmission of virulent Newcastle disease virus from 2018–2019 California outbreak and related viruses in young and adult chickens. *Virology* 531: 203–218.

8 Crawshaw, G.J. and Boycott, B.R. (1981). Infectious laryngotracheitis in peafowl and pheasants. *Avian Dis.* 26 (2): 397–401.

9 Menendez, K.R., Garcia, M., Spatz, S. et al. (2014). Molecular epidemiology of infectious laryngotracheitis a review. *Avian Pathol.* 43 (2): 108–117.

10 Cavanaugh, D., Mawditt, K., Welchman, D.B. et al. (2002). Coronaviruses from pheasants (*Phasianus colchicus*) are genetically closely related to coronaviruses of domestic fowl (infectious bronchitis virus) and turkeys. *Avian Pathol.* 31 (1): 81–93.

11 Jack, S.W., Reed, W.M., and Burnstein, T. (1994). The pathogenesis of quail bronchitis. *Avian Dis.* 38 (3): 548–556.

12 Reece, R.L., Ireland, L., and Barr, D.A. (1986). Infectious sinusitis associated with *Mycoplasma gallisepticum* in game-birds. *Aust. Vet. J.* 63 (5): 167–168.

13 Benčina, D., Mrzel, I., Rojas Zorman, O. et al. (2003). Characterization of Mycoplasma gallisepticum strains involved in respiratory disease in pheasants and peafowl. *Vet. Rec.* 152 (8): 230–234.

14 Catania, S., Gobbo, F., Rodio, S. et al. (2014). First isolation of Mycoplasma iowae in grey partridge flocks. *Avian Dis.* 58 (2): 323–325.

15 Einum, P., Kiupel, M., and Bolin, C. (2003). An outbreak of fowl cholera in ring-necked pheasants (*Phasianus cholchicus*). *Avian Dis.* 47 (3): 777–780.

16 Gregg, D.A., Olson, L.D., and McCune, E.L. (1974). Experimental transmission *of Pasteurella multocida* from raccoons to turkeys via bite wounds. *Avian Dis.* 18 (4): 559–564.

17 Glisson, J.R. (1998). Bacterial respiratory diseases of poultry. *Poult. Sci.* 77 (8): 1138–1142.

18 Reece, R.L., Barr, D.A., and Owen, A.C. (1981). The isolation of *Haemophilus paragallinarum* from Japanese quail. *Aust. Vet. J.* 57 (7): 350–351.

19 Welchman, D.B., Ainsworth, H.L., Jensen, T.K. et al. (2013). Demonstration of *Ornithobacterium rhinotracheale* in pheasants (*Phasianus colchicus*) with pneumonia and airsacculitis. *Avian Pathol.* 42 (2): 171–178.

20 Fulton, R.M. (2021). Common diseases of Michigan gamebirds: a retrospective study. *Avian Dis.* 65 (1): 26–29.

21 Máca, O. and Pavlásek, I. (2015). First finding of spontaneous infections with *Cryptosporidium baileyi* and *C. meleagridis* in the red-legged partridge *Alectoris rufa* from an aviary in the Czech Republic. *Vet. Parasitol.* 209 (3–4): 164–168.

22 Baines, D., Newborn, D., and Richardson, M. (2020). Correlates of pathological lesions associated with respiratory cryptosporidiosis prevalence in shot red grouse *Lagopus lagopus* scotica. *Avian Pathol.* 49 (1): 74–79.

23 Murakami, S., Miyama, M., Ogawa, J. et al. (2002). Occurrence of conjunctivitis, sinusitis and upper region tracheitis in Japanese quail (*Coturnix coturnix japonica*), possibly caused by *Mycoplasma gallisepticum* accompanied by *Cryptosporidium* sp. infection. *Avian Pathol.* 31 (4): 363–370.

24 Cacciuttolo, C., Rossi, S., Nardoni, S. et al. (2009). Anatomorphological aspects of avian aspergillosis. *Vet. Res. Commun.* 33 (6): 521–527.

25 Simpson, V. (2011). Spinal aspergillosis in pheasants. *Vet. Rec.* 169 (21): 562.

11

Gamebird Digestive Diseases
Robert E. Porter, Jr and Teresa Y. Morishita

A healthy digestive tract is essential for all aspects of gamebird production, from early growth to feathering and conformation at maturity, and reproduction. The digestive tract acts as a selective barrier between ingested feed and the internal organs. The digestive tract has physical, chemical, immunologic, and microbiologic components that can be altered by the ration, infectious disease, flock environment and a variety of management factors. Any change in the delicate balance of components in the avian digestive tract can alter nutrient absorption to affect growth rate and feed conversion [1].

The components of avian intestinal health have mostly been studied in commercial poultry, such as chickens and turkeys, but the relationships between these components in gamebirds are undoubtedly similar. Without question, diseases of the digestive tract play a significant role in impairing all aspects of gamebird production. In some instances, management decisions can reduce the risk of digestive tract disease; for example, enteric parasites and bacterial enteritis can generally be reduced in young gamebirds by raising them on wire rather than on soil or litter, but this may not be an effective strategy for the producer. Styles of management are not the same for all flocks, but must be altered to fit the climate, environment, housing, species of gamebirds, and feed available in a particular region. The management style can influence which infectious agents will pose a challenge to a given flock.

There are a variety of diseases of the digestive tract that have been documented in gamebirds in detail and these are highlighted in this chapter.

11.1 Conditions of the Oral Cavity, Esophagus, and Crop

11.1.1 *Candida* sp. Infection (Crop Mycosis)

Infection with an overgrowth of *Candida* sp. (synonyms candidiasis, crop mold, thrush) is common and affects the upper digestive tract in a wide variety of birds, especially young birds. The most common species is *Candida albicans*, although a variety of other species (*C. tropicalis, C. glabrata, C. parapsilosis, C. krusei, C. lusitaniae*) have been identified and these all have similar growth characteristics in culture (Sabouraud dextrose agar, 37 °C for 3–5 days) [2, 3]. *Candida* infection of the upper digestive tract has been well characterized in commercial chickens and turkeys, and described in pheasants, quail, guineafowl, peafowl, and partridges [3–6]. Although candidiasis is common, it is generally not a major clinical problem and usually occurs secondary to another underlying disease or condition; in fact, it is often caused by an extended use of oral antibiotics administered in the feed or drinking water.

Risk factors for *Candida* overgrowth include prolonged administration of antibiotics, malnutirion, poor flock hygiene, and immunosuppression from stress [2]. Most antibiotics in feed or drinking water have a label to use for less than 4–6 days. The infection most often affects the oral cavity, esophagus, and crop.

Candida is a ubiquitous yeast organism and can be part of the normal microflora; overgrowth is usually controlled by the normal bacterial microflora. When other diseases, such as those of the respiratory or digestive tract, are treated long term with antibiotics, the normal inhibitory microflora of upper digestive tract can be reduced to allow for yeast overgrowth. The organism can also be transmitted in contaminated drinking water, and infected adults that feed their precocial young can directly transmit the organisms [3].

Clinical signs are nonspecific because birds are often ill from some unrelated condition. Birds may appear unthrifty or have other more significant diseases being treated with oral antibiotics. Lesions appear grossly as a fine, white "pseudomembrane" or lining in the crop, upper esophagus or oral cavity (Figure 11.1). In the digestive tract, *Candida* growth starts as budding yeasts (blastospores) on the surface of the mucosa and progresses as branching, septate chains or pseudohyphae that extend into the deeper tissue (Figure 11.2). The condition may not be recognized until affected birds are examined by necropsy. The white membrane can be scraped or peeled off the mucosa. Gross and histopathologic lesions will confirm the diagnosis, although fungal culture can also be considered if speciation is necessary. The crop lesions when observed in gamebirds should be differentiated from *Capillaria* infection (crop worms).

The condition is often reversible by eliminating the primary disease condition, removing antibiotics and improving husbandry, but specific treatments such as copper sulfate solution (0.05%) in drinking water for several days [7] or addition of nystatin (100 g/ton) to feed [2] have been described. Prevention of this condition focuses on good husbandry, sanitary conditions, and

Figure 11.1 The open crop from a 2-week-old chukar partridge is lined by a white, friable pseudomembrane typical of *Candida albicans* overgrowth.

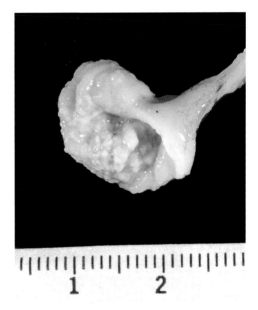

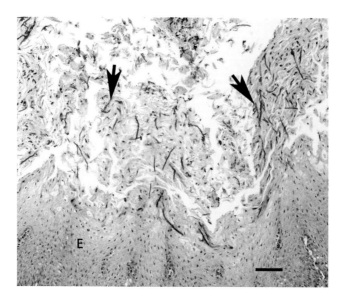

Figure 11.2 Candidiasis of partridge crop. There is epithelial hyperplasia and the crop epithelium (E) is infiltrated with linear pseudohyphae (arrows) consistent with *C. albicans*. PAS stain, bar = 20 μm.

reduction of primary stressors and infectious diseases in the flock. Judicious use of antibiotics is warranted, especially in young birds.

11.1.2 Capillariasis (Crop Worms, Threadworm)

There are multiple species of nematodes (family Capillariidae) that infect the digestive tract of pheasant, quail, partridge, and guineafowl (Table 11.1). Crop and small intestine are most often affected depending on the species of Capillaria, which are speciated based on the (i) morphology of the genitalia of the adult nematodes and (ii) location of infection in the host [14]. The nematode ova are distinctly bioperculate.

The most common Capillaria in gamebirds are *Capillaria (Eucoleus) annulatus* and *Capillaria (Eucoleus) contortus*, which infect the crop. These nematodes are long and slender and less than 60 mm long. *Capillaria* are shorter and thinner than *Heterakis* and *Ascaridia* (cecal worms and roundworms). There is generally a 30-day life cycle from ova to adult. Adults embedded in the crop mucosa or small intestine produce ova that are shed in the feces. The ova of most *Capillaria* species require an arthropod or earthworm intermediate host for transmission, but *Chaetoceros contortus* can also be transmitted directly through consumption of the ova [31]. *C. annulatus* and *C. contortus* are embedded in the crop mucosa in large numbers, and the affected birds can be depressed, weak and emaciated, often dying without premonitory signs. Birds might occasionally gasp if agitated because of respiratory difficulty. When pressing on the crop of an infected live bird, one might express white to gray opaque crop fluid into the oral cavity [15].

In mild infections the crop mucosa can be covered with a thin, white film, while in heavy infections the entire crop wall can be thickened and fluid-filled, with a rough, irregular mucosa covered by a thick white, fibrinonecrotic exudate (Figure 11.3). The infection can extend beyond the crop into adjacent regions of the esophagus. In species affecting the small intestine and cecum, such as *C. caudinflata* and *C. phasianina*, respectively, the affected organ can be distended with mucus and have a tan pseudomembrane or pointpoint ulcers on the mucosa [15].

Table 11.1 Infection sites and hosts for the life cycle of various *Capillaria* species.

Capillaria species	Infection sites	Intermediate host	Definitive host
C. (Eucoleus) annulatus	Esophagus, crop	Earthworm	Pheasant [8, 9] Partridge [10, 11] Quail [12] Guineafowl [13]
C. (Eucoleus) contortus	Esophagus, crop	None or earthworm	Pheasant [14–16] Partridge [17] Quail [18] Peafowl [19] Guineafowl [13]
C. anatis	Cecum	None	Pheasant [20] Partridge [17]
C. (Aonchotheca) bursata	Small intestine	Earthworm	Pheasant [8, 21]
C. caudinflata	Small intestine	Earthworm	Pheasant [15, 16] Partridge [11, 22] Quail [23] Guineafowl [24, 25]
C. (Baruscapillaria) obsignata	Small intestine	None	Pheasant [14, 26] Partridge [11, 27] Quail [14, 23] Guineafowl [24]
C. phasianina	Cecum, small intestine	Not reported	Pheasant [8, 14, 16] Partridge [28]
C. perforans	Esophagus, crop	Not reported	Pheasant [9, 29] Partridge [28, 29] Guineafowl [29, 30]

Diagnosis can be made by examining mucosal scrapings or washings under a microscope to view the nematodes and distinctive bioperculate ova (Figure 11.4) or by histopathology of the affected segment of the digestive tract. *Capillaria* nematodes have distinctive histologic morphologic features (coelomyarian-polymarian musculature and bacillary bands in hypodermis), including the distinctive bioperculate ova in the reproductive tract. Capillarid adults, depending on the species of nematode, burrow into the mucosa of the crop or deep into the glands of the small intestine to induce necrosis and heterophilic to granulomatous inflammation [13, 15].

Fenbendazole, mebendazole, and tramisole (levamisole) as off-label medications are effective treatment for *Capillaria* in poultry [32–34], including peafowl [35]. Infections are most severe in birds raised on soil or floor because of the greater opportunity for fecal–oral transmission. Raising smaller gamebirds (quail, partridge) on wire at early ages can decrease the buildup of *Capillaria* ova. Rotating the use of pens or moving the flight pens intermittently will decrease the buildup of ova in the soil. Keep the soil dry and well drained to decrease the number of earthworms. Intermittent tilling of the soil may help cover manure to reduce exposure to nematode ova.

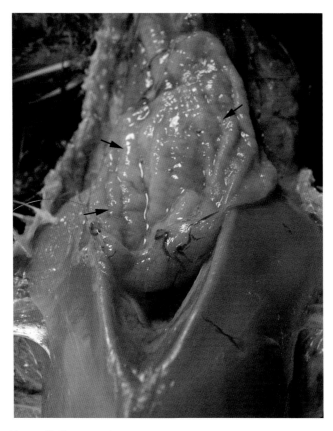

Figure 11.3   Bobwhite quail. The opened crop has white, rugated, thickened mucosa (arrows) caused by *Capillaria* nematodes embedded in the crop wall.

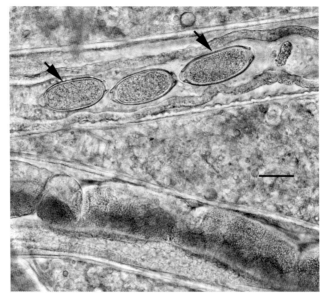

Figure 11.4   Mucosal scraping of crop mucosa reveals *Capillaria* nematodes containing distinctive bioperculate ova (arrows). Bar = 50 μm.

11.1.3 Trichomoniasis

Members of the protozoal family Trichomonadidae, mainly *Trichomonas gallinae* and *Tetratrichomonas gallinarum*, are digestive tract parasites in birds; infections have been described worldwide, most commonly affecting passerines, pigeons, raptors, chickens, and turkeys, among others. The condition is known as "canker" in pigeons and doves and as "frounce" in raptors and passerine birds.

Trichomonad infections have been described in pheasants, partridge, quail, and guineafowl. First, *T. gallinae* is more pathogenic than *Tetratrichomonas gallinarum* [36]. Infections are often worse and more extensive in birds that have concomitant infections and are raised under poor conditions. Fecal–oral spread and consumption of contaminated water and feed are the likely routes of transmission, but some authors have suggested retrograde infection of colon as an alternative route [37], particularly with *Te. gallinarum*. Infected birds excrete live parasites as soon as 2 days post infection, as demonstrated by experimental infection [38]. Field surveys of wild bobwhite quail failed to find *T. gallinae*, suggesting that either the infection is more common in farm-raised birds or the route of transmission is hindered in nature [39].

Clinical signs associated with avian trichomoniasis are loss of appetite, vomiting, ruffled feathers, diarrhea, dysphagia, dyspnea, weight loss, increased thirst, inability to stand or to maintain balance, and a pendulous crop [38]. *T. gallinae* has been well described in Columbidae (pigeons) with necrotizing lesions in the upper digestive tract. *Te. gallinarum* can also cause typhlohepatitis in galliform and anseriform birds [38].

Trichomonads have been described in a variety of gamebirds. *Trichomonas phasiani* has long been associated with mortality in young pheasants, with yellow, fluid-filled ceca containing the protozoa [40]. Wichmann and Bankowski described young chukar partridges with fatal *Te. gallinarum* infection, as confirmed by wet-mount preparations collected from multifocal necrotic lesions in the cecum and liver [37]. Other trichomonas infections have been described in quail. *Tritrichomonas gigantica* caused mortality in coturnix quail [41], and a unique *Tritrichomonas* species has been described in a single coturnix quail [42].

Trichomonads colonize specific regions of the digestive tract after infection. *T. gallinae* occurs in the mouth, pharynx, esophagus, and crop, with the parasite rarely found posterior to the proventriculus. *T. gallinae* causes inflammation of the mucosa and accumulation of caseous exudate, which can block the esophagus and subsequently kill the host through starvation (Figure 11.5). Trichomonads can survive in a moist environment for 4–5 days [39]. Lesions associated with *Te. gallinarum* occur most often in the cecum and colon and can be variable in extent, often manifested as dilated fluid-filled intestines. *Te. gallinarum* has caused fatal typhlocolitis in the red-legged partridge with histopathologic evidence of necrotic foci containing intralesional protozoa in the cecum, liver, and spleen [36]. It appears that in many instances, *Te. gallinarum* can be present without clinical signs or gross lesions, but the protozoa can contribute to disease in birds with other enteric infections, including *Salmonella*, *Spironucleus*, and *Blastocystis* sp.

Diagnosis of trichomoniasis is based on gross lesions and observation of the protozoa through histology or cytologic wet mounts. Histopathology of *Te. gallinarum* can be based on protozoa situated in the mucosal glands or there can be moderate diffuse lymphocytic infiltration of the cecal or colonic mucosa associated with a large number of protozoa within the lumen. Live trichomonads can be observed on direct microscopic observation of motile protozoa via wet-mount preparation (mucosal scraping placed on a wet glass slide) from a live or recently euthanized bird. Sample material can be obtained via swabbing the cloacae for *Te. gallinarum* [43] or the oral cavity for *T. gallinae* [44]. Trichomonads appear as elongated, oval shapes, which move briskly. The

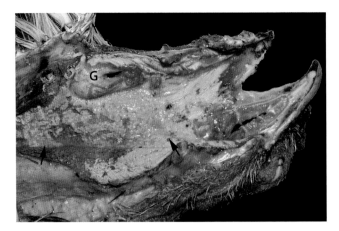

Figure 11.5   *Trichomonas* infection is often observed as white to yellow pseudomembrane (arrows) in the oral cavity and esophagus, as shown in this galliform bird. G, glottis.

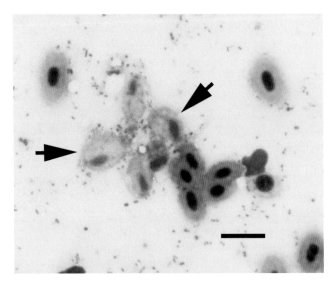

Figure 11.6   Cytologic imprint of oral mucosa of racing pigeon with *Trichomonas gallinae* infection. Note the cluster of five ovoid protozoa (arrows) with multiple anterior flagella. The field also contains erythrocytes and bacteria. Diff-Quik stain, bar = 10 μm.

wet-mount sample smeared on a glass slide can be stained with Wright-Giemsa to demonstrate protozoal detail [45]. The oval to pear-shaped protozoa are 4–6 μm by 8–14 μm. They contain a single axostyle, a 1–2 μm diameter parabasal body and multiple anterior flagella (Figure 11.6).

Treatment can be challenging because of the lack of approved antiprotozoal drugs. Various nitroimidazoles, including metronidazole, dimetridazole, ronidazole, and carnidazole, have been considered the standard treatment for avian trichomoniasis [38, 46, 47], but these products are no longer approved for meat-type birds. Prevention should be the major focus. Trichomonads have limited survival in a dry environment. Because trichomonads can be harbored in wild birds, strict biosecurity should prevent entry of wild carrier birds into pens and buildings, particularly those harboring gamebird chicks. Routine cleaning and disinfection of brooding pens between grow-outs are essential.

11.2 Conditions of the Proventriculus and Gizzard

11.2.1 Dispharynx Nasuta (Proventricular and Gizzard Worm)

Dispharynx nasuta, a spirurid nematode, has been recognized in wild passerine and galliform birds, including upland gamebirds, for many years. It appears to be present most often in wild-caught upland gamebirds, but the risk for domestic birds remains. *Dispharynx* has been reported in pheasants [21], partridges [48], quail [49], peafowl [50, 51] and guineafowl [52]. *D. nasuta* adults reside in the proventriculus, and less often the esophagus or gizzard, of infected birds. The life cycle is often indirect with an invertebrate intermediate host. Adult nematodes produce eggs that are shed in host feces.

Birds become infected by consuming an isopod intermediate host that has eaten the nematode ova. The most common intermediate hosts involved with the indirect life cycle are isopod crustaceans – pillbugs (*Armadillidium vulgare*) and sowbugs (*Porcellio scaber*). Larvae develop to the infective stage in the intermediate host within 26 days and are viable in this host for up to 6 months. When the isopod is ingested by a bird host, the infective larvae then escape and migrate/attach to the proventriculus or gizzard lining where they develop into adults within 27 days [53].

The parasitic infections are often subclinical, but if infection is severe with a high parasite load, the birds can become emaciated, weak, and anemic from blood loss in the proventriculus. The proventriculus is distended with mucus and the proventricular walls are thickened. Numerous 5–8 mm long, white, coiled nematodes can be observed adhered to the mucosal lining (Figure 11.7) [21]. In light infections, inflammation and hypertrophy of the mucosa occur. In heavy infections, the adult worms penetrate the mucosa, creating deep ulcers, glandular hyperplasia, and thickening of the mucosal layer.

Numerous classic broad-spectrum anthelmintics are effective against *Dyspharynx* nematodes, including several benzimidazoles (albendazole, fenbendazole, flubendazole, mebendazole, oxfendazole, etc.), levamisole, and macrocyclic lactones (e.g., ivermectin) [31].

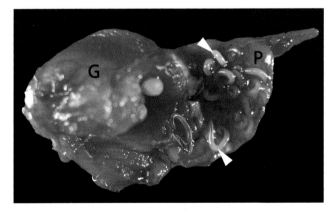

Figure 11.7 The proventriculus (P) of a passerine bird contains numerous adult *Dispharynx nasuta* nematodes (arrowheads). G, gizzard. Source: Photo used by permission of Dr Arno Wuenschmann, University of Minnesota.

11.2.2 Tetrameridosis (*Tetrameres* sp.)

This condition encompasses nematode parasitism associated with three genera of the family tetrameridae: Tetrameres, Microtetrameres, and Geopetitia. Adult nematodes are often embedded in the proventricular glands, with or without associated clinical signs. The condition is characterized in both aquatic and terrestrial birds, including pigeons [54]. The nematode infection has been reported in gamebirds, including ring-necked pheasants [21], partridges [17], quail [55, 56], guineafowl [57–59] and peafowl [60]. In the literature, the species of *Tetrameres* is not always determined, but *T. americana* and *T. pattersoni* have been reported in bobwhite quail [55]. *Tetrameres fissipina* was reported in ring-necked pheasants [21] and *T. numida* is described in helmeted guineafowl [59].

Tetramerid nematodes show sexual dimorphism. Both the female and smaller male nematodes are often in copulation within the proventricular glands. In the life cycle involving terrestrial bird hosts, gravid female nematodes residing in the proventricular glands lay eggs that are shed in the feces and ultimately consumed by intermediate hosts, such as grasshoppers, cockroaches or earthworms, depending on the genus or species of nematode [54]. The cycle is completed following consumption of the intermediate host.

Because this parasite is relatively rare in gamebirds, clincal signs are poorly described; however, in the authors' experience, these nematode parasites are usually a secondary, subclinical finding. Fecal flotation is generally not useful for diagnosis and necropsy/histopathology is suggested. Gross lesions of tetrameridosis are usually observed when the birds are necropsied for other primary conditions. The female nematodes appear as dark, red 2–4 mm diameter nodules within the wall of the proventriculus (Figure 11.8). Histopathology is confirmatory and reveals cross-sections of female and male nematodes within dilated proventricular glands with or without glandular atrophy and minimal inflammation. The need for treatment is unlikely, but control should be based on reducing exposure to the intermediate host in the soil by maintaining dry soil and practicing insect control.

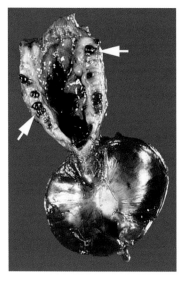

Figure 11.8   The proventriculus of pigeon contains multiple dark, round foci (arrows) corresponding to female *Tetrameres* sp. embedded in the wall.

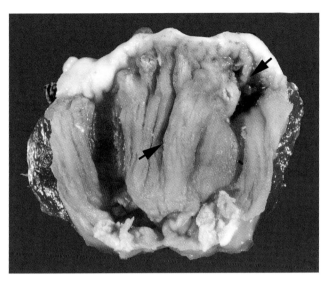

Figure 11.9   The gizzard of a 2-week-old bobwhite quail has a thick, brown to yellow koilin layer, which is distorted by pits and linear erosions (arrows). Fowl adenovirus 1 was isolated from the gizzard.

11.2.3   Miscellaneous Gizzard Conditions

Factors associated with gizzard erosion and ulceration in domestic poultry include bacterial infection, histamine, gizzerosine, mycotoxins, and vitamin deficiencies [61, 62]. Affected gizzards usually have a thickened, dark tan to gray lining with multiple linear erosions and ulcerations (Figure 11.9). Additionally, koilin erosion and ulceration is commonly observed in young gamebirds with paratyphoid *Salmonella* infection or pica/litter consumption, resulting in litter accumulation in gizzard. In these instances, the damage to the koilin layer is caused by bacterial overgrowth and direct invasion of koilin by bacterial colonies.

Gizzard koilin erosions associated with infection with fowl adenovirus 1 (FAdV-1) have been reported in coturnix quail [63] and bobwhite quail [64]. In the latter report, the 2-week-old bobwhite quail were depressed with loose droppings and increased mortality. The only lesions were observed in gizzards. Histologically, gizzards are inflamed with multifocal koilin degeneration and fragmentation, epithelial degeneration and necrosis, and infiltration of inflammatory cells. Necrotic epithelial cells contained large, basophilic intranuclear inclusions, and FAdV-1 was isolated from affected gizzards. The lesions resembled those reported in broiler chickens infected with FAdV-1. Both vertical and horizontal transmission were reported as important routes for the spread of FAdVs [65].

Gizzard "impaction," more accurately referred to as litter eating, is common in young, commercial gallinaceous birds that are brooded on litter, such as wood shavings, straw, or peanut hulls. Young, curious birds raised on sawdust, sand or small particle size straw may consume the litter to excess, resulting in accumulation of the coarse material in the gizzard (Figure 11.10). Litter consumption may not affect the health of the birds, but it can reduce feed efficiency and promote bacterial enteritis. Alternatively, litter consumption is often a necropsy finding in birds that have been ill with a digestive tract disorder or have no access to feed because of lameness or malfunction of the feeder system. In these cases, the consumption of litter is not the primary issue, but it is a symptom of a larger management issue.

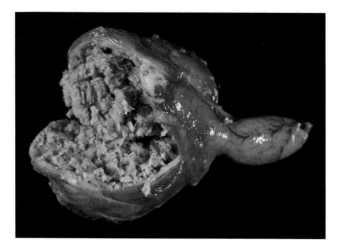

Figure 11.10   The gizzard from a 3-week-old partridge was filled with litter. The condition of litter eating was a complication of marked coccidiosis in the flock.

11.3   Conditions of the Intestine and Cecum

11.3.1   Salmonellosis

A variety of bacteria from the Enterobacteriaceae family can affect the digestive tract of birds, but *Salmonella* is recognized as the most important aerobic bacterial pathogen of the gamebird digestive tract. *Salmonella* sp. are Gram-negative bacterial rods that can infect all types of birds and mammals. In gamebird chicks, *Salmonella* most often infects the digestive tract and yolk sac. It can also be harbored in the intestine of adult birds with no clinical signs. *Salmonella* infection in gamebirds is primarily a problem of young birds, although the adults (breeders) can still be involved as carriers and periodic shedders of bacteria. The veterinary literature distinguishes between avian Salmonellae that are largely avian-adapted serovars – *Salmonella pullorum* and *S. gallinarum*, the causes of pullorum disease and fowl typhoid, respectively – and 200 other serovars (paratyphoid species) of *Salmonella* that are not avian adapted and can occur in a variety of species. These avian-adapted and paratyphoid *Salmonella* serovars will be addressed separately.

Fowl typhoid and pullorum disease are caused by two different biovars of *S. enterica* subsp. *enterica serovar gallinarum*, a Gram-negative bacterial rod in *Salmonella* serogroup D (nonflagellated organisms with O antigens 1, 9, and 12) in the family Enterobacteriaceae. *S. enterica* subsp. *enterica serovar gallinarum biovar gallinarum*, which causes fowl typhoid, is usually abbreviated as *S. gallinarum*, and *S. enterica* subsp. *enterica ser. fallinarum biovar pullorum* as *S. pullorum* [66]. Recently, *S. pullorum* (pullorum disease) and *S. gallinarum* (fowl typhoid) were taxonomically assigned to a single serovar (*S. pullorum-gallinarum*), but because the microorganisms are both biochemically and genetically distinguishable, they are often referred to as separate species and conditions.

Salmonella pullorum and *S. gallinarum* are nonmotile and tend to be specific for birds, while the motile paratyphoid serotypes can infect a wide variety of birds and mammals. These have been described in most upland gamebirds.

Salmonella pullorum and *S. gallinarum* (*S. pullorum-gallinarum*) are relatively nonmotile and are generally considered to be species specific for birds. Disease with typhoid has been described in pheasants, partridges, quail, peafowl, and guinea hens, as well as chickens and turkeys [66–69].

S. pullorum-gallinarum can be harbored in adult birds and cause little to no clinical signs, but these microorganisms can be vertically transmitted from the ovary of the hen into the egg and then to hatchling chicks. Chicks can appear normal at hatch, but they can transmit *Salmonella* laterally and experience heavy mortality during the next 3 weeks, with death in the early brooding stages. For reasons previously stated, both *S. pullorum* and *S. gallinarum* are regularly monitored in US commercial poultry breeder flocks that participate in the National Poultry Improvement Plan (NPIP) [66].

Clinical signs of pullorum disease, apart from sudden mortality of hatchlings, are nonspecific. In one study, bobwhite quail infected with *S. pullorum* were depressed with closed eyes, ruffled feathers, profuse white diarrhea, and 75% mortality from hatch to 16–17 days of age [69]. There is delayed resorption of the yolk sac in chicks, with inflammatory foci, sometimes forming large nodules, in liver, heart, kidney, spleen, pancreas, intestine, and articular joints [66]. Fowl typhoid affects both young and old birds. As with pullorum disease, chicks with fowl typhoid may be found dead soon after hatching while depression, decreased appetite, weight loss, dehydration, ruffled feathers, and watery to mucoid yellowish diarrhea can be observed in live birds. In some instances, breeders infected with *S. gallinarum* will have decreased egg production as well. In one study, Japanese quail chicks infected with *S. gallinarum* had enlarged livers and spleens with pale, necrotic foci as well as similar foci in kidney and heart. Histologic evidence of sepsis with necrotic foci and intralesional bacteria is observed in a variety of internal organs, particularly liver and spleen [70].

Diagnosis of pullorum disease can be confirmed by assessment of clinical signs, gross and histologic lesions and bacterial culture. The whole-blood plate test is routinely used to assess breeder flocks for the presence of antibodies (reactors) to *S. pullorum* or *S. gallinarum*, which are antigenically similar. Salmonellae can be isolated by recommended procedures [71]. Veterinarians or diagnostic labs that suspect a flock is infected with pullorum disease or fowl typhoid should contact their NPIP office or state veterinarian immediately. There is no antibiotic treatment for pullorum or fowl typhoid as the entire exposed flock will face euthanasia in an eradication effort as determined by the state veterinarian.

There are over 2000 serovars of paratyphoid *Salmonella* and about 10% of these have been described in poultry. A variety of paratyphoid *Salmonella* has been described in gamebirds, guineafowl, and peafowl. For example, there are reports of *Salmonella derby* and *S. anatum* in chukar partridge chicks [72], *S. typhimurium* in bobwhite quail [73], *S. typhimurium*, *S. kentucky*, and *S. enteritidis* in golden pheasants in a zoological exhibit [74]. Gross lesions of paratyphoid *Salmonella* in gamebirds are most prominent in chicks and include dehydration, distended abdomens, enlarged liver and spleen, dark or hemorrhagic yolk sacs and increased mucus and frothy fluid in the intestine (Figure 11.11) [73]. Gamebird chicks can pile in the corners of the pen. Dead chicks often have enlarged livers and spleens with caseous, white to tan exudate in the cecum (Figure 11.12). Birds can have a variety of histologic lesions indicative of sepsis, including interstitial pneumonia, necrotizing hepatitis and splenitis, and fibrinonecrotic typhlitis.

Diagnosis of paratyphoid *Salmonella* infections is readily made on gross and microscopic lesions and culture of the causative agent. Antibiotic treatment should be based on culture and sensitivity, but few antibiotics are approved for use in poultry. Paratyphoid infections can be treated with antibiotics in feed or drinking water, but affected chicks will continue to die because they are usually not eating or drinking ("starve-outs"). Walking the house or running the feeder may stimulate chick activity. Antibiotics can help the birds in the pen that are least affected and most susceptible to contracting the infection. Because of a diminishing supply of approved antibiotics, some

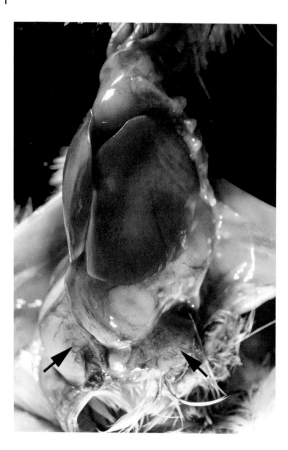

Figure 11.11 A ring-necked pheasant chick with paratyphoid *Salmonella* (Group B). Note the enlarged liver with impressions from ribs and keelbone, and the hemorrhages on the yolk sac (arrows).

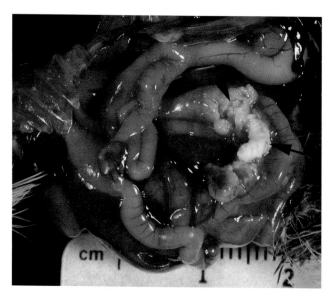

Figure 11.12 A ring-necked pheasant chick infected with paratyphoid strain of *Salmonella* (*S. kentucky*). The cecum contains caseous exudate (arrows).

operations are looking at alternative therapies such as essential oils, probiotics, berry extracts, and organic acids [75].

Strong biosecurity is key in preventing the infection from getting into the farms and flocks. Several species of paratyphoid Salmonellae, such as *S. enterica serovar enteritidis* [76], can enter the egg before hatch while others infect the chick in the pen through shell contamination or lateral transmission in feces. Employees who have contact with infected birds can introduce the infection into a clean flock. A comprehensive biosecurity program should cover all potential sources of poultry farm contamination. Sources of *Salmonella* contamination include the following [72, 77, 78].

1. Infected breeder flock
2. Soiled or manure-contaminated hatching eggs
3. Contaminated byproducts in feed
4. Feces of other infected chicks
5. Hatchery contamination
6. Vectors: mice, rats, insects, and wild birds
7. Dirty litter or poorly disinfected flooring, feeders, drinkers
8. Young and old birds in close proximity
9. Vehicle traffic (delivery and feeder trucks) on the farm
10. Human foot traffic

11.3.2 Ulcerative Enteritis (Quail Disease)

Ulcerative enteritis (UE) or "quail disease" is a severe bacterial disease produced by *Clostridium colinum* that is highly contagious and produces high mortality in bobwhite quail (*Colinus virginianus*) [79, 80]. *C. colinum* is a Gram-positive, spore-forming, anaerobic bacterial rod and, based on 16S rRNA sequencing, it is closely related to *C. piliforme*, the causative agent for Tyzzer disease [81]. The organism is hardy in the environment. More recently, other Clostridia, such as *C. perfringens* type A and *C. sordellii*, have been determined to cause similar lesions in the intestines of quail [82, 83]. UE is diagnosed most often in bobwhite quail, and has been reported in other upland gamebirds (pheasants, grouse, partridges, California quail), as well as young turkeys and white leghorn pullets. UE appears typically between 4 and 20 weeks of age with a mortality rate of up to 50% or more in untreated flocks [84–86]. The lesions are characterized by multifocal discoid ulcers in the small intestine and multifocal hepatic necrosis.

The microorganism spreads rapidly from bird to bird via the fecal–oral route. It is shed in the feces of infected birds and is hardy, persisting in the soil or litter for several months. UE is rare in quail raised on wire. The infection can be spread in contaminated feces by flies.

Quail are usually 4–10 weeks of age at sudden death associated with white, watery diarrhea. Birds that do not die suddenly will be depressed with closed eyes, ruffled feathers, and bloody diarrhea. Infected birds are thirsty and will huddle around the drinkers. The course of disease is about two weeks and can result in nearly 100% mortality in bobwhite quail [87].

Necropsy findings are consistent. Crops can be distended with fluid. Affected birds have deep, punctate to discoid, tan to yellow ulcers along the small intestine (Figures 11.13 and 11.14). The ulcers often penetrate the entire wall of the intestine to result in peritonitis and adherence of intestinal loops. The liver may or may not have pale foci of necrosis on the capsule and on cut surfaces. Histologic lesions are further supportive of the diagnosis and in the intestine consist of severe multifocal mucosal to transmural necrosis with numerous inflammatory cells and large Gram-positive

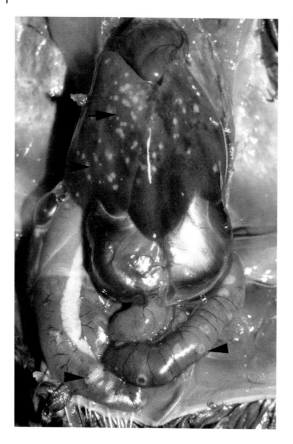

Figure 11.13 Four-week-old bobwhite quail with ulcerative enteritis. Note the multifocal punctate ulcers in the liver (arrows) and small intestine (arrowheads).

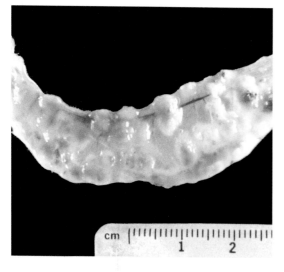

Figure 11.14 Small intestine of 4-week-old bobwhite quail with ulcerative enteritis. Multifocal punctate, transmural ulcers (arrows) on the serosa and mucosa are typical of this condition.

bacterial rods. Peritonitis with serosal fibrosis can occur adjacent to the transmural lesions. The liver has acute, moderate to marked, multifocal hepatocellular necrosis with fibrin exudation and varying numbers of intralesional rod-shaped Gram-positive bacteria [86]. The flock history along with the gross and histologic lesions are usually diagnostic.

The microorganism can be cultured from liver and intestine, but culture of the agent from typical lesions can be challenging because of fastidious growth requirements [80, 88]. Culture can be important if one is differentiating UE (*C. colinum*) from necrotic enteritis (*C. perfringens*) [89]. Polymerase chain reaction (PCR) testing for *C. colinum* has been reported, but the assay is not readily available for laboratory diagnosis [90].

Clostridium colinum is sensitive to a wide range of antimicrobials including penicillin, oxytetracycline, monensin, and bacitracin [88]. Bacitracin is generally the antibiotic of choice at 100–200 g/ton of feed for 7–10 days, or in the water at 0.25–0.50 g per gallon of water for 7–10 days. Antibiotics may not be successful if birds are not eating or drinking; workers should walk the pens and run the feeders and drinkers to encourage bird activity. UE rarely occurs in quail raised on wire, although the microorganism can be spread by flies. Rotation of pens on a regular basis can reduce exposure to *Clostridium* spores.

11.3.3 Enteric Viruses

The role that viruses play in gamebird enteric disease is poorly characterized. In the authors' diagnostic experience, the most common viruses detected by electron microscopy of the feces of pheasants, partridges, and quail are rotavirus, reovirus, and adenovirus. Calicivirus has also been associated with enteritis in gamebirds and will be described below.

Because commercial gamebirds are grown in a concentrated confinement setting prior to release, one would expect them to have enteric viral diseases that are similar to those of other intensively farmed poultry; however, studies on the viral agents producing digestive disease in gamebirds are limited. Additionally, in the field, these various enteric viruses are often found in association with other infectious agents, such as coccidia and *Salmonella* sp. Therefore, the role of these viruses may be additive at best.

To characterize the effect of enteric viruses in a diagnostic setting, it is essential to receive freshly dead or euthanized birds to reduce autolysis artifact in microscopic sections of digestive tract. Bacterial culture, virus isolation, electron microscopy on negatively stained feces, and, for some viruses, PCR analysis of intestine or feces are part of a thorough enteric virus workup.

11.3.3.1 Enteric Rotavirus

Rotavirus is a nonenveloped, icosahedral, double-stranded RNA virus of the reovirus family. The virus replicates in and destroys intestinal enterocytes to cause villus blunting, resulting in malabsorption and diarrhea. The nucleocapsid (genetic core) contains 11 segments of double-stranded RNA. Each gene segment encodes a different viral protein to create the entire virus [91]. The virus must invade intestinal epithelial cells to survive in vivo.

Rotavirus was first identified in the diarrheic feces of turkey poults [92], and different strains of rotaviruses have been identified in turkeys, pigeons, chickens, guineafowl, lovebirds, partridges, and pheasants. In gamebirds, the virus typically causes diarrhea in pheasant and partridge chicks [93]. Avian rotaviruses can be characterized into different groups by serum neutralization, enzyme-linked immunosorbent assay (ELISA) and by migration patterns on polyacrylamide gel electrophoresis [94]. Type A, D, F, and G rotaviruses have been detected in birds, and type A and D have been characterized in pheasants. By genetic analysis, pheasant rotaviruses are only distantly related to other poultry rotaviruses [95]. Most human rotaviruses are type A, but there is no evidence that avian rotaviruses can be transmitted to people; these viruses are antigenically and genetically dissimilar [96]. Avian rotaviruses have not been detected in humans and human rotaviruses have not been detected in birds.

Large numbers of rotaviruses are shed in the feces of infected birds. The virus is then contracted by swallowing contaminated manure which may be on the soil, feeder, drinker or equipment, shoes and clothing of workers. There is no evidence that rotavirus can be transmitted inside eggs. The virus must multiply in mature enterocytes at the tips (apices) of intestinal villi rather than the deeper crypts [97]. Damage to enterocytes with blunting of the villi will impair the absorption of fluid and nutrients, resulting in diarrhea with increased fluid in the intestinal lumen. Virus can be observed by electron microscopy of feces or intestinal contents [98, 99].

Clinical signs of rotavirus infection in pheasants and partridges usually start as early as 4–14 days of age, but signs can be observed in birds as old as 6 weeks. Clinical signs include death without pre-monitory signs, depression, huddling, piling in corners, decreased feed consumption, discomfort as evidenced by chirping and consumption of litter, and diarrhea or wet litter. Rotavirus infection in gamebird chicks is often complicated by *Salmonella* or *Escherichia coli* infection, and the virus can be apathogenic as a solitary infection [91]. Gross necropsy reveals dehydrated carcasses, fecal pasting of the vent feathers, pale viscera and small intestine, and ceca dilated with yellow frothy fluid (Figure 11.15) [94]. Gizzards can contain litter.

11.3.3.2 Enteric Reovirus

Avian reoviruses (ARVs) are one of the 15 members of the genus *Orthoreovirus* in the family Reoviridae. ARVs are nonencapsulated and contain 10 double-stranded RNA segments [100]. An estimated 85–90% of ARVs are nonpathogenic while the pathogenic ARVs cause lameness, immune dysfunction and infection of liver, heart, and intestine. These viruses can be isolated from the tissues or organs of affected birds [101, 102] and from the gastrointestinal and respiratory tracts of clinically healthy birds [103]. The clinical disease is dependent upon the host's age and immune status, virus

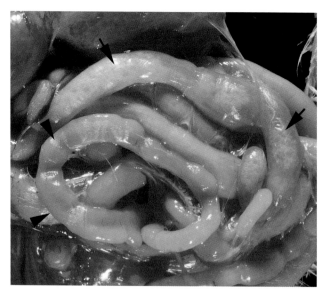

Figure 11.15 Nine-day-old pheasant chick with rotaviral enteritis. The small intestines (arrowhead) and ceca (arrows) are pale and distended with clear, frothy fluid.

pathotype, and route of exposure [104, 105]. In commercial chickens and turkeys, economic losses are a result of decreased livability, diminished weight gains, poor feed efficiency, uneven growth rate, nonuniformity of the flock, and reduced marketability owing to downgraded carcass quality at slaughter [106, 107].

Mutlu et al. observed green, watery diarrhea and increased mortality associated with reovirus infection in a pheasant flock; the birds had catarrhal enteritis from which reovirus was isolated [108]. In another report, both rotavirus and reovirus were isolated from feces of 7-week-old ring-necked pheasants with ruffled feathers, increased water consumption, diarrhea, and mortality. Phylogenetic analyses of this pheasant reovirus revealed a reassortant virus with gene segments shared by chicken, partridge, and turkey reoviruses [109]. Kugler et al. characterized a reovirus isolated from gray partridges as showing genetic sequences that were similar to those of chicken enteric reovirus; however, the partridge virus was isolated from the respiratory tract rather than digestive tract [110]. Magee et al. [111] described depression and death in 10–14-day-old quail with necrotizing hepatitis; reovirus was isolated and the condition was experimentally reproduced. Both coccidia and adenovirus were sometimes isolated from these field cases [111]. In an additional study, reovirus and *Cryptosporidium* oocysts were identified in intestinal contents of 5-day-old commercial bobwhite quail with severe enteritis, hepatic necrosis, and mortality; however, experimental oral inoculation of quail with reovirus alone caused no clinical signs, while inoculation with both reovirus and *Cryptosporidium* resulted in severe enteritis and mortality. These results indicated that *Cryptosporidium* was the primary pathogen, and reovirus served only to exacerbate the protozoal infection in quail [112].

From the above reports, it is evident that the role of reovirus as a primary digestive tract pathogen in gamebirds is tentative and that the virus may play a role in enteric disease with multifactorial causes.

11.3.3.3 Other Enteric Viruses

Coronaviruses are enveloped, positive sense, single-stranded RNA viruses in the subfamily Orthocoronavirinae, family Coronaviridae. These viruses have a wide range of hosts and have been associated with enteritis in quail and guineafowl. In one report, farm-reared coturnix quail showed depression, diarrhea, and reduced growth rate, with the most severe mortality in the youngest birds (3 weeks). The prominent lesion in the quail was enteritis, with coronavirus observed in intestinal contents by electron microscopy [113]. Sequence analysis of the virus revealed genetic similarities to turkey coronavirus. Similarly, Japanese quail with high mortality had histologic lesions of decreased villous length, increased crypt depth, and lymphoplasmacytic infiltrates in the lamina propria of small intestine [114]. Metagenomic analysis of intestinal contents from the quail revealed predominantly coronavirus with a lesser percentage of picornavirus. The coronavirus shared genetic similarity to turkey enteric coronavirus and infectious bronchitis virus [114].

In France, there are reports of a novel avian coronavirus implicated as one of the causes of an enteric condition of guineafowl known as "fulminating disease." Clinical signs of the fulminating disease of guineafowl were prostration, decreased water and feed consumption, with mortality reaching as high as 20% per day. Lesions of enteritis and an enlarged, white pancreas (pancreatic degeneration) were observed. In most instances, a coronavirus was identified by electron microscopy of intestinal contents, immunohistochemistry, PCR or whole-genome sequencing [115, 116]. This novel virus has been sequenced and renamed as guineafowl coronavirus, a gammacoronavirus [117].

Caliciviruses are in the family Caliciviridae and are small, nonenveloped, single-stranded RNA viruses with distinct cup-shaped surface structures [118]. Gough et al. described calicivirus in the feces of 3–4-week-old pheasant chicks with mild enteritis, inappetence, and weight loss with eventual loss of 25% of the flock [119]. Similarly, in another report, 3–4-week-old farm-reared ring-necked pheasants had high mortality from enteritis, preceded by depression and dehydration. These chicks had histological evidence of hepatic necrosis and severe enteritis, and the predominant virus observed in feces by electron microscopy was calicivirus, although parvovirus and reovirus were also observed [120]. In another report, calicivirus was observed in the cecal contents of 6–16-day-old guineafowl keets with acute, 50% mortality and prominent lesions of typhlitis [121].

Astroviruses are nonenveloped, 28–30 nm diameter, positive-sense, single-stranded RNA viruses that infect both mammals and birds [122]. Farmed guineafowl experiencing enteritis and mortality were found by molecular analysis to contain astrovirus in their feces [123, 124], and cross-species transmission between turkeys and guineafowl was suspected [123]. Experimental oral inoculation of both 5-day-old guineafowl and turkey poults with the astrovirus resulted in reduced weight gain, ruffled feathers, depression, and diarrhea of 5–6 days duration, accompanied by histologic lesions of enteritis and bursa atrophy [125].

Picorna-like viruses have been detected from feces of both quail and guineafowl. Picornaviruses are small nonenveloped viruses with single-stranded, positive-sense genomic RNA [126]. Quail deaths were observed without clinical signs and the feces consistently contained picornavirus; however, the presence of enteritis was not established [127]. Picornavirus, along with coronavirus, was isolated from guineafowl with high mortality and enteritis and may play a role in the enteritis associated with the previously described guineafowl fulminating disease [116].

Finally, viruses morphologically resembling parvovirus were associated with anorexia, depression, and sudden, high mortality in captive-farmed 15–25-day-old Mongolian pheasants. The pheasant chicks had both catarrhal enteritis and necrotizing hepatitis, and parvo-like virus was observed in tissues by electron microscopy [128].

11.3.3.4 Treatment of Enteric Viruses

Treatment of enteric viruses should focus on prevention because antibiotics are not effective and there are no commercial vaccines for enteric viruses of gamebirds. Although enteric viruses cannot be killed by antibiotics, the antibiotics can help to prevent secondary bacterial infection. Farms with a history of viral enteritis in successive grow-outs might consider the use of probiotics in healthy chicks. Increase the temperature under the brooder for chilled birds and walk the pen several times a day to stimulate the birds to move, eat, and drink. An inactive gamebird chick will not survive. Avoid contact with other gamebird flocks and do not visit other farms or pens if you are working with sick chicks.

Because most of the RNA enteric viruses do not possess a lipid envelope, they are not readily killed by detergents and can be resistant to some disinfectants. Generic disinfectants that should be effective against enteric viruses include oxine, glutaraldehyde, hydrogen peroxide, sodium hypochlorite (bleach), phenol, and chlorhexidine [129]. In the face of an enteric virus outbreak or when the house is empty between flocks, one should replace litter, thoroughly dry clean floors, walls, drinkers, and feeders and then wet clean with detergent followed by disinfection. Sunlight and downtime in the brooder pen are also effective in reducing the load of bacteria and viruses. More aggressive disinfection might be needed if the brooder pen contains irregular or creviced surfaces such as wood, soil, and concrete.

Enhanced chick-rearing biosecurity is important to reduce the opportunity for introduction of infectious agents. Chicks raised on wire flooring at early ages generally have fewer outbreaks of rotavirus, *Salmonella*, and coccidiosis.

In summary, it may be impossible to eliminate an enteric virus from a premises once it has been introduced, but one can reduce the viral load to which new chicks will be exposed. There are no commercial vaccines for prevention of enteric viruses in gamebirds.

11.3.4 Ascarids (Roundworms)

Ascaridia is a genus of nematode residing in the small intestine and the larval stages migrate in other soft tissues during the life cycle. A summary of ascarid species described in gamebirds is given in Table 11.2.

The life cycle of *Ascaridia galli* is well documented in the chicken and likely reflects the cycle of other *Ascaridia*. The cycle is direct (no intermediate host) and takes about 28–30 days to complete, beginning with nematode ova that are shed in feces into the environment. The ova can remain viable and infectious in the environment for 1–3 years and are resistant to low temperatures [139]. After being shed into the soil or litter, ova must mature or embryonate to be infectious, and this process take 10–12 days. Embryonation occurs faster if the ova are in a moist and warm environment. In some circumstances, ascarids such as *A. galli* can be consumed by earthworms, which then serve as a transport host. In chickens, ingested *A. galli* ova hatch in the lumen of the proventriculus or gizzard, releasing third-stage larvae (L3) that live in the intestinal lumen for 8–10 days. The larvae then burrow into the intestinal mucosa, remaining there for about 17 days before returning to the intestinal lumen to mature. In some instances, the larvae can exhibit ectopic migration and briefly

Table 11.2 Ascarid species referenced in gamebirds, guineafowl, and peafowl.

Ascarid species	Avian host	Reference
Ascaridia galli	Ring-necked pheasant	Gilbertson and Huggins [130]
	Chukar partridge	Tibbits and Babero [131]
	Blood pheasant	Baylis and Daubney [132]
	Barbary partridge	Foronada et al. [11]
	Bobwhite quail	Cram et al. [23]
	Helmeted guineafowl	Ayeni [24]
	Indian peafowl	Yamaguti [133]
Ascaridia compar	Ring-necked pheasant	Barus [134]
	Chukar partridge	Canavan [135]
	Bobwhite quail	Barus [134]
	Coturnix quail	Weatherbee [136]
	Rock partridge	Baylis and Daubney [132]
	Helmeted guineafowl	Cram et al. [23]
Ascaridia numidae	Chukar partridge	Canavan [135]
	Rock partridge	Avcioglu et al. [137]
	Vulturine guineafowl	Barus [134]
	Helmeted guineafowl	Avcioglu et al. [137]
	Crested guineafowl	Skrjabin et al. [138]
Ascaridia cordata	Scaled quail	Cram et al. [23]
Ascaridia columbae	Indian peafowl	Skrjabin et al. [138]

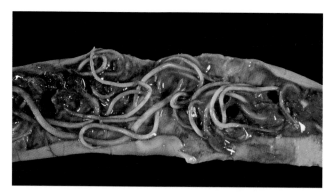

Figure 11.16 The small intestine of a 7-month-old peacock is distended with adult ascarids (*Ascaridia* sp.).

infiltrate viscera in the coelomic cavity, causing a variable degree of tissue damage depending on the nematode load in the host [140, 141].

Clinical signs will correlate with the overall ascarid egg and worm burden on the farm. Infected birds can show no clinical signs, but they serve as a continual source of environmental contamination with ascarid ova. Birds can die acutely from an impaction of large numbers of ascarids in the small intestinal lumen. Other birds, particularly young, can be depressed with decreased feed consumption, weight loss, diarrhea, decreased growth, and poor feathering. *A. galli* can decrease body weight and egg production in laying chickens [141] and similar effects are likely to be observed in gamebird breeder flocks. In severe cases, dead birds can have hundreds of adult nematodes obstructing the small intestine. Carcasses can be dehydrated and emaciated with atrophy of breast muscle and decreased body fat. In other instances, with fewer numbers of nematodes, there will be reddening of the intestinal mucosa with increased mucus. The adult nematodes are narrow, white to yellow, and 5–11 cm long, depending on the species (Figure 11.16).

The diagnosis can be made on gross necropsy findings or fecal flotation (eggs float in zinc sulfate or sodium nitrate solution). On microscopic evaluation, ascarid ova are round to oval (50–100 μm in diameter) and have a chitinous, homogenous shell [140, 141]. Ova from fecal samples or intestinal contents will have early, single cell embryos. Historically, treatments for ascarids have included piperazine, levamisole, and fenbendazole [33, 141, 142]. Several medicinal plant extracts have been shown to have significant anthelmintic activity against *A. galli* in vitro and in vivo. Extracts from *Psorelia corylifolia*, *Piper betle*, *Pilostigma thonningi*, *Caesalpinia crista*, *Ocimum gratissimum*, and *Anacardium occidentale* were effective for reducing *A. galli* numbers in chickens in a dose-dependent manner [142].

For prevention in large flocks, the emphasis should be on reducing the ova burden in the environment. Rotating brooding pens and raising small birds on wire can reduce the initial fecal–oral transmission of nematode ova. Floor-raised chicks should be on deep (3–4 in.) litter with proper cleanup between brooder flocks to reduce exposure to parasite ova. Young birds should be medicated before they are transferred to a larger outdoor flight pen.

11.3.5 *Heterakis gallinarum* (Cecal Worm)

Heterakis sp., the cecal worm, has been described in a variety of gamebirds. *Heterakis gallinarum* has been described in the ring-necked pheasant, blood pheasant, blue-eared pheasant, brown-eared pheasant, cheer pheasant, copper pheasant, gray peacock pheasant, green pheasant, golden pheasant, Kalij pheasant, Lady Amherst's pheasant, silver pheasant, Barbary partridge, chukar partridge, crested partridge, gray partridge, hill partridge, red-legged partridge, rock partridge, coturnix quail, bobwhite quail, helmeted guineafowl, vulturine guineafowl, green peafowl, and Indian peafowl [11, 23, 130, 133, 143–145]. *Heterakis isolonche* has been described in the ring-necked pheasant, golden pheasant, brown-eared pheasant, gray peacock-pheasant, and bobwhite quail [23, 143, 146].

Heterakis adults are attached to the superficial cecal mucosa and are generally considered to be nonpathogenic for most poultry. However, the protozoan *Histomonas meleagridis* (blackhead of turkeys) can be harbored in eggs of the cecal worm, which is the probable source of infection of the protozoan for pheasants. Additionally, *Heterakis* adults can sometimes invade deeper into the mucosa to induce granulomatous inflammation in the cecal wall.

The complete life cycle of *Heterakis* takes 30 days or less, depending on how quickly the eggs embryonate in the environment. Unembryonated ova are shed in the feces of infected birds into the environment, where complete embryonation takes 10–12 days. The embryo can be protected by the thick shell of the ovum for 3 years or more in soil and feces. When the ovum is directly consumed by the avian host, it will hatch in the intestines. Alternatively, the ova can be consumed by an earthworm paratenic host and the larvae can remain in an arrested state indefinitely until the earthworm is consumed by the avian host. Larvae are then released and reach the ceca as early as 8.5 hours after ingestion, and burrow into the cecal mucosa where the L1 stage will undergo two successive molts (L2, L3) in 10 days. Migration of larvae into internal organs is either minimal or rarely occurs. Larvae reach sexual maturity by day 14 after ingestion and produce ova by day 25 [147].

Adult *Heterakis* can observed in slightly gas-distended ceca and are often adhered to the wall (Figure 11.17). The adult nematodes, which are shorter than ascarids, are observed in the cecum as thin, white and 0.5–1.5 cm long with an undulating shape [147]. The adults burrow slightly into the mucosa of the cecum. In some instances, the cecal wall can be thickened with granulomas caused by adult nematodes burrowing deep into the mucosa (Figure 11.18) [148]. Diagnosis can be confirmed by histopathology of the cecum, flotation of ova by placing feces in zinc sulfate or sodium sulfate, or by viewing a direct mucosal scraping from the cecum (Figure 11.19). The anthelmintic

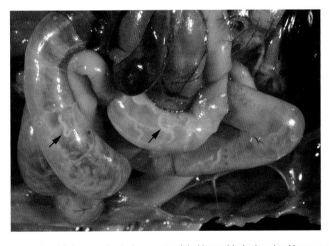

Figure 11.17 Fifteen-week-old ring-necked pheasant with *Heterakis isolonche*. Narrow, undulating adult nematodes (arrows) can be observed through the wall of the gas-filled ceca.

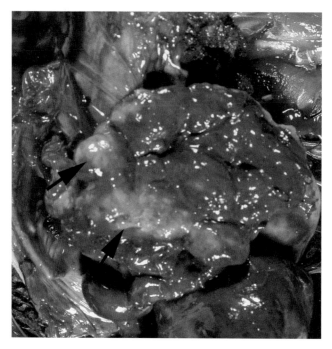

Figure 11.18 The opened cecum of an adult pheasant contains mural granulomas (arrows) caused by burrowing of *Heterakis isolonche* into the wall.

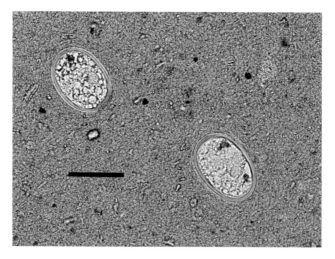

Figure 11.19 The oval ova of *Heterakis* can be observed microscopically in a cecal mucosal scraping or by fecal flotation. Bar = 50 μm.

piperazine is approved by the USDA for treatment of ascarids, but is not effective against *Heterakis*. Benzimidazoles, such as an oral drench of fenbendazole, can reduce the number of intestinal *Heterakis* and *Ascaridia* adults by 90% in egg-laying chickens and by 70–80% in turkeys [33]. Research with medicinal plants is incomplete, but *Aloe ferox*, *Agave sisalana*, and *Gunnera perpensa* have all been shown to reduce the numbers of *H. gallinarum* eggs shed in the feces of infected chickens by more than 90% [149].

11.3.6 Cestodes (Tapeworms)

Cestodes are parasitic flatworms with multiple segments (proglottids), each segment representing a complete organism unit that is capable of absorbing nutrients from the host and producing eggs. Most avian cestodes infect the intestine of birds. Mature, gravid proglottids break off the adult chain and are shed into the intestinal lumen to be shed in feces. The elongated, adult parasites are white and attach to the intestinal mucosa by an anterior end (scolex) bearing multiple burrowing hooks. Some species also possess circular suckers on the scolex to aid attachment to the intestinal mucosa. Mature cestodes survive in the intestine through attachment and direct absorption of nutrients.

The parasites have an indirect life cycle with at least one intermediate host to complete the larval stage of development. These intermediate hosts are flies, beetles, and snails. Birds shed gravid proglottids in their feces, and the eggs within the proglottids are consumed by insects, slugs and snails, and eventually reach the larval stage. Naïve birds can then contract the parasitic infection by eating the invertebrate intermediate host [150]. Mature cestodes in the intestinal lumen are recognized by their unique segmented appearance (Figure 11.20). The literature on cestodes in gamebirds is somewhat limited, but *Raillietina echinobothria* has been described in young partridges and pheasants [151]. *Choanotaenia infundibulum*, *Skrjabinia bolivari*, and *Rhabdometra nigropunctata* have also been described in partridges [152].

There is no specific treatment available for intestinal cestodes, but their presence indicates the need for control of flies and beetles in the poultry house. Diligent sanitation and manure management are also essential.

11.3.7 Coccidiosis (*Eimeria* sp.)

Gamebirds are readily susceptible to infection with coccidia, which are protozoan parasites of the intestinal tract [153]. This remains one of the most common causes of mortality in young game birds 1–5 weeks of age despite improvements in chemotherapy and husbandry. The species of coccidia that infect pheasants, chukars or quail differ from each other (Table 11.3) as well as from those that infect turkeys and chickens. Cross-protection against coccidial species is rare, with birds recovering from infection with one species generally being susceptible to infection with other novel species.

The most pathogenic species of coccidia for gamebirds are *Eimeria colchici* and *E. legionensis* in the ceca of pheasants and partridges, respectively. *Eimeria duodenalis* and *E. phasiani*, which infect

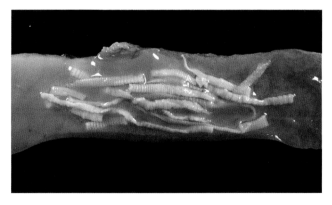

Figure 11.20   The opened intestine of a 1-year-old bantam chicken contains segmented proglottids of adult cestodes (not speciated).

Table 11.3 *Coccidia* species referenced in gamebirds, guineafowl, and peafowl.

Avian	Eimeria species	Reference
Pheasant	*E. cholchici*	Liou et al. [154]
	E. duodenalis	Norton et al. [155]
	E. dispersa	Tyzzer [156]
	E. gennaeuscus	Ray and Hiregaudar [157]
	E. langeroni	Yakimoff and Matschoulsky [158]
	E. megalosomata	Ormsbee [159]
	E. pacifica	McQuistion [160]
	E. picta	Bhatia [161]
	E. phasiani	Norton et al. [155]
	E. tatartoomia	Gassal and Schmaschke [9]
Partridge	*E. caucasica*	Gerhold et al. [162]
	E. innocua	Hafeez et al. [163]
	E. kofoidi	Naciri et al. [164]
	E. legionensis	Fernandez-Alvarez [165]
	E. procera	Naciri et al. [164]
	E. rhynchoti	Freitas et al. [166]
	E. schneider	Goldová et al. [167]
	E. teetari	Bhatia et al. [168]
Quail	*E. batari*	Shah et al. [169]
	E. colini	Gerhold et al. [170]
	E. dispersa	Ruff et al. [171]
	E. innocua	Hafeez et al. [163]
	E. lettyae	Ruff [172]
	E. tahamensis	Amoudi [173]
	E. taldykurganica	Ruff et al. [171]
	E. tsunodai	Rao et al. [175]
	E. urzura	Tsutsumi et al. [174]
Peafowl	*E. arabica*	Amoudi [176]
	E. pavoaegyptica	El-Shahawy [177]
	E. pavonina	Hauck et al. [178]
	E. pavonis	Titilincu et al. [179]
	E. patnaiki	Titilincu et al. [179]
	E. mandalin	Banik and Ray [180]
	E. riyadhae	Amoudi [176]
	Isospora mayurai	Williams [181]
Guineafowl	*E. gorakhpuri*	Long and Millard [182]
	E. grenieri	Harkirat et al. [183]
	E. numidae	Bhatia et al. [184]

the small intestine of pheasants, are less pathogenic than those that cause lesions in the ceca. Additionally, the coccidian life cycle involves both sexual and asexual phases that can affect enterocytes in different segments of intestine. For example, *E. colchici* infection in pheasants begins with the asexual phases in the small intestine while the sexual phase occurs in the ceca. *E. duodenalis* of pheasants has both asexual and sexual phases of replication occurring along the proximal small intestine [185].

The life cycle for most avian enteric coccidia is similar and can be completed in less than 1–2 weeks if the birds are raised on warm, moist soil or litter [186]. Based on the species of *Eimeria*, the number of asexual divisions and the time required for each developmental stage can differ. Infection is initiated by ingestion of sporulated oocysts (eggs). Mature or sporulated *Eimeria* oocysts contain four sporocysts, and each sporocyst contains two sporozoites. Ingested oocysts are subject to the grinding action of the gizzard, releasing the sporocysts and eventually the sporozoites into the intestinal lumen. Sporozoites then course along the intestine to invade preferred enterocytes at various segments, depending on the *Eimeria* species [187]. Asexual division (schizogony or merogony) occurs for 2–4 generations (*Eimeria* species dependent) to produce numerous crescent-shaped intracellular schizonts (or meronts). The enterocytes are then destroyed, releasing many schizonts that reenter enterocytes for the asexual cycle or for the sexual phase. During the reproductive phase, the schizonts form either small, round microgametes (male) or larger macrogametes (female) within enterocytes. Microgametes are eventually released from enterocytes and migrate to fertilize the macrogametes to form a zygote that will mature into an oocyst. The cycle of infectivity is completed when oocysts are shed through feces into the environment, where oocyst sporulation may require 1–3 days, depending on ambient temperature and moisture. The shed oocysts are resistant to chemical and mechanical damage and can persist in the environment for 1–2 years [167, 187, 188].

Young birds that are raised on soil or litter will have increased risk for coccidiosis; brooding chicks on wire can reduce transmission through feces. Clinical signs can resemble those caused by other intestinal protozoa. Sudden death and history of piling may be the only signs, but birds can exhibit ruffled feathers, shivering, weight loss, depression, and blood in droppings (Figure 11.21). Because of diarrheic feces, the feet of chicks are often crusted with feces (Figure 11.22). Susceptible breeder

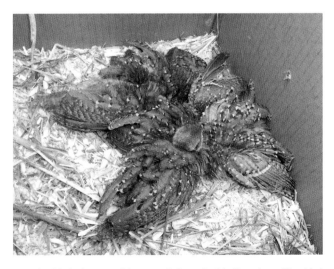

Figure 11.21   Three-week-old chukar partridges are infected with *Eimeria* sp. The birds are depressed with ruffled feathers and huddle or pile.

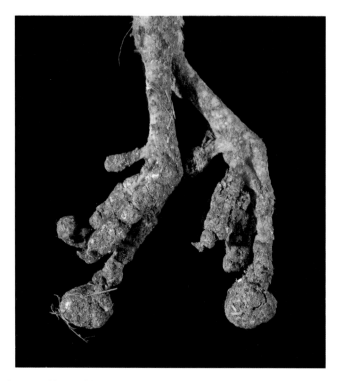

Figure 11.22 Chukar partridges with severe coccidiosis have feet and toes covered with adherent feces, which is a common finding in young birds affected with diarrhea from *Eimeria* infection.

birds infected at maturity can have decreased egg production. Necropsy lesions vary depending on which species of *Eimeria* are involved [187]. Affected birds are often dehydrated and the intestines or ceca are distended with either clear to green fluid to resemble viral enteritis or tan to white caseous exudate (Figure 11.23).

Rapid diagnosis can be made by fecal flotation of feces or by lightly scraping the mucosa of affected intestines with a histology glass coverslip and then placing on a glass slide for microscopic examination. Mucosal scrapings from birds dying from coccidiosis will often contain large numbers of ovoid, thick-walled oocysts that are 10–30 μm long (Figure 11.24) [189]. Histopathology of intestinal tract or cecum will reveal hemorrhagic to necrotic enteritis with large numbers of oocysts, sexual and asexual *Eimeria* stages in both enterocytes and the lumen [188].

The key to coccidiosis control is to reduce oocyst production or the exposure of birds to oocysts. Examples include the following. (i) Reduce stocking density of birds. (ii) Periodically apply antic-occidial chemicals that kill (coccidiocidal) or decrease the growth rate (coccidiostat) of coccidia at days 1–4 of infection; [190] these anticoccidials can be rotated in the flock during the year to minimize accumulation of drug-resistant coccidia strains. Additionally, there are a variety of natural products, such as fats, antioxidants, and essential oils, that are purported to have anticoccidial activity [187]. (iii) Reduce exposure to feces and oocysts in the environment by maintaining deep (3 in.), dry litter or dry soil with good drainage, or brooding chicks on wire. (iv) Kill oocysts in the environment by using a mechanical poultry floor flame sanitizer between grow-outs. (v) Promote flock immunity to coccidia by vaccinating with attenuated, live oocysts; [191] however, commercial anticoccidial vaccines are not available for upland gamebirds as they are in chickens and turkeys.

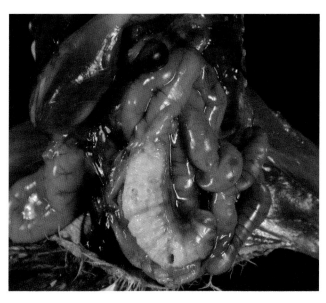

Figure 11.23   Three-week-old chukar partridge with cecal coccidiosis (*Eimeria sp.*). Note the pale, caseous exudate distending the ceca. This cecal lesion must be differentiated from *Salmonella* infection.

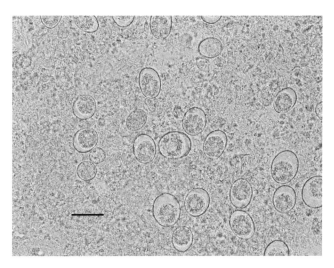

Figure 11.24   Fresh fecal or intestinal oocysts of *Eimeria* sp. as observed on a mucosal scraping are thick-walled, ovoid, nonsporulated and 10–30 μm in length (bar = 10 μm).

A variety of drugs have been used for treatment and prevention of *Eimeria* infection in poultry, including gamebirds, particularly pheasants, quail, and partridge. Treatments and prevention programs should be planned with the advice of a veterinarian to ensure that approved compounds are administered properly and judiciously. Sulfanilamides were one of the first compounds shown to be effective against coccidia [190]. Sulfa drugs, such as sulfadimethoxine, have long been used in the field for treatment of *Eimeria* in gamebirds, with varying efficacy. Patton et al. demonstrated that amprolium, a pyrimidine derivative, was effective for the control of *Eimeria colchici*, *E. duodenalis*, and *E. phasiani* in pheasants [192].

Additionally, a variety of polyether ionophores have been used in shuttle programs in chickens; two different compounds (ionophore and a chemical coccidiostat) are administered at different timepoints during the grow-out in order to reduce drug resistance and maintain product efficacy [190]. These ionophores have been assessed in gamebirds as well. Ruff et al. demonstrated that the ionophores monensin and salinomycin were superior to amprolium in reducing oocyst numbers shed in the feces of captive bobwhite quail [193]. Fuller et al. indicated that the ionophore lasalocid was highly effective in pheasants when challenged with a variety of field isolates of *Eimeria*; [194] these results were supported by the work of McQuiston who found lasalocid and salinomycin to be superior to monensin for reducing fecal shedding of *Eimeria* oocysts in pheasants [160].

Additionally, other compounds have been assessed as anticoccidials in gamebirds. Gerhold et al. determined that the most effective anticoccidials for treatment of *Eimeria* in bobwhite quail were clopidol, decoquinate, diclazuril, lasalocid, narasin, nicarbazine, and robenidine; these compounds were superior to amprolium and roxarsone [195]. Sokol et al. found totrazuril to be an effective treatment against coccidia in Japanese quail [196]. Norton and Wise reported that clopidol and the coccidiostat arprinocid protected pheasants against challenge with *E. colchici*; halofuginone and monensin were less effective, while amprolium and sulphaquinoxaline were ineffective [155]. Finally, Gerhold et al. assessed a variety of anticoccidials (placed in feed) against *Eimeria kofoidi* infection in partridges [162]. They determined that rofenaid, robenidicne, diclazuril, and decoquinate were highly effective in reducing infection and severity of lesions, while the ionophores lasalocid, monensin, salinomycin, and semduramicin showed moderate effectiveness.

11.3.8 Cryptosporidiosis (Enteric Form)

Cryptosporidiosis is a common protozoan infection that has been described as a respiratory or gastrointestinal pathogen in a variety of domestic animals and over 30 species of birds, plus it has zoonotic potential. The genus *Cryptosporidium* is in the phylum Apicomplexa, class Sporozoasida [197]. *Cryptosporidium meleagridis* and *C. baileyi*, and to a lesser extent *C. parvum*, have been documented in turkeys and chickens [198]. Both *C. meleagridis* and *C. parvum* have been linked to human infections, resulting in gastrointestinal disease [198].

Natural infection with *Cryptosporidium* spp. has been described in ring-necked pheasants [199, 200], red-legged and chukar partridges [201, 202], peafowl [203], bobwhite quail [204], and Japanese quail [205]. These natural infections in quail, peafowl, partridge, and pheasants can result in primary respiratory or GI disease or both. This chapter will focus on GI infection since respiratory cryptosporidiosis has been described in Chapter 10.

Shaapan et al. found native Egyptian quail (bobwhite and brown quail) to be natural reservoirs of three *Cryptosporidium* species (*C. meleagridis, C. baileyi, C. galli*) [206]. In addition to those three species, *C. avium, C. andersoni,* and *C. parvum* have also been isolated from wild birds. These birds pose a risk for contamination of gamebird premises, hence the need for farm biosecurity [207]. Both *C. baileyi* and *C. meleagridis* have been identified as causing respiratory and intestinal disease in the red-legged partridge [201]. *C. meleagridis* tends to be located primarily in the intestine while *C. baileyi* is isolated most often from trachea, esophagus, and bursa of Fabricius [208, 209]. Lindsey and Blagburn noted that pheasant, partridge, and guineafowl were susceptible to oral infection with *Cryptosporidium* oocysts originating from chickens [210]. There are similar findings in which bobwhite and Japanese quail were successfully infected with chicken fecal oocysts [211–213]. Conversely, chickens have been successfully infected with fecal *Cryptosporidium* oocysts from pheasants and quail [202, 205]. Finally, chicken fecal *Cryptosporidium* oocysts have been experimentally transmitted to guineafowl [210]. In summary, it is clear that multiple cryptosporidial species, particularly *C. meleagridis*, are cross-transmissible between poultry species and also pose a zoonotic risk [206].

Infection generally occurs by ingesting feces or contaminated water and feed [206]. The enteric life cycle of *Cryptosporidium* sp. includes both sexual and asexual development stages that involve a single host. Ingested oocysts reach the small intestine whereupon the cyst wall is dissolved and infective sporozoites are released. Sporozoites then attach to the surface of enterocytes, become enclosed in parasitophorous vacuoles and are then referred to as trophozoites, which will undergo one or more asexual divisions (merogony). Type I meronts form eight merozoites which are liberated from the parasitophorous vacuole when mature. There can be 1–3 type I meront generations depending on the host and the species of *Cryptosporidium* [209]. Merozoites will either invade other enterocytes to undergo another cycle of type I merogony or develop into type II meronts.

The type II meronts form four merozoites, which enter the sexual reproductive stages (gametogony). Both microgamonts (male) and macrogamonts (female) are produced during gametogony. The macrogamonts are fertilized by the smaller microgametes to form zygotes. Further development of zygotes results in the production of thick-walled oocysts that contain four sporozoites. Oocysts are eventually released from enterocytes and will be shed in the feces [211]. The prepatent period (time between infection and oocyst excretion) ranges from 2 to 14 days in most domestic animal species. Infections can be short-lived or may persist for months, resulting in prolonged shedding of oocysts [209]. Oocysts shed into the environment can survive for months.

Clinical signs in infected quail and partridges consist of diarrhea, reduced weight gain, lethargy, and sporadic mortality [112, 201, 205]. Most reports of *Cryptosporidium* in pheasants refer to respiratory signs, although the organism is readily detected in intestine [214]. Ritter et al. reported quail with white, watery diarrhea, dehydration, and death [199]. The birds had infected intestines and ceca distended with clear to brown, foamy fluid. Microscopic lesions in intestine consist of shortened or fused villi with detached apical enterocytes. In one report, red-legged partridges had large numbers of *Cryptosporidium* trophozoites colonizing the surface of intestinal enterocytes with no overt clinical signs [201].

On both light and electron microscopy, the development stages of *Cryptosporidium* can be observed on the luminal surface of enterocytes [199, 204]. These organisms can also be observed in the esophagus and bursa of Fabricius, and microscopic evidence of lymphofollicular atrophy and epithelial hyperplasia can be observed in the latter organ [205]. In the authors' experience, inflammatory cells in the intestine are not commonly observed. With hematoxylin and eosin stain, the protozoa appear as small, often numerous, circular, basophilic bodies (2–6 µ diameter) that protrude from the cell surface. Electron microscopy shows these protozoa in a characteristic intracellular, extracytoplasmic location beneath the enterocyte plasma membrane. The ovoid, thick-walled ocysts vary from 4 to 8 µ wide and 4–8 µ in length, depending on the species [215].

Diagnosis is based on gross lesions, histopathologic findings, and positive identification of cryptosporidial trophozoites or oocysts. Clinical signs of digestive disease can be confused with other parasites, enteric viruses, *Salmonella* and *E. coli* [215]. For example, cryptosporidial enteritis of bobwhite quail is most severe with greater mortality if the infection is complicated by reovirus [112]. Because the gross lesions in the digestive tract alone are nonspecific and can have multiple causes, one should always collect feces and intestine for bacterial culture and enteric virus testing. Autolysis will impair the ability to observe cryptosporidia on enterocytes in histologic sections, so intestine from recently euthanized or dead carcasses should be collected and fixed in formalin as soon as possible. Acid-fast stain (Ziehl–Neelsen), auramine phenol and immunofluorescence have been applied to fecal smears for identification of *Cryptosporidium* oocysts [216]. The oocysts cannot be speciated based on morphology or immunologic assays, but molecular analysis of DNA amplified by PCR can be used to characterize most species of *Cryptosporidium* [217]. Nevertheless, the diagnosis of avian cryptosporidiosis and the approach to treatment and prevention can be made without speciation of the protozoan.

There are no commercial vaccines for *Cryptosporidium* in poultry. Additionally, an effective medication for the treatment and prevention of cryptosporidiosis in birds is lacking [215]. Prevention of exposure or infection is the best measure. The emphasis should be on reducing oocyst contamination in feed and water. *Cryptosporidium* is a significant protozoal contaminant in natural water sources [218]. Fortunately, conventional treatment (sedimentation and filtration) of sewage surface waters and public drinking water sources can eliminate most of the *Cryptosporidium* oocysts. Both chlorine and ozone, as water treatments, are very effective in destroying oocysts and can serve as useful adjuncts to filtration [218]. *C. baileyi* can infect a wide variety of bird species, thus wild birds pose a risk of infection and must be kept out of the brooder and flight pens [215]. Rodents (mice, rats, voles) may be susceptible to infection with *Cryptosporidium*, while insects (e.g., darkling beetles and flies) may also serve as vectors for the oocysts; hence, well-managed insect and rodent control programs are essential for disease control. Additionally, stressors such as high stocking density, environmental contamination with oocysts, seasonality or primary diseases could act as stressors to promote immune suppression and facilitate infection with *Cryptosporidium* oocysts.

11.3.9 *Spironucleus (Hexamita) meleagridis* Infection

This enteric protozoal organism was described as early as 1939 in young pheasants and quail, but partridge chicks are also affected [219–221]. Affected chicks are usually less than 2 weeks old and are depressed with reduced feed consumption. Gross findings include dehydration, and small intestines and ceca dilated with yellow fluid and gas. In fresh specimens, cytologic preparations of intestinal mucus will reveal both cysts and trophozoites, the latter being 8–10 μm long, elongate, ovoid to pear-shaped protozoa with eight flagella [220]. Histology will reveal numerous flagellated protozoa in the intestinal lumen and deep within crypts of the duodenum and jejunum [221]. Concomitant infections with *Cryptosporidium*, coccidia, rotavirus and *Salmonella* have been described and result in greater mortality. Raising chicks on wire in early stages can help to reduce lateral transmission.

There is no effective or approved medication for treatment. Infected birds that survive can serve as potential carriers so prevention should focus on eliminating direct exposure of young birds to older birds, not reusing litter in the brooder pen, and thorough cleaning and disinfection of feeders and drinkers between flocks.

11.3.10 Histomoniasis (Blackhead, Infectious Enterohepatitis, *Histomonas meleagridis* Infection)

Infection with the protozoan *H. meleagridis* can cause high mortality in poultry flocks, and treatment is complicated by the fact that nitroimidazole products have been taken off the US market. *H. meleagridis* is a protozoan that infects the cecum and liver of gallinaceous birds. The protozoan is pleomorphic, possessing a single flagellum in the cecal lumen, and assumes a nonflagellated ameboid form in the liver and other soft tissues. The disease is diagnosed most often in turkeys and chickens, but also in peafowl, guineafowl, pheasants, partridge, and quail [222–226].

Within the cecal lumen, *H. meleagridis* has a single flagellum (sometimes two during cell division) and is usually 8–12 μm diameter. *Histomonas* assumes a 10–15 μm diameter, pure ameboid form as trophozoites in the liver and other soft tissues. Birds are most often infected with *H. meleagridis* by ingesting the ova of the cecal worm, *Heterakis gallinarum*. *Histomonas* is harbored within ova of the cecal worm. In the cecal lumen, *Heterakis* enters the cecal worm reproductive tract to gain entry to the nematode ova. *Heterakis* ova that are shed into the feces will protect the fragile ameba from dessication in the environment. Earthworms in the soil serve as a paratenic host by consuming the embryonated *Heterakis* ova [226]. The bird is exposed to *Histomonas* by ingesting embryonated cecal worm eggs or earthworms. *Heterakis* larvae hatch from the ova in the cecum and assume a flagellated form to infiltrate the cecal mucosa to cause a thick-walled, fibrinonecrotic typhlitis. The histomonads enter the portal circulation and shower the liver, resulting in multifocal hallmark necrotic "target" lesions [225]. A variety of soft tissues in the coelomic cavity can be infected with protozoa, but the liver is the most common.

The cecal worm was long considered to be a required intermediate host for *Histomonas* transmission, but research indicates that the protozoan can be spread directly between turkeys, in the absence of cecal worms and earthworms, through the phenomenon of cloacal drinking, by which contaminated fecal material in the soil is carried into the colon by rhythmic contractions of the cloaca or vent. Lesions can be observed in ceca at 8 days post infection while liver lesions are present by 10 days post infection.

Clinical signs develop 7–10 days after infection and include depression, closed eyes, huddling, anorexia, ruffled feathers, and yellow feces that can contain flecks of blood. Birds can die suddenly in good condition or exhibit progressive wasting. On gross necropsy, the hallmark lesions are in liver and cecum (Figure 11.25). The ceca are enlarged, thick-walled and contain hemorrhagic,

Figure 11.25 Eight-week-old pheasant with *Histomonas meleagridis*. Note the multifocal discoid, pale necrotic foci in liver (arrows) and the enlarged, thick-walled cecum (arrow heads) containing fibrinonecrotic exudate.

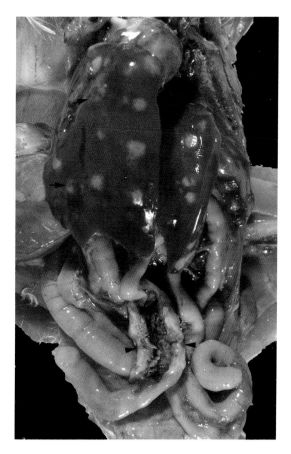

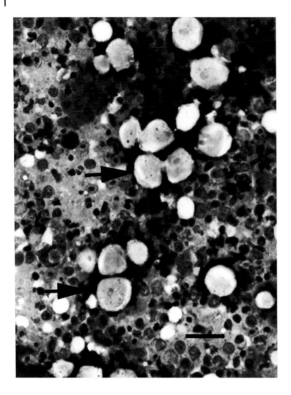

Figure 11.26 Cytologic impression of liver infected with *Histomonas* reveals round, 10–20 μm diameter ameboid trophozoites (arrows) with a single nucleus. Wright–Giemsa stain, bar = 20 μm.

fibrinonecrotic (caseous) exudate. Peritonitis can be present if inflammation penetrates the cecal wall. Enlarged livers contain multifocal, circular, concentric, pale necrotic foci ("target lesions"). Stained cytologic touch impressions of liver in acute to subacute stages of infection will contain round, 10–20 μm diameter trophozoites (Figure 11.26). Similarly, histology of the liver reveals well-demarcated necrotic foci (corresponding to target lesions) bordered by epithelioid macrophages and lesser numbers of heterophils, lymphocytes, and plasma cells. Varying numbers of round (10–20 μm diameter) trophozoites are both free in the necrotic centers as well as inside macrophages. The cecum has transmural fibrinonecrotic typhlitis with similar trophozoites both free in the necrotic cecal wall and within macrophages [227].

Histomoniasis was historically controlled by chemical and environmental management. Nitroimidazole drugs (e.g., dimetridazole and ipronidazole) were widely used in commercial turkeys for prevention and treatment; [228] however, due to concerns about tissue residues, the products are no longer approved for production birds [229]. Arsenicals (e.g., nitarsone, Histostat®-50) used for protozoal control are no longer approved for use in poultry feed [230]. There are no commercial vaccines for *Histomonas*.

With a lack of available chemotherapeutics, the key for *Histomonas* control should be to reduce the opportunity for protozoal transmission through early diagnosis, reduce cecal worm populations, maintain birds on dry, clean litter in pens or on dry, well-draining soil in flight pens to reduce exposure to earth worms, and reduced stocking density. Reduction of cecal worm infections with anthelmintics (e.g. fenbendazole and Hygromycin-B) can be effective to reduce the transmission cycle. Ring-necked pheasants have been shown to support replication of *Heterakis* in greater numbers compared to Japanese quail, bobwhite quail, Hungarian partridge, chukar partridge, and guineafowl [231]. Hygromycin-B is currently not available in the US. Liver lesions caused by *Histomonas* are exacerbated by concomitant parasitic and bacterial infections, so one should implement a strong husbandry program to reduce bacterial, viral, and coccidial disease.

References

1 Yegani, M. and Korver, D. (2008). Factors affecting intestinal health in poultry. *Poult. Sci.* 87 (10): 2052–2063.

2 Dhama, K., Chakraborty, S., Verma, A.K. et al. (2013). Fungal/mycotic diseases of poultry-diagnosis, treatment and control. *Pak. J. Biol. Sci.* 16 (23): 1626–1640.

3 Ibrahim, Z.Y., Ali, B.H., Ali, R.K. et al. (2020). Avian candidiasis: a review. *Int. J. Pharmaceut. Res.* 12 (1): 1088–1091.

4 Hamet, N. and Corbel, A.M. (1983). Guinea fowl candidiasis: description, reproduction trial of the disease. *Bull d'Inform Statiion Exper d'Avicult de Plouf.* 23 (4): 169–173.

5 Sampurnanand, C., Lakshmana Char, N., and Rao, R.K. (1990). Candidiasis in peacocks (Pavo cristatus). *Indian Vet. J.* 67 (1): 79–80.

6 Asrani, R.K., Paul Gupta, R.K., Sadana, J.R. et al. (1993). Experimental candidiasis in Japanese quail: pathological changes. *Mycopathologia* 121 (2): 83–89.

7 Asfaw, M. and Dawit, D. (2017). Review on major fungal disease of poultry. *Br, J. Poult. Sci.* 6 (1): 16–25.

8 Tampieri, M.P., Galuppi, R., and Rugna, G. (2005). Survey on Helminthofauna in pheasants from Eastern Europe. *Parasitologia* 47 (2): 241–245.

9 Gassal, S. and Schmäschke, R. (2006). The helminth and coccidial fauna of pheasants (*Phasianus colchicus*) in view of the specific environmental conditions in pheasantries and in the wild. *Berl. Munch. Tierarztl. Wochenschr.* 119 (7–8): 295–302.

10 Cram, E.B. (1936). Species of the upper digestive tract of birds. USDA Technical Bulletin No. 516. USDA: Washington, D.C, pp. 1–28.

11 Foronada, P., Casanova, J.C., Figueruedo, E. et al. (2005). The helminth fauna of the barbary partridge *Alectoris Barbara* in Tenerife, Canary Islands. *J. Helminthol.* 79 (2): 133–138.

12 Thomas, E.F. (1937). *Capillaria annulata* in quail. *J. Am. Vet. Med. Assoc.* 76: 95.

13 De Rosa, M. and Shivaprasad, H.L. (1999). Capilliariasis in a vulture Guinea fowl. *Avian Dis.* 43 (1): 131–135.

14 Sakaguchi, S., Yunus, M., Sugi, S. et al. (2020). Integrated taxonomic approaches to seven species of capillariid nematodes (Nematoda: Trichocephalida: Trichinelloidea) in poultry from Japan and Indonesia, with special reference to their 18S rDNA phylogenetic relationships. *Parasitol. Res.* 119 (3): 957–972.

15 Bickford, A.A. and Gaafar, S.M. (1966). Multiple capillariasis in game-farm pheasants. *Avian Dis.* 10 (4): 428–437.

16 Kellog, F.E. and Prestwood, A.K. (1968). Case report and differentiating characteristics of *Capillaria phasianina* from pen-raised pheasants of Maryland. *Avian Dis.* 12 (3): 518–522.

17 Calvete, C., Estrada, R., Lucientes, J. et al. (2003). Correlates of helminth community in the red-legged partridge (*Alectoris rufus L.*) in Spain. *J. Parasitol.* 89 (3): 445–451.

18 Davis, R.B., Good, R.E., Tumlin, J.T. et al. (1969). An effective anthelmintic in treatment of quail infected with *Capillaria contorta*. *Avian Dis.* 13 (3): 690–691.

19 Ravipati, V. (2012). Infection of *Capillara contoarta* in peafowl. *Zoo's Print J.* 27 (7): 21.

20 Wojcik, A.R., Wasielewski, L., Grygon-Franckiewicz, B. et al. (1999). Economic losses in pheasant breeding evoked with endoparasites. *Wiad. Parazytol.* 45 (3): 3634–3368.

21 Pinto, R.M., Menezes, R.C., and Gomes, D.G. (2004). First report of five nematode species in *Phasianus colchicus* Linnaeus (Aves, Galliformes Phasianidae). *Rev. Brasil de Zool.* 21 (4): 961–970.

22 Fanelli, A., Menardi, G., Chiodo, M. et al. (2020). Gastroenteric parasite of wild Galliformes of the Italian Alps: implication for conservation management. *Parasitology* 147 (4): 471–477.

23 Cram, E.B., Jones, M.B., and Allen, E.A. (1931). Internal parasites and parasitic diseases of the bobwhite. In: *The Bobwhite Quail its Habits, Preservation and Increase* (ed. H.L. Stoddard), 229–313. New York: Charles Scribner's Sons.

24 Ayeni, J.S.O., Dipeolu, O.O., and Okaeme, A.N. (1983). Parasitic infections of the grey-breasted helmet guineafowl (*Numica meleagris galeata*) in Nigeria. *Vet. Parasitol.* 12 (1): 59–63.

25 Carerra-Jativa, P.D., Morgan, E.R., Barrows, M. et al. (2020). Free-ranging avifauna as a source of generalist parasites for captive birds in zoological settings: an overview of parasite records and potential for cross-transmission. *J. Adv. Vet. Anim. Res.* 7 (3): 482–500.

26 Gurler, A.T., Bolukbas, C.S., Pekmezci, G.Z. et al. (2012). Helminths of pheasant (Phasianus cholchicus) detected by necropsy and fecal examination in Samsun, Turkey. *Turkeiye Parazitol. Derg.* 36 (4): 222–227.

27 Park, S. and Shin, S.S. (2010). Concurrent Capilliaria and Heterakis infections in zoo rock partridges (*Alectoris graeca*). *Korean J. Parasitol.* 48 (3): 253–257.

28 Maca, O. and Pavlasek, I. (2020). Protozoan and helminth infections of aviary-reared *Alectoris rufa* (Galliformes: Phasianidae) before releasing for hunting in the Czech Republic: infection dynamic and potential risks. *J. Parasitol.* 106 (4): 439–443.

29 Baruš, V. and Sergejeva, T.P. (1989). Capillariids parasitic in birds in the Palaearctic region (2): genera Eucoleus and Echinocoleus. *Acta Sci. Nat. Brno.* 23 (6): 1–47.

30 Itagaki, H., Watanabe, T., and Kobara, J. (1974). Studies on *Capillaria perforans* Kotlán et Orosz, 1931 from the Guinea fowl I. morphology. *Bull. Azabu Vet. Colloids* 28: 77–82.

31 Perman, A. and Hansen, J.W. (1998). Epidemiology, diagnosis and control of poultry parasites. *FAO Anim. Health Manual* 4: 1–160.

32 Kirsch, R. (1984). Treatment of nematodiasis in poultry and game birds with fenbendazole. *Avian Dis.* 28 (2): 311–318.

33 Yazwinski, T.A., Andrews, P., Holtzen, H. et al. (1986). Dose-titration of fenbendazole in the treatment of poultry nematodiasis. *Avian Dis.* 30 (4): 716–718.

34 Pavlovic, I., Jakic-dimic, D., Kulisic, Z. et al. (2003). Frequent nematode parasites of artifially raised pheasants (*Phasianus colchicis L.*) and measures for their control. *Acta Vet.* 53 (5–6): 393–398.

35 Ashraf, M., Wataich, N., Ahmad, I.G. et al. (2002). Chemotherapy of gastrointestinal nematodes in common peafowl (*Pavo cristatus*). *Pakistan Vet. J.* 22 (2): 91–93.

36 Liebhart, D., Neale, S., Garcia-Rueda, C. et al. (2014). A single strain of *Tetratrichomonas gallinarum* causes fatal typhlohepatitis in red-legged partridges (*Alectoris rufa*) to be distinguished from histomonosis. *Avian Pathol.* 43 (5): 473–480.

37 Wichmann, R.W. and Bankowski, R.A. (1956). A report of *Trichomonas gallinarum* infection in chukar partridges (*Alectoris graeca*). *Cornell Vet.* 46 (3): 367–369.

38 Amin, A., Bilic, I., Liebhart, D., and Hess, M. (2014). Trichomonads in birds – a review. *Parasitology* 141 (6): 733–747.

39 Bruno, A., Fedynich, A., Purple, K. et al. (2015). Survey for *Trichomonas gallinae* in northern bobwhites (*Colinus virginianus*) from the Rolling Plains ecoregion, Oklahoma and Texas, USA. *J. Wildl. Dis.* 51 (3): 780–783.

40 Pennycott, T.W. (1996). Effect of four therapeutic agents on *Trichomas phasiani* carriage in pheasants. *Vet. Rec.* 139 (9): 214–215.

41 Navarathnam, E.S. (1970). A new species of *Tritrichomonas* from the caecum of the bird *Coturnix coturnix Linneaus*. *Riv. Parasitol.* 31 (1): 9–14.

42 Mostefl, M.M., Richter, B., Nedorost, N. et al. (2012). Identification of a putatively novel trichomonad species in the intestine of a common quail (*Coturnix coturnix*). *Vet. Parasitol.* 183 (3–4): 369–372.

43 Allen, A. (1941). Macroscopic differentiation of lesions of histomoniasis and trichomoniasis in turkeys. *Am. J. Vet. Res.* 2: 214–217.

44 Honigberg, B.M. (1978). Trichomonads of importance in human medicine. In: *Parasitic Protozoa* (ed. J.P. Kreier), 275–454. New York: Academic Press.

45 Borji, J., Razmi, G.H., Movassaghi, A.H. et al. (2011). Prevalence and pathological lesions of *Trichomonas gallinae* in pigeons of Iran. *Parasitol. Dis.* 35 (2): 186–189.

46 Dalton, P. (1996). Use of dimetridazole in gamebirds. *Vet. Rec.* 139 (16): 399.

47 Hussain, A.Z. (2001). Morphometric evaluation of the small intestines and caeca of pheasants infected with *Hexamita* and *Trichomonas* species. *Vet. Rec.* 148 (15): 484–485.

48 Madsen, H. (1941). The occurrence of helminths and coccidia in partridges and pheasants in Denmark. *J. Parasitol.* 27 (1): 29–34.

49 Moore, J., Freehling, M., and Simberloff, D. (1986). Gastrointestinal helminths of the northern bobwhite in Florida: 1968 and 1983. *J. Wildl. Dis.* 22 (4): 497–501.

50 Goble, F.C. and Kutz, H.L. (1945). The genus *Dispharynx* (Nemadoa: Acuariidae) in galliform and passeriform birds. *J. Parasitol.* 31 (5): 323–331.

51 Gomez-Puerta, L., Enciso, M.A., and Rojas, G. (2009). Natural parasitism by *Synhimantus (Dispharynx) nasuta* (Nematoda: Acuariidae) in captive common peafowl (Pavo cirstatus). *Rev Peruana de Biol.* 16 (1): 121–123.

52 Vassilev, G.D. and Jooste, R. (1991). Pathology and taxonomy of *Synhimantus* (*Dispharynx*) *nasuta* infesting bantams and Guinea-fowl in Zimbabwe. *Bull. Anim. Health Prod. Africa* 39 (1): 27–30.

53 Hwang, J.C., Tolgay, N., Shalkop, W.T. et al. (1961). Case report – *Dispharynx nasuta* causing severe proventriculitis in pigeons. *Avian Dis.* 5 (1): 60–65.

54 Flatt, L.E. and Nelson, L.R. (1969). *Tetrameres americana* in laboratory pigeons (*Columba livia*). *Lab. Anim. Care* 19 (6). 853–856.

55 Calpin, J.P. (1971). A checklist of diseases reported from the bobwhite quail. *Avian Dis.* 15 (4): 704–715.

56 Davidson, W.R., Kellog, F.E., and Doster, G.L. (1980). Seasonal trends of helminth parasites of bobwhite quail. *J. Wildl. Dis.* 16 (3): 367–375.

57 Appleton, C.C. (1983). Tetrameriasis in creasted guineafowl from Natal. *Ostrich* 54 (4): 238–240.

58 Junker, K. and Boomker, J. (2007). Helminths of guineafowls in Limpopo Province, South Africa. *Onderstepoort J. Vet. Res.* 74 (4): 265–280.

59 Junker, K. and Boomker, J. (2007). *Tetrameres numida* n. sp. (Nematoda: Tetrameridae) from helmeted guineafowls, *Numida meleagris* (Linnaeus, 1758), in South Africa. *Onderstepoort J. Vet. Res.* 74 (2): 115–128.

60 Chertkova, A.N. (1953). A new nematode *Tetrameres* (*Petrowimeres*) pavonis nov. subgen., nov. sp., from peacocks. In: *Contributions to Helminthology on the 75th birthday of Academician K. I. Skrjabin* (ed. A.M. Petrov), 812. Moscow: lzdatel'stvo Akademii Nauk S.S.S.R.

61 Gjevre, A.G., Kaldhusdal, M., and Eriksen, G.S. (2013). Gizzard erosion and ulceration syndrome in chickens and turkeys: a review of causal or predisposing factors. *Avian Pathol.* 42 (4): 297–303.

62 Grafl, B., Prokofieva, I., Wernsdorf, P. et al. (2015). Clinical signs and progression of lesions in the gizzard are not influenced by inclusion of ground oats or whole wheat in the diet following experimental infection with pathogenic fowl adenovirus serotype 1. *Avian Pathol.* 44: 230–236.

63 Tsai, S.S., Chang, T.C., Chang, G.N. et al. (1998). Naturally-occurring adenovirus-associated gastrointestinal lesions in Coturnix (*Coturnix coturnix*) quail. *Avian Pathol.* 27 (6): 641–643.

64 Kumar, R., Sturos, M., Porter, R.E. et al. (2021). An outbreak of fowl Aviadenovirus A-associated gizzard erosion and ulceration in captive bobwhite quail (*Colinus virginianus*). *Avian Dis.* 65 (1): 52–58.

65 Hess, M. (2013). Aviadenovirus infection. In: *Diseases of Poultry*, 13e (ed. D.E. Swayne, J.R. Glisson, L.R. McDonald, et al.), 290–300. Hoboken, NJ: Wiley-Blackwell.

66 Spickler, A.R. (2019). Fowl Typhoid and Pullorum Disease. www.cfsph.iastate.edu/Factsheets/pdfs/fowl_typhoid.pdf (accessed February 2022).

67 Cass, J.S. and Williams, J.E. (1947). *Salmonella pullorum* recovered from a wild pheasant in Minnesota. *J. Am. Vet. Med. Assoc.* 111 (847): 282.

68 Sharp, M.W. and Lang, P.W. (1980). *Salmonella pullorum* infection and pheasants. *Vet. Rec.* 107 (18): 431.

69 Buchholz, P.S. and Fairbrother, A. (1992). Pathogenicity of *Salmonella pullorum* in northern bobwhite quail and mallard ducks. *Avian Dis.* 36 (2): 304–312.

70 Casagrande, R.A., Angelica, A.B., Wouters, T.B. et al. (2014). Fowl typhoid (*Salmonella gallinarum*) outbreak in Japanese quail (*Coturnix coturnix japonica*). *Avian Dis.* 58 (3): 491–494.

71 USDA, APHIS (2019). National Poultry Improvement Plan Standards. US Government Printing Office, Washington, D.C.

72 Francis, D.W., Campbell, H., and Newton, G.R. (1963). A study of a *Salmonella* infection in a flock of chukar partridges. *Avian Dis.* 7 (4): 501–506.

73 Helm, J.D., Hines, R.K., Hill, J.E. et al. (1999). Multiple drug-resistant *Salmonella* typhimurium DT104 and DT104b isolated in bobwhite quail (*Colinus virginianus*). *Avian Dis.* 43 (4): 788–791.

74 Milton, A.A.P., Agarwal, R.K., Priya, G.B. et al. (2018). Occurrence, antimicrobial susceptibility patterns and genotypic relatedness of *Salmonella* spp. isolates from captive wildlife, their caretakers, feed and water in India. *Epidemiol. Infect.* 146 (12): 1543–1549.

75 Diarra, M.S. and Malouin, F. (2014). Antibiotics in Canadian poultry productions and anticipated alternatives. *Front. Microbiol.* 5 (282): 1–15.

76 Lister, S.A. (1990). *Salmonella enteritidis* infection in pheasants. *Vet. Rec.* 126 (2): 148.

77 O.I.E (2021). Prevention, detection and control of *Salmonella* in poultry. In: *O.I.E. – Terrestrial Animal Health Code*, 29e. France: World Organization for Animal Health (OIE) www.oie.int/en/what-we-do/standards/codes-and-manuals/terrestrial-code-online-access. (accessed February 2022).

78 Sander, J., Hudson, C.R., Dufour-Zavala, L. et al. (2001). Dynamics of *Salmonella* contamination in a commercial quail operation. *Avian Dis.* 45 (4): 1044–1049.

79 Berkhoff, G.A. and Campbell, S.G. (1974). Etiology and pathogenesis of ulcerative enteritis ("quail disease"). The experimental disease. *Avian Dis.* 18 (2): 205–212.

80 Berkhoff, G.A., Campbell, S.G., Naylor, H.B. et al. (1974). Etiology and pathogenesis of ulcerative enteritis ("quail disease"). Characterization of the causative anaerobe. *Avian Dis.* 18 (2): 195–204.

81 Feldman, S.H., Kiavand, A., Seidelin, M. et al. (2006). Ribosomal RNA sequences of *Clostridium piliforme* isolated from rodent and rabbit: re-examining the phylogeny of the Tyzzer's disease agent and development of a diagnostic polymerase chain reaction assay. *J. Am. Assoc. Lab. Anim. Sci.* 45 (5): 65–73.

82 Shivaprasad, H.L., Uzal, F., Kokka, R. et al. (2008). Ulcerative enteritis-like disease associated with *Clostridium perfringens* Type A in bobwhite quail (*Colinus virginianus*). *Avian Dis.* 52 (4): 635–640.

83 Crespo, R., Franca, M., and Shivaprasad, H.L. (2013). Ulcerative enteritis-like disease associated with *Clostridium sordellii* in quail. *Avian Dis.* 57 (3): 698–702.

84 Buss, I.O., Conrad, R.D., and Reilly, J.R. (1958). Ulcerative enteritis in the pheasant, blue grouse and California quail. *J. Wildl. Manage.* 22 (4): 446–449.

85 Harris, A.H. (1961). An outbreak of ulcerative enteritis amongst bobwhite quail (*Colinus virginanus*). *Vet. Rec.* 73 (1): 11–13.

86 Davis, R.B. (1973). Ulcerative enteritis in chickens: coccidiosis and stress as predisposing factors. *Poult. Sci.* 52 (4): 1283–1287.

87 Beltran-Alcrudo, D., Cardona, C., McLellan, L. et al. (2013). A persistent outbreak of ulcerative enteritis in bobwhite quail (*Colinus virginianus*). *Avian Dis.* 57 (3): 698–702.

88 Kondo, F., Tottori, J., and Soki, K. (1988). Ulcerative enteritis in broiler chickens caused by *Clostridium colinum* and in vitro activity of 19 antimicrobial agents in tests on isolates. *Poult. Sci.* 67 (10): 1424–1430.

89 Cooper, K.K., Songer, J.G., and Uzal, F.A. (2013). Diagnosing clostridial enteric disease in poultry. *J. Vet. Diagn. Invest.* 25 (3): 314–327.

90 Bano, L., Drigo, I., Macklin, K.S. et al. (2008). Development of a polymerase chain reaction assay for specific identification of *Clostridium colinum*. *Avian Pathol.* 37 (2): 179–181.

91 Yason, C.V. and Schat, K.A. (1985). Isolation and characterization of avian rotaviruses. *Avian Dis.* 29 (2): 499–506.

92 Bergeland, M.E., McAdaragh, J.P., Stolz, I. (1977). Rotaviral enteritis in turkey poults. In: *Proceedings of the 26th Western Poultry Disease Conference*. University of California, Davis, California. pp. 129–130.

93 Gough, R.E., Collins, M.S., Alexander, D.J. et al. (1990). Viruses and virus-like particles detected in samples from diseased game birds in Great Britain during 1988. *Avian Pathol.* 19 (2): 331–342.

94 Legrottaglie, R., Rizzi, V., and Agrimi, P. (1997). Isolation and identification of avian rotavirus from pheasant chicks with signs of clinical enteritis. *Comp. Immunol. Microbiol. Infect. Dis.* 20 (3): 205–210.

95 Ursu, K., Kisfali, P., Rigo, D. et al. (2009). Molecular analysis of the VP7 gene of pheasant rotaviruses identifies a new genotype, designated G23. *Arch. Virol.* 154 (8): 1365–1369.

96 Schumann, T., Hotzel, H., Otto, P., and Johne, R (2009). Evidence of interspecies transmission and reassortment among avian rotaviruses. *Virology* 386 (2): 334–343.

97 Hayes, J.S., Reynolds, D.L., Fagerlund, J.A. et al. (1994). Morphogenesis of enteric lesions induced by group D rotavirus in ringneck pheasant chicks (*Phasianus colchicus*). *Vet. Pathol.* 31 (1): 74–81.

98 Reynolds, D.L., Saif, Y.M., and Theil, K.W. (1987). Enteric viral infectious of Turkey poults: incidence of infection. *Avian Dis.* 31 (2): 272–276.

99 Yason, C.V. and Schat, K.A. (1986). Experimental infection of specific-pathogen-free chickens with avian rotaviruses. *Avian Dis.* 30 (3): 551–556.

100 Benavente, J. and Martinez-Costas, J. (2007). Avian reovirus: structure and biology. *Virus Res.* 123 (2): 105–119.

101 Jones, R.C. (2000). Avian reovirus infections. *Rev. Sci. Tech.* 19 (2): 614–625.

102 Van der Heide, L. (2000). The history of avian reovirus. *Avian Dis.* 44 (3): 638–641.

103 Rosenberger, J.K., Sterner, F.J., Botts, S. et al. (1989). In vitro and in vivo characterization of avian reoviruses. I. Pathogenicity and antigenic relatedness of several avian reovirus isolates. *Avian Dis.* 33 (3): 535–544.

104 Davis, J.F., Kulkami, A., and Fletcher, O. (2012). Myocarditis in 9- and 11-day-old broiler breeder chicks associated with a reovirus infections. *Avian Dis.* 56 (4): 786–790.

105 Troxler, S., Rigomier, P., Bilic, I. et al. (2013). Identification of a new reovirus causing substantial losses in broiler production in France, despite routine vaccination of breeders. *Vet. Rec.* 172 (21): 556–556.

106 Dobson, K.N. and Glisson, J.R. (1992). Economic impact of a documented case of reovirus infection in broiler breeders. *Avian Dis.* 36 (3): 788–791.

107 Jones, R.C., Al-Afaleq, A., Savage, C.E. et al. (1994). Early pathogenesis in chicks of infection with a trypsin-sensitive avian reovirus. *Avian Pathol.* 23 (4): 683–692.

108 Mutlu, O.F., Grund, C., and Coven, F. (1998). Reovirus infection of pheasants (*Phasianus colchicus*). *Tierarztl. Prax. Ausg. G Grosstiere Nutztiere* 26 (2): 104–107.

109 Farkas, S.L., Varga-Kugler, R., Ihasz, K. et al. (2021). Genomic characterization of avian and neoavian orthoreoviruses detected in pheasants. *Virus Res.* 297: 198349.

110 Kugler, R., Dnadar, E., Feher, E. et al. (2016). Phylogenetic analysis of a novel reassortant orthoreovirus strain detected in partridge (*Perdix perdix*). *Virus Res.* 215: 99–103.

111 Magee, D.L., Montgomery, R.D., Maslin, W.R. et al. (1993). Reovirus association with excessive mortality in young bobwhite quail. *Avian Dis.* 37 (4): 1130–1135.

112 Guy, J.S., Levy, M.G., Ley, D.H. et al. (1987). Experimental reproduction of enteritis in bobwhite quail (*Colinus virginianus*) with Cryptosporidium and reovirus. *Avian Dis.* 31 (4): 713–722.

113 Circella, E., Camarda, A., Martella, V. et al. (2005). Coronavirus associated with an enteric syndrome on a quail farm. *Avian Pathol.* 36 (3): 251–258.

114 Kim, H.-R., Jang, I., Kim, S.-H. et al. (2021). Viral metagenomic analysis of Japanese quail (*Coturnix japonica*) with enteritis in the Republic of Korea. *Avian Dis.* 65 (1): 40–45.

115 Liais, E., Croville, G., Marriette, J. et al. (2014). Novel avian coronavirus and fulminating disease in Guinea fowl, France. *Emerg. Infect. Dis.* 20 (1): 105–108.

116 Courtillon, C., Briand, F.-X., Allee, C. et al. (2021). Description of the first isolates of Guinea fowl corona and picornaviruses obtained from a case of Guinea fowl fulminating enteritis. *Avian Pathol.* 21: 1–35.

117 Ducatez, M., Liais, E., Croville, G. et al. (2015). Full genome sequenced of Guinea fowl coronavirus associated with fulminating disease. *Virus Genes* 50 (3): 514–517.

118 Poet, S.E., Skilling, D.E., Megyesi, J.L. et al. (1996). Detection of non-cultivable calicivirus from the white tern (*Gygis Alba Rothschildi*). *J. Wildl. Dis.* 32 (3): 461–467.

119 Gough, R.E., Drury, S.E.D., Bygrave, A.C. et al. (1992). Detection of caliciviruses from pheasants with enteritis. *Vet. Rec.* 131: 290–291.

120 Toffan, A., Bano, L., Montesi, F. et al. (2005). Detection of caliciviruses in young pheasants (*Phasianus cholchicus*) with enteritis in Italy. *Ital. J. Anim. Sci.* 4 (3): 300–302.

121 Gough, R.E. and Spackman, D. (1981). Virus-like particles associated with disease in Guinea fowl. *Vet. Rec.* 109 (22): 497.

122 Roach, S.N. and Langlois, R.A. (2021). Intra- and cross-species transmission of astroviruses. *Viruses* 13 (6): 1127–1138.

123 Cattoli, G., De Battisti, C., Toffan, A. et al. (2007). Co-circulation of distinct genetic lineages of astroviruses in turkeys and Guinea fowl. *Arch. Virol.* 152 (3): 595–602.

124 De Battisti, C., Salviato, A., Jonassen, C.M. et al. (2021). Genetic characterization of astroviruses detected in Guinea fowl (*Numida meleagridis*) reveals a distinct genotype and suggests cross-species transmission between Turkey and Guinea fowl. *Arch. Virol.* 157 (7): 1329–1337.

125 Toffan, A., Catania, S., Salviato, A. et al. (2012). Experimental infection of poults and Guinea fowl with genetically distinct avian astroviruses. *Avian Pathol.* 41 (5): 429–435.

126 Zell, R. (2018). Picornaviridae – the ever-growing virus family. *Arch. Virol.* 163 (2): 299–317.

127 Pankovics, P., Boros, A., and Reuter, G. (2012). Novel picornavirus in domesticated common quail (*Coturnix coturnix*) in Hungary. *Arch. Virol.* 157 (3): 525–530.

128 Gelmetti, D., Fabbi, M., Sironi, G. et al. (1996). Identification of parvovirus-like particles associated with three outbreaks of mortality in young pheasants (*Phasianus colchicus*). *J. Vet. Diagn. Invest.* 8 (1): 108–112.

129 Heit, M.C. and Rivere, J.E. (1995). Antiseptics and disinfectants. In: *Veterinary Pharmacology and Therapeutics* (ed. R.H. Adams), 741–752. Ames, IA: Iowa State Press.

130 Gilbertson, D. and Hugghins, E.J. (1964). Helminth infections in pheasant from Brown County, South Dakota. *J. Wildl. Manage.* 28 (3): 543–546.

131 Tibbits, F.D. and Babero, B.B. (1969). *Ascaridia galli* (Schrank, 1788) from the chukar partridge, *Alectoris chukar* (Gray), in Nevada. *J. Parasitol.* 55 (6): 1252.

132 Baylis, H.A. and Daubney, R. (1922). Report on the parasitic nematodes in the collection of the zoological survey of India. *Memoirs Indian Museum* 7: 263–347.

133 Yamaguti, S. (1961). The nematodes of vertebrates, part. 1. In: *Systema Helminthum*, vol. 3, 197–331. New York: Interscience Publishers.

134 Barus, V. (1966). Some remarks on nematodes of the genus *Ascaridia Dujardin*, 1845 from birds in Czechoslovakia. *Folia Parasitol.* 13: 170–181.

135 Canavan, W.P.N. (1929). Nematode parasites of vertebrates in the Philadelphia Zoological Garden and vicinity. *J. Parasitol.* 21 (1–2): 63–102.

136 Wetherbee, D.K. (1961). Investigations in the life history of the common coturnix. *Am. Midl. Nat.* 65 (1): 168–186.

137 Avcioglu, H., Burgu, A., and Bolukbas, C.S. (2008). Ascaridia numidae (Leiper, 1908; Travassos, 1913) in Rock Partridge (Alectoris chukar) in Turkey. *Parasitol. Res.* 102 (2): 527–530.

138 Skrjabin, K.I., Shikhobalova, N.P., and Mozgovi, A.A. (1951). Key to parasitic nematodes. In: *Oxyurata and Ascaridata*, vol. 2. New Dehli, India: Amerind Publishing.

139 Christenson, R.O., Earle, H.H., Butler, R.L. Jr., et al. (1942). Studies on the eggs of *Ascaridia galli* and *Heterakis gallinae*. *Trans. Am. Microsc. Soc.* 61 (2): 191–205.

140 Anderson, R.C. (2000). *Nematode Parasites of Vertebrates: Their Development and Transmission*, 2e. New York: CABI Publishing.

141 Sharma, N., Hunt, P.W., Hine, B.B. et al. (2019). The impacts of Ascardia galli on performance, health and immune response of laying hens: new insights into an old problem. *Poult. Sci.* 98 (12): 6517–6526.

142 Raza, A., Muhammad, F., Bashir, S. et al. (2016). In-vitro and in-vivo anthelmintic potential of different medicinal plants against *Ascaridia galli* infection in poultry birds. *World Poult. Sci. J.* 72 (1): 115–124.

143 Cram, E.B. (1927). Bird parasites of the Nematode Suborders Strongylata, Ascaridata, and Spirurata. Smithonian Institute, US National Museum Bulletin 140. US Government Printing Office: Washington, D.C.

144 Madsen, H. (1941). Studies on species of *Heterakis* (Nematodes) in birds. *Danish Rev. Game Biol.* 1 (3): 1–42.

145 Maplestone, P.A. (1932). The genera *Heterakis* and *Pseudaspidodera* in Indian hosts. *Indian J. Med. Res.* 20: 403–420.

146 Griner, L.A., Migaki, G., Penner, L.R. et al. (1977). Heterakidosis and nodular granuloma caused by Heterakis isolonche in the ceca of gallinaceous birds. *Vet. Pathol.* 14 (6): 582–590.

147 Cupo, K.L. and Beckstead, R.B. (2019). *Heterakis gallinarum*, the cecal nematode of gallinaceous birds: a critical review. *Avian Dis.* 63 (3): 381–388.

148 Menezes, R.C., Tortelly, R., Gomes, D.C. et al. (2003). Nodular typhlitis associated with the nematodes *Heterakis gallinarum* and *Heterakis isolonche* in pheasants: frequency and pathology with evidence of neoplasia. *Meoria do Instituto Oswaldo Cruz.* 98 (8): 1011–1016.

149 Mwale, M. and Masika, P. (2015). In vivo anthelmintic efficacy of *Aloe ferox*, *Agave sisalana*, and *Gunnera perpensa* in village chickens naturally infected with *Heterakis gallinarum*. *Trop. Anim. Health Prod.* 47: 131–138.

150 McLaughlin, J.D. (2008). Cestodes. In: *Parasitic Diseases of Wild Birds* (ed. T.C. Atkinson, N.J. Thomas and B.D. Hunter), 261–276. Hoboken, NJ: Wiley-Blackwell.

151 Shillinger, J.E., Morley, L.C. (1937). Diseases of Upland Game Birds. USDA Farmers' Bulletin No. 1781. US Government Printing Office: Washington, D.C. pp. 19–26.

152 Millan, J. (2009). Diseases of the red-legged partridge (*Alectoris rufa* L.): a review. *Wildl. Biol. Pract.* 5 (1): 70–88.

153 Chapman, H.D. (2014). Milestones in avian coccidiosis research: a review. *Poult. Sci.* 93 (1): 501–511.

154 Liou, C.T. (2001). Immunization against coccidiosis in pheasants with low-dose live sporulated oocysts of *Eimeria colchici*. *Avian Pathol.* 30 (4): 283–295.

155 Norton, C.C. and Wise, D.R. (1981). Anticoccidial drugs for preventive therapy in intensively reared pheasants. *Vet. Rec.* 109 (25–26): 554–556.

156 Tyzzer, E.E. (1929). Coccidiosis in gallinaceous birds. *Am. J. Hyg.* 10 (2): 269–307.

157 Ray, H.N. and Hiregaudar, L.S. (1959). Coccidia from some birds at the Calcutta zoo. *Bull. Calcutta Sch. Trop. Med.* 7: 111–112.

158 Yakimoff, W.L. and Matschoulsky, S.N. (1937). Nouvelle coccidia du faisan. *Ann. Parasitol. Hum. Comp.* 15: 162.

159 Ormsbee, R.A. (1939). Field studies on coccidiosis in the ring-neck pheasants of eastern Washington. *Parasitology* 31 (3): 389–399.

160 McQuiston, T.E. (1987). Efficacy of ionophorous anticoccidial drugs against coccidian in farm-reared pheasants (*Phasianus colchicus*) from Illinois. *Avian Dis.* 31 (2): 327–331.

161 Bhatia, B.B. (1968). A new and two known eimerian species from gallinaceous birds. *Indian J. Microbiol.* 8 (4): 239–244.

162 Gerhold, R.W., Fuller, A.L., and McDougald, L.R. (2016). Coccidiosis in the chukar partridge (*Alectoris chukar*): a survey of coccidiosis outbreaks and a test of anticoccidial drugs against *Eimeria kofoidi*. *Avian Dis.* 60 (4): 752–757.

163 Hafeez, M.A., Vrba, V., and Barta, J.R. (2015). The complete mitochondrial genome sequence of Eimeria innocua (Eimeriidae, Coccidia, Apicomplexa). Mitochondrial DNA A DNA Mapp. *Seq. Anal.* 27 (4): 2805–2806.

164 Naciri, M., Fort, G., Briant, J. et al. (2014). Incidence of single and mixed infections with *Eimeria kofoidi*, *E. caucasica* and *E. legionensis* on the health of experimentally infected red-legged partridges (*Alectoris rufa*). *Vet. Parasitol.* 205 (1–2): 77–84.

165 Fernandez-Alvarez, A., Modry, D., and Foronada, P.A. (2016). New species of *Eimeri schneider*, 1875 (Apicomlexa : Eimeriidae) from *Alectoris Barbara* (Aves: Phasianidae) from the Canary Islands (Spain). 115 (5): 1817–1825.

166 Freitas, F.L., Almeida, K.d.S., do Nascimento, A.A. et al. (2006). An outbreak of coccidiosis in partridge (*Rhynchotus rufescens*), reared in captivity, by *Eimeria rhynchoti* Reis and Nobrega, 1936 (Apicomplexa: Emeriidae). *Rev. Bras. Parasitol. Vet.* 15 (2): 85–87.

167 Goldová, M., Letková, V., and Csiszmárová, G. (2000). Life cycle of Eimeria procera in experimentally infected grey partridges (*Perdix perdix*). *Vet. Parasitol.* 90 (4): 255–263.

168 Bhatia, B.B., Pandey, T.P., and Pande, B.P. (1966). *Eimeria teetarisn*. Sp. (Eimeriidae. Sporozoa) in Indian partridges. *Acta Vet. Acad. Sci. Hung.* 16 (3): 329–333.

169 Shah, H.L. and Johnson, C.A. (1971). *Eimeria bateri* Bhatia, Pandey and Pande, 1965 from the Hungarian quail *Coturnix c. coturnix* in the United States and its attempted transmission to the chicken. *J. Protozool.* 18 (2): 219–220.

170 Gerhold, R.W., Guven, E., and McDougald, L.R. (2011). Oocyst production of Eimeria lettyae in northern bobwhites following low-dose inoculations. *J. Parasitol.* 97 (3): 525–526.

171 Ruff, M.D., Fagan, J.M., and Dick, J.W. (1984). Pathogenicity of coccidia in Japanese quail (*Coturnix coturnix japonica*). *Poult. Sci.* 63 (1): 55–60.

172 Ruff, M.D. (1985). Life cycle and biology of *Eimeria lettyae sp. n.* (Protozoa: Eimeriidae) from the northern bobwhite, *Colinus virginianus. J. Wildl. Dis.* 21 (4): 361–370.

173 Amoudi, M.A. (1987). *Eimeria tahamensis N. sp.* (Apicomplexa: Eimeriidae) from the Arabian quail (*Coturnix delegorguei arabica*). *J. Protozool.* 34 (4): 455–456.

174 Tsutsumi, Y. and Tsunoda, K. (1972). Pathogenicity of *Eimeria tsunodai* for Japanese quails (*Coturnis coturnix japonica*) and susceptibility of the coccidium to some drugs. *Nihon Juigaku Zasshi* 34 (3): 115–120.

175 Rao, J.R., Sharma, N.N., and Johri, T.S. (1995). Influence of dietary aflatoxin on *Eimeria uzura* infection in Japanese quail (*Coturnix coturnix japonica*). *Vet. Parasitol.* 56 (1–3): 17–22.

176 Amoudi, M.A. (1988). Two new species of *Eimeria* from peacocks (Pavo cirstatus) in Saudi Arabia. *J. Protozool.* 35 (4): 546–548.

177 El-Shahawy, I.S. (2010). *Eimeria pavoaegyptica* sp. nov. (Apicomplexa: Eimeriidae) in faeces of Indian peacocks, *Pavo cristatus* Linnaeus, 1758 (Galliformes: Phasianidae) from Egypt. *Mem. Inst. Oswaldo Cruz* 105 (8): 965–969.

178 Hauck, R. and Hafez, H.M. (2012). Description of *Eimeria pavonina* (coccidia) of peafowl in Germany. *Avian Dis.* 56 (1): 238–242.

179 Titilincu, A., Mircean, V., Bejan, A. et al. (2009). Preventa endoparazitozelor la Pauni (*Pavo cristatus*). *Sci. Paratisol.* 1-2: 101–105.

180 Banik, D.C. and Ray, H.N. (1964). On a new coccidium, *Eimeria mandalin n. sp.* from peacock. *Bull. Calcutta Sch. Trop. Med.* 12 (1): 27.

181 Williams, R.B. (1978). Notes on some coccidia of peafowl, pheasants and chickens. *Vet. Parasitol.* 4 (2): 193–197.

182 Long, P.L. and Millard, B.J. (1978). Studies on *Eimeria grenieri* in the Guinea fowl (*Numida meleagris*). *Parasitology* 76 (1): 1–9.

183 Harkirat, S., Mishra, A., and Rao, J.R. (2006). Occurrence of coccidian infections in turkeys and Guinea fowls. *J. Vet. Parasitol.* 20 (2): 153–154.

184 Bhatia, B.B. and Pande, B.P. (1967). A new eimerian species from Guinea fowl. A preliminary note. *Acta Vet. Acad. Sci. Hung.* 17 (4): 359–361.

185 Norton, C.C. (1976). Coccidia of the pheasant. *Folia Vet. Lat.* 6 (3): 218–238.

186 Canning, E.U. and Anwar, M. (1969). Studies on meiotic division in coccidial and malarial parasites. *J. Protozool.* 15 (2): 290–298.

187 Quiroz-Castaneda, R.E. and Dantan-Gonzalez, E. (2015). Control of avian coccidiosis: future and present natural alternatives. *Biomed. Res. Int.* 2015: 1–11.

188 Yabsley, M.J. (2008). Eimeria. In: *Parasitic Diseases of Wild Birds* (ed. T.C. Atkinson, N.J. Thomas and B.D. Hunter), 162–180. Hoboken, NJ: Wiley-Blackwell.

189 Musaev, M., Gaibova, G., Ismailova, G. et al. (1998). The coccidia of gallinaceous birds in Azerbaijan. *Trop. J. Vet. Am. Sci.* 22 (5): 409–413.

190 Chapman, H.D. (2009). A landmark contribution to poultry science – prophylactic control of coccidiosis in poultry. *Poult. Sci.* 88 (4): 813–815.

191 Danforth, H.D. (1998). Use of live oocyst vaccines in the control of avian coccidiosis: experimental studies and field trials. *Int. J. Parasitol.* 28 (7): 1099–1109.

192 Patton, W.H., Schwartz, L.D., Babish, J.G. et al. (1984). Use of amprolium for the control of coccidiosis in pheasants. *Avian Dis.* 28 (3): 693–698.

193 Ruff, M.D., Wilkins, G.C., and Chute, M.B. (1987). Prevention of coccidiosis in bobwhites by medication. *Poult. Sci.* 66 (9): 1437–1445.

194 Fuller, L., Griffith, R., and McDougald, L.R. (2000). Efficacy of lasalocid against coccidiosis in Chinese ring-necked pheasants. *Avian Dis.* 52 (4): 632–634.

195 Gerhold, R.W., Fuller, A.L., Lollis, L. et al. (2011). The efficacy of anticoccidial drugs against Eimeria spp. in northern bobwhites. *Avian Dis.* 55 (1): 59–64.

196 Sokol, R., Gesak, M., Ras-Norynaka, M. et al. (2014). Titrazuril (Baycox) treatment against coccidiosis caused by Eimeria sp. in Japanese quail (*Coturnix coturnix* japonica). *Pol. J. Vet. Sci.* 17 (3): 465–468.

197 OIE. Cryptosporidiosis. In: OIE Terrestrial Manual www.oie.int/fileadmin/Home/eng/Health_standards/tahm/3.10.02_CRYPTO.pdf (accessed February 2022).

198 Kabir, B.M.H., Han, Y., Lee, S.H. et al. (2020). Prevalence and molecular characterization of cryptosporidium species in poultry in Bangladesh. *One Health* 9 (00122).

199 Ritter, G.D., Ley, D.H., Levy, M. et al. (1986). Intestinal cryptosporidiosis and reovirus isolation from bobwhite quail (*Colinus virginianus*) with enteritis. *Avian Dis.* 30 (3): 603–608.

200 Maca, O. and Pavlasek, I. (2016). Cryptosporidium infections of ring-necked pheasants (*Phasianus colchicus*) from an intensive artificial breeding programme in the Czech Republic. *Parasitol. Res.* 115 (5): 1915–1922.

201 Maca, O. and Pavlasek, I. (2015). First finding of spontaneous infections with *Cryptosporidium baileyi* and *C. meleagridis* in the red-legged partridge *Alectoris rufa* from an aviary in the Czech Republic. *Vet. Parasitol.* 209 (3–4): 164–168.

202 O'Donoghue, P.J., Tham, V.L., de Saram, W.G. et al. (1987). Cryptosporidium infections in birds and mammals and attempted cross-transmission studies. *Vet. Parasitol.* 26 (1): 1–11.

203 Mason, R.W. and Hartley, W.J. (1980). Respiratory cryptosporidiosis in a peacock chick. *Avian Dis.* 24 (3): 771–776.

204 Hoerr, F.J., Current, W.L., and Haynes, T.B. (1986). Fatal cryptosporidiosis in a quail. *Avian Dis.* 30 (2): 421–425.

205 Tham, V.L., Kniesberg, S., and Dixon, B.R. (1982). Cryptosporidiosis in quails. *Avian Pathol.* 11 (4): 619–626.

206 Shaapan, R.M., Khalil, F.A.M., and Abu El Ezz, M.T. (2011). Cryptosporidiosis and Toxoplasmosis in native quails of Egypt. *Res. J. Vet. Sci.* 4 (2): 30–36.

207 Wang, Y., Zhang, K., Chen, Y. et al. (2021). *Cryptosporidium* and cryptospordiosis in wild birds: One Health perspective. *Parasitol. Res.* 120 (9): 3035–3044.

208 Upton, S.J., McAllister, C.T., Freed, P.S., and Barnard, S.M. (1989). *Cryptosporidium spp.* in wild and captive reptiles. *J. Wildl. Dis.* 25 (1): 20–30.

209 O'Donoghue, P.J. (1995). *Cryptosporidium* and cryptosporidiosis in man and animals. *Int. J. Parasitol.* 25 (2): 139–195.

210 Lindsay, D.S. and Blagburn, B.L. (1990). Cryptosporidiosis in birds. In: *Cryptosporidiosis of Man and Animals* (ed. J.P. Dubey, C.A. Speer and R. Fayer), 125–148. Boston, MA.: CRC Press.

211 Current, W.L., Upton, S.J., and Haynes, T.B. (1986). The life cycle of *Cryptosporidium baileyi n.sp.* (Apicomplexa, Cryptosporidiidae) infecting chickens. *J. Protozool.* 33 (2): 289–296.

212 Fujino, T. (1996). Infectivity and immunogenicity to Japanese quails (*Coturnix coturnix japonica*) of *Cryptosporidium sp.* isolated from chickens in Japan. *Jpn. J. Parasitol.* 45 (3): 139–143.

213 Fujino, T. (1996). Infectivity of *Cryptospordiium sp.* isolated from chickens in Japan to turkeys, bobwhite quails and several kinds of experimental animals. *Jpn. J. Parasitol.* 45 (4): 295–298.

214 Whittington, R.J. and Wilson, J.M. (1985). Cryptosporidiosis of the respiratory tract in a pheasant. *Aust. Vet. J.* 62 (8): 284–285.

215 Sreter, T. and Varga, I. (2000). Cryptosporidiosis in birds – a review. *Vet. Parasitol.* 87 (4): 261–279.

216 Nakamura, A.A. and Meireles, M.V. (2015). *Cryptosporidium* infections in birds – a review. *Rev. Braz. Parasitol. Vet.* 24 (3): 253–267.

217 El-Alfy, E.S. and Nishikawa, Y. (2020). *Cryptosporidium* species and cryptosporidiosis in Japan: a literature review and insights into the role played by animals in its transmission. *J. Vet. Med. Sci.* 82 (8): 1051–1067.

218 Rose, J.B. (1997). Environmental ecology of *Cryptosporidium* and public health considerations. *Annu. Rev. Public Health* 18 (1): 135–161.

219 McNeil, E., Platt, E.D., and Hinshaw, W.R. (1939). *Hexamita sp.* from quail and from chukar partridges. *Cornell Vet.* 29 (3): 330–333.

220 Wood, A.M. and Smith, H.V. (2005). Spironucleosis (Hexamitiasis, Hexamitosis) in the ring-necked pheasant (*Phasianus colchicus*): detection of cysts and description of *Spironucleus meleagridis* in stained smears. *Avian Dis.* 49 (1): 138–143.

221 Cooper, G.L., Charlton, B.R., Bickford, A.A. et al. (2004). *Hexamita meleagridis* (*Spironucleus meleagridis*) infection in chukar partridges associated with high mortality and intracellular trophozoites. *Avian Dis.* 48 (4): 706–710.

222 Ashlund, E.E. and Chute, A.M. (1971). Bobwhite, *Colinus virginianus*, as host for *Heterakis* and *Histomonas*. *J. Wildl. Dis.* 7 (1): 70–75.

223 Lund, E.E. and Chute, A.M. (1971). Histomoniasis in the chukar partridge. *J. Wildl. Manage.* 35 (2): 307–315.

224 Lund, E.E. and Chute, A.M. (1972). The ring-necked pheasant (*Phasianus colchicus toryuatus*) as a host for *Heterakis gallinarum* and *Histomonas meleagridis*. *Am. Midland Nat.* 87 (1): 1–7.

225 McDougald, L.R. (2005). Blackhead disease (Histomoniasis) in poultry: a critical review. *Avian Dis.* 49 (4): 462–476.

226 Lund, E.E., Wehr, E.E., and Ellis, D.J. (1966). Earthworm transmission of *Heterakis* and *Histomonas* to turkeys and chickens. *J. Parasitol.* 52 (5): 899–902.

227 Clarke, L.L., Beckstead, R.B., Hayes, J.R. et al. (2017). Pathologic and molecular characterization of histomoniasis in peafowl (*Pavo cristatus*). *J. Vet. Diagn. Invest.* 29 (2): 237–241.

228 Chute, M.B., Chute, A.M., and Wilkins, G.C. (1978). Effect of dimetridazole on transmission of *Histomonas meleagridis* by *Heterakis gallinarum*. *Parasitology* 77 (1): 41–48.

229 National Toxicology Program (NTP) (2014). NTP Report on Carcinogens, 13. National Institute of Environmental Health Sciences, Research Triangle Park, NC.

230 Clark, S. and Kimminau, E. (2017). Critical review: future control of blackhead disease (histomoniasis) in poultry. *Avian Dis.* 61 (3): 281–288.

231 Lund, E.E. and Chute, A.M. (1974). The reproductive potential of *Heterakis gallinarum* in various species of galliform birds: implications for survival of *H. gallinarum* and *Histomonas meleagridis* to recent times. *Int. J. Parasitol.* 4 (5): 455–461.

12

Gamebird Musculoskeletal and Neurologic Diseases
Daniel P. Shaw

Gamebirds can be afflicted with musculoskeletal and neurologic diseases that are similar to those found in domestic poultry species.

12.1   Diseases Affecting the Extremities

12.1.1   Bacterial Osteomyelitis

The condition tends to be seen mainly in meat birds, such as broilers and turkeys, during the growing period. It can, however, occur in any class of gamebirds and poultry. The condition develops when bacteria enter the bloodstream and lodge in the tiny capillaries of the bone, particularly in the growth plate. In this location, they can grow and damage bone by inducing inflammation. Bone tissue is difficult for the body to defend effectively. Once injured by infection, the damaged bone breaks down. This results in lameness if a leg bone is involved, or impairment of the use of the wings.

12.1.1.1   Clinical Signs
Lameness becomes noticeable when body weight increases because the damaged bone bulges and stimulates the pressure receptors in the periosteum. This is interpreted as pain and causes limping. There are several bacteria that can cause the infection.

12.1.1.2   Diagnosis
At necropsy, the ends of the affected long bones, such as the proximal tibia, should be sectioned sagittally to reveal the growth plate area. The gross changes can be subtle but if several birds are examined, there will be at least a few that have obvious damage, such as accumulation of caseous tan material in the center of the growth plate area. Bacterial culture of the damaged bone is required for identification of the causative organism. Extensive bone damage may occur in chicks from a flock that had septicemia from infection with *Salmonella* sp. Infection with *Escherichia coli* is a common cause of osteomyelitis in birds of various ages.

12.1.1.3   Treatment and Prevention
There is a poor prognosis for affected birds. Broad-spectrum antibiotic treatment should be administered to the flock to try to protect the birds that do not have yet osteomyelitis. It may also help

Gamebird Medicine and Management, First Edition. Edited by Teresa Y. Morishita and Robert E. Porter, Jr.
© 2023 John Wiley & Sons, Inc. Published 2023 by John Wiley & Sons, Inc.

some of the less severely affected birds in the flock. Prognosis is poor for birds that have bone damage. Even if the bacteria are killed by the antibacterial therapy, it is unlikely that the damage can be repaired.

Maintaining good sanitation is important in preventing this disease.

12.1.2   *Mycoplasma synoviae* Infection

Mycoplasma synoviae (MS) is a unique, fragile bacterium that lacks a cell wall. It is very fastidious in its growth requirements on artificial media and can be difficult to isolate from infected birds. It can be transmitted vertically, from an infected hen to her chick through the egg. It can also be transmitted horizontally, between birds. Natural infection occurs in ducks, geese, guineafowl, pigeons, Japanese quail, pheasants, red-legged partridge, chickens, and turkeys [1]. There is variation in pathogenicity of different strains of the bacterium, but infection can cause synovitis and arthritis. The organism can be carried between groups of birds on shoes, hands, and clothing.

12.1.2.1   Clinical Signs

Lame birds with swollen hocks and foot pads will appear. The swollen hocks and foot pads contain inflammatory exudate. The affected birds are reluctant to move, have a limping gait, and develop breast blisters. Younger birds are more severely affected and may develop bone deformities. Some of the infected chicks may also develop airsacculitis.

12.1.2.2   Diagnosis

Several different agents may cause synovitis and swollen foot pads. Laboratory workup is required to identify the cause. Many veterinary diagnostic laboratories offer a very sensitive and specific PCR assay that is performed on preparations of tracheal or pharyngeal swabs. Affected joints from at least a few birds should be cultured to determine if some other bacterium is present. Serologic tests for detection of antibody are available specifically for chickens and turkeys but should function well enough for gamebird species. These include the enzyme-linked immunosorbent assay (ELISA), serum plate agglutination (SPA), and hemagglutination inhibition (HI). The detection of antibody indicates that the bird has been exposed to the organism at least 1.5 weeks previously. The primary immune response requires 10–14 days for development.

12.1.2.3   Treatment and Prevention

This is a chronic condition and infected birds are carriers for life. Administration of an appropriate antibiotic in the water or feed often decreases the severity of clinical signs but is unlikely to eliminate the organism from an infected flock. Prevention requires that chicks be purchased from breeding flocks that are free of the organism. The National Poultry Improvement Program (NPIP) promotes and manages a program aimed at prevention and elimination of this organism in poultry species. Chicks specifically certified by NPIP against the presence this organism are derived from breeding stock that is free of it.

12.1.3   Pododermatitis

Pododermatitis is also known as bumblefoot and affects the bottom of the footpad [2]. It appears as varying degrees of irritation, up to and including the formation of a large thick ulcerated area. It can affect any species of gamebird at any age. The cause can be obvious, such as injury from overly rough bedding or excessively moist litter, or obscure. The source of the problem, however, is not always apparent.

12.1.3.1 Clinical Signs

Affected birds may be reluctant to walk. While walking, affected gamebirds may display lameness. The footpad is often reddened and swollen in the early stages. Without intervention, this lesion can progress to formation of an ulcerated sore that is covered by a mat of necrotic exudate. There is often an underlying cavity filled with thick exudate. It can progress deeper into underlying tissue and involve the tendon sheaths.

12.1.3.2 Diagnosis

The condition is readily identified with physical examination. Several birds should be examined to determine the extent of the problem in the flock.

12.1.3.3 Treatment and Prevention

It is helpful to find the cause of the irritation which often arises from wet litter or overly rough flooring surfaces. Jumping from high perches to rough flooring may also be suspected as a cause. Sometimes, dietary deficiencies can cause weakness in the skin of the ball of the foot and predispose it to secondary infection. The lesion can be cultured to identify the causative bacterium, but the area is usually so contaminated that it is difficult to isolate the original inciting agent. Broad-spectrum antibiotics can be administered through the water or feed to help prevent the infection developing in other members of the flock. The poor blood circulation in the foot impairs healing and delivery of antibiotics to the affected area. Topical administration of antibacterial agents and bandaging may be helpful in treating individual cases. Steps should be taken to improve the condition of the flooring to prevent injury to the feet of other birds in the group [3].

12.1.4 Marek Disease

Marek disease (MD) is a neoplastic disease of the lymphocytes caused by infection with a specific herpesvirus. It is primarily a disease of chickens but it can also infect pheasants, quail (coturnix and bobwhite), domestic turkeys, and crested partridges [4–9]. The neoplastic lymphocytes proliferate and form tumors in different organs, including liver, spleen, proventriculus, and kidneys. Tumors may also form in the skin (skin leukosis). The neoplastic lymphocytes from MD also typically infiltrate peripheral nerves and the central nervous system (CNS) and cause impairment of their function.

12.1.4.1 Clinical Signs

The incubation period can be as short as 5 days. In chickens, outbreaks usually occur after 8–9 weeks of age. The disease in quail tends to produce tumors in visceral organs and nerves are not as commonly involved. Pheasants appear to be more susceptible to the neurologic form of the disease but also develop tumors in visceral organs. Signs of the neurologic form include paralysis of a limb or torticollis (twisted neck), depending on which nerves are affected by the infiltrating neoplastic lymphocytes. Other signs are dependent on which internal organs are involved.

12.1.4.2 Diagnosis

Diagnosis is based on gross and microscopic changes in tissues. Grossly, the tumors in visceral organs are soft, tan-white, and variable in size and shape. In addition, the neoplastic lymphocytes of MD invade the nervous system. Peripheral nerves may be grossly enlarged and have a yellowish discoloration. The eyeball may be involved, causing the iris to be discolored and the pupil misshapen. Microscopically, the neoplastic lymphocytes are visible invading nerves, brain, or eye [9, 10]. In the internal organs, the neoplastic lymphocytes form sheets that invade the structures of the affected organ.

12.1.4.3 Treatment and Prevention

There is no treatment for the disease. Vaccines are available to prevent the development of tumors in chickens. The vaccine, however, does not prevent infection with the virus. There are no vaccines available for gamebirds. Typical of herpesviruses, once infected, a bird is a carrier for life and can shed the virus periodically. The virus itself is delicate. It is transmitted via the airborne route in the feather follicle dander which protects it. It can remain viable in poultry house dust for several months at 20–25 °C and for years at 4 °C. It is, therefore, important to clean and disinfect between broods to eliminate the virus or, at least, reduce the level of exposure for new chicks.

12.1.5 Crooked Toes

Occasionally, gamebirds have been observed to have crooked toes. The condition is also known as curly toe paralysis or curled-toe paralysis. It is caused by a deficiency of vitamin B2 (riboflavin) in young chicks [3, 11]. Any species of gamebirds or poultry can be affected [9]. The deficiency causes damage to the nerves that control the legs and toes.

12.1.5.1 Clinical Signs

Affected chicks are reluctant to walk. When forced to walk, they may walk on their hocks. When examined, the toes of affected chicks curl medially (inward). One or both legs may be affected. Many of the chicks may have paralysis of the legs. In advanced stages, they lie with their legs sprawled out. Depending on the severity of the deficiency, the flock may be unthrifty and the chicks stunted. Diarrhea may develop by 2 weeks of age.

Breeding hens fed a deficient diet will have decreased egg production, poor embryo survival, and decreased hatchability. The embryos that fail to hatch are dwarfed and have "clubbed" down. "Clubbed" down results from failure of the down feathers to rupture the feather sheaths, causing them to coil in a characteristic way.

12.1.5.2 Diagnosis

The clinical signs are typical for crooked toes. Microscopic examination will reveal the damage to the sciatic, cervical, and lumbar spinal nerves characterized by axonal swelling and demyelination [9]. There is also atrophy of the muscles in the legs.

12.1.5.3 Treatment and Prevention

If this condition is suspected, it is important to add a water-soluble B vitamin supplement that contains riboflavin to the drinking water and supply new fresh starter feed. It is uncommon for feed to be deficient in vitamin B2 due to errors in mixing or formulation. The vitamin is, however, susceptible to degradation when stored for long periods of time or in adverse conditions of heat and humidity. Hence, it is important to provide fresh feed for baby chicks. It is also necessary to feed a balanced, age-appropriate, and species-specific formulated ration as gamebird species require higher levels of several nutrients than chickens. Gamebirds do not do well on rations formulated for chickens. If the deficiency has been of long standing, the damage will be permanent.

12.1.6 Perosis

Perosis is also known as splay leg or slipped tendon. It is associated with a deficiency of manganese, choline, or other B vitamins [3, 9]. It is usually seen in young growing birds. Most species of poultry and gamebirds are susceptible. Due to the nutritional deficiency, the groove at the end of the tibiotarsus (back of the hock) is malformed and shallow. This defect allows the gastrocnemius (Achilles) tendon to slip out of the groove. When this occurs, the muscle attached the tendon loses its fulcrum and cannot extend the leg. The condition can affect one or both legs.

12.1.6.1 Clinical Signs
Affected chicks are unable to extend the affected leg and cannot support weight on that leg (Figure 12.1a) [3].

12.1.6.2 Diagnosis
This condition is easily detected on physical examination of live birds or during necropsy of dead birds (Figure 12.1b) [9].

12.1.6.3 Treatment and Prevention
There is a poor prognosis for affected birds. The addition of water-soluble vitamins and minerals in the drinking water for 1 week to prevent this disease in the rest of the flock is recommended. It is important to feed a balanced ration appropriate for the species. The only species that does well on chicken feed is chickens. Gamebird species have higher nutrient requirements as supplied in specialized rations or in turkey feed formulations. Hence, it is crucial that gamebirds be fed diets formulated specifically for gamebirds.

(a)
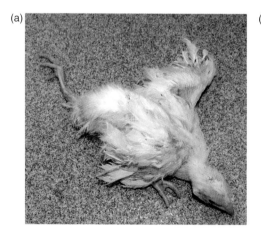
(b)
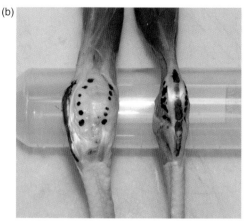

Figure 12.1 Perosis. (a) White pheasant chick cannot extend right leg due to lateral dislocation of the gastrocnemius tendon. (b) Partially dissected legs. On the left, the abnormal left hock has a gastrocnemius tendon (marked in blue) that is dislocated laterally from groove (bordered with black dots) of the distal tibiotarsus. On the right, the gastrocnemius tendon (marked in blue) of the normal leg extends over the caudal aspect of the hock joint (groove in distal tibiotarsus is marked as the space between the two lines of black dots).

12.1.7   Rickets

Rickets is caused by a deficiency of calcium, phosphorus, or vitamin D, or an imbalance in the calcium/phosphorus ratio in the feed [9, 10]. It is seen in young growing birds and is associated with weakness, inability to stand, and excessive death loss in the flock. Adults develop soft bones (osteomalcia) [9].

12.1.7.1   Clinical Signs
The joints of affected chicks are enlarged, especially noticeable in the hocks. The chicks are reluctant or unable to stand. The bones may be soft and rubbery. In fact, these soft bones can often be flexed with minimal discomfort to the affected chick.

12.1.7.2   Diagnosis
The diagnosis may be obvious on physical examination of live or dead chicks. At necropsy, the long bones and ribs are softer than expected or rubbery. There may be thickening of the junctions of the ribs with the sternum and spinal column (beading) Deformities of the long bones, sternum, or spinal column may also be present. The long bones can be sectioned sagittally and the growth plate will appear as a wide zone of cartilage (Figure 12.2). The accumulation of cartilage is due to failure of mineralization of the cartilage model in the growth plate. The diagnosis can be confirmed by microscopic examination of the growth plate area [9, 10].

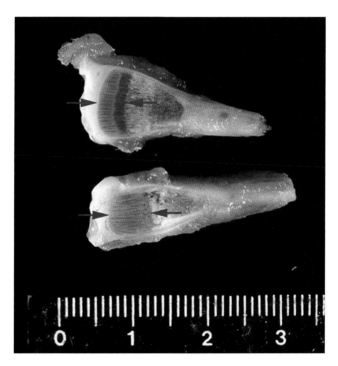

Figure 12.2   Rickets. The proximal tibiotarsal bones have been sectioned sagittally. The normal bone (upper) has a growth plate (arrows) of normal length. The rachitic bone (lower) has a growth plate (arrows) that is abnormally elongated.

12.1.7.3 Treatment and Prevention

Treatment includes adding water-soluble vitamin D to the drinking water as prescribed in the label directions. The feed can be top dressed with a calcium supplement. Because of their tiny size, baby chicks do not eat very much feed very quickly. It is possible for the ration, if improperly stored, to become stale and the vitamin D degraded. It should also be noted that baby chicks are kept inside to facilitate brooding and thus they do not have exposure to sunlight. Sunlight activates the sterols in the dander and the bird ingests the vitamin when it preens. Birds that have access to direct sunlight, therefore, are unlikely to develop a vitamin D deficiency.

12.2 Diseases Affecting the Head

12.2.1 Bacterial Infection of the Brain

Bacterial infection of the brain is often manifest as meningitis with perivascular infiltration by inflammatory cells in the encephalon. It can be caused by infection with several different bacteria including *E. coli*, *Pasteurella multocida*, *Salmonella* sp., *Riemerella anatipestifer* (ducks and turkeys), and *Listeria monocytogenes* [9, 12–15]. It may occur as a primary infection or as part of a general infection. It may also be secondary to airsacculitis.

12.2.1.1 Clinical Signs
Affected birds display listlessness, ataxia, torticollis, tremors of head and neck, and depression.

12.2.1.2 Diagnosis
There may not be very many gross changes visible in the brains of affected birds. If present, though, the meninges appear wet and cloudy. The underlying structures of the brain, such as the cerebellar folia, may be obscured because of the inflammatory reaction in the meninges. Blood vessels in the meninges and brain may be engorged with blood and edged by white caused by cuffing with inflammatory cells. There may be a thick layer of soft tenacious exudate over the meninges in severe cases. Other systems such as the respiratory tract may also be involved. Microscopically, the meninges contain fibrin and infiltration by large numbers of heterophils and macrophages [10]. Heterophils and macrophages form cuffs around blood vessels and capillaries in the encephalon. The ventricles of the brain may contain inflammatory exudate. Bacterial colonies may be visible among the inflammatory cells and fibrin.

Bacterial culture of brains is required for identification of the causative organism, keeping in mind that some of the bacteria may have special requirements for robust growth and detection on artificial media.

12.2.1.3 Treatment and Prevention
Antibiotic therapy is indicated. Ideally, it is based on the results of susceptibility testing but a broad-spectrum antibiotic can be administered in the water to help slow the spread in the flock while laboratory workup is in progress. Severely affected birds are unlikely to recover. Prevention requires provision of optimal air quality and environment conditions that reduce dust and bacterial load in the air.

12.2.2   Mycotic Encephalitis

Mycotic encephalitis is a fungal infection of the brain. The most common fungi associated with infections are *Aspergillus fumigatus* and *A. flavus* [16]. Any species of bird can be affected, and it tends to be seen in young birds. These fungi are more often associated with infections of the lung and air sacs in various ages of poultry and gamebirds. *Ochroconis gallopava* (formerly known as *Dactylaria gallopava*) is a different fungus that is an occasional cause of encephalitis in chickens, turkeys, and quail [16]. *Aspergillus* sp. are the most common fungi in the air and litter in poultry facilities [9]. The fungi pose greater problems in confinement where stress factors and poor air quality are present or when moldy litter or feed is present.

12.2.2.1   Clinical Signs
Fungal infection of the brain causes neurologic signs including torticollis or lack of equilibrium.

12.2.2.2   Diagnosis
Gross lesions in the brain include discolored areas of malacia and hemorrhage. Microscopically, there are multiple foci of hemorrhage and necrosis in the brain [10, 16]. The fungi grow in the walls of blood vessels and capillaries, causing thrombosis that leads to infarction of the areas supplied by those vessels (Figure 12.3a). The fungal hyphae are often visible in sections stained with hematoxylin and eosin (HE). Gomori's methamine silver (GMS) or periodic acid–Schiff (PAS) stains highlight the presence of fungal hyphae in tissue sections, making them easier to detect (Figure 12.3b). The affected tissue can be cultured for the fungi, but this is not usually necessary for diagnosis.

12.2.2.3   Treatment and Prevention
There is no effective treatment for aspergillosis. Ventilation and dust control should be enhanced to reduce the concentration of mold spores in the air. The facility should be checked for the presence of moldy materials, which should be removed if found. Birds will pant if the ambient temperature is too high. Once they open their mouths to breathe, they bypass the filtration mechanisms of the upper respiratory system and have increased chances of inhaling the fungal spores.

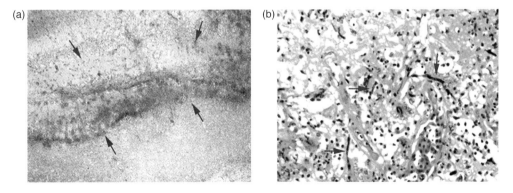

Figure 12.3   Mycotic encephalitis photomicrographs. (a) Low magnification of area of necrosis and hemorrhage in cerebellum (arrows) (H&E stain, 40×). (b) High magnification of section stained with GMS showing the fungal hyphae (arrows) (40×).

12.2.3 Arboviruses

The members of this group of viruses cause fatal infection in the CNS in susceptible species of birds and mammals. The term "arbovirus" is short for *ar*thropod-*bo*rne *virus*. These viruses are transmitted by mosquitos and other blood-sucking insects. The arboviruses are a large diverse group composed of 12 families [17]. Only the families Togaviridae and Flaviviridae contain viruses that cause disease in poultry and gamebirds. The family Togaviridae contains eastern equine encephalitis virus (EEE), western equine encephalitis virus (WEE), and Highlands J virus (HJV). The family Flaviviridae contains West Nile virus (WNV).

12.2.4 Eastern Equine Encephalitis

Eastern equine encephalitis occurs most commonly as a disease of horses but is also the cause of many outbreaks in farm-raised pheasant [17, 18]. It occurs only sporadically in other species of poultry and gamebirds, such as chukar partridge, pigeons, turkeys, and ducks. The disease occurs primarily in eastern parts of the United States and Canada. It is also present in Central America, the Caribbean, and eastern parts of South America. Wild birds, primarily the smaller passerine birds, are the principal vertebrate hosts and rarely become sick from infection. They develop viremia that can last up to 14 days. The virus is transmitted primarily by mosquitoes but has been identified in mites, lice, simuliid flies, and culicoides. It can also be transmitted directly as a result of feather picking and cannibalism.

12.2.4.1 Clinical Signs

The virus infects the CNS. In pheasants and chukar partridges, it causes listlessness, somnolence, leg paralysis, torticollis, and tremors [9]. Death loss can range up to 80% in infected flocks of pheasants and chukar partridge. Additionally, EEE infection may produce visceral infections with little or no involvement of the CNS.

12.2.4.2 Diagnosis

The infection does not produce gross lesions. Microscopically, there is perivascular cuffing by lymphocytes, patchy necrosis, neuronal degeneration, and meningitis in the brain and spinal cord [9, 10]. These findings are very suggestive of a viral infection in the CNS and, combined with the history (season and presence of mosquitoes), provide the basis of a presumptive diagnosis. Several techniques can be used to identify the presence of the virus, including isolation and identification of the agent, antigen capture ELISA, immunohistochemistry, reverse transcription-polymerase chain reaction (RT-PCR), and serologic testing. Not all veterinary diagnostic laboratories have the capability to identify the virus but may be able to send specimens out to a laboratory that has the testing available.

12.2.4.3 Treatment and Prevention

There is no effective treatment for EEE. Prevention and control are best achieved through reducing vector populations through management of the habitat that produces them.

12.2.5 Western Equine Encephalitis and Highlands J Virus

Western equine encephalitis virus shares many of the characteristics of the EEE virus. It is, however, rarely associated with disease in avian species [17]. It is present mainly in the western parts of the USA. A few outbreaks have been reported in domestic turkeys and caused high mortality; the affected turkeys had somnolence, tremors, and leg paralysis. Laboratory diagnosis is accomplished using the same techniques as for EEE.

The Highlands J virus is antigenically closely related to the WEE virus. It is likely to be the cause of disease outbreaks in the eastern US attributed to WEE [17]. Experimental inoculation of chukar partridge with Highlands J virus has induced somnolence, recumbency, and death. Grossly, the spleen may be swollen and mottled and the heart pale (due to necrosis of myocardial fibers). Microscopically, there is nonsuppurative encephalitis, myocardial necrosis, enteritis with necrosis of the gut-associated lymphoid tissue, and lymphoid depletion and necrosis in the bursa of Fabricius, spleen, and thymus [9]. It has also been associated with drops in egg production in domestic turkeys. It is only mildly pathogenic for young turkeys. The laboratory diagnosis is accomplished using the same techniques as for EEE.

12.2.6 West Nile Virus

West Nile virus was first detected in the USA in 1999 and is now considered endemic [17, 19]. It infects a variety of avian and mammalian species, including humans. Infection causes clinical signs only in certain species. Humans and horses may be severely affected. Among avian species, crows, jays, raptors, sage grouse, ruffed grouse, ostrich, waterfowl, sea birds, and others are particularly severely affected [17, 20–22]. Even though ducks, chukar partridge, red-legged partridge, and pheasants are susceptible, reports of clinical signs and death from naturally occurring infection are rare [9, 18, 21, 23, 24].

12.2.6.1 Clinical Signs
Affected birds display recumbency, asymmetric leg or wing paralysis, incoordination, torticollis, and opisthotonos [17, 24].

12.2.6.2 Diagnosis
Few gross changes are usually present in gamebirds. Microscopically, there is often nonsuppurative encephalitis. Inflammatory lesions may also be found in the heart and intestine. It is notable that brains of gamebirds may have no lesions [19, 24]. The virus is found in several different organs besides the brain and heart [17, 19, 22]. History and clinical signs combined with microscopic changes in brain are suggestive of WNV [10, 17]. The PCR assay is sensitive and widely available in veterinary diagnostic laboratories. Immunohistochemical staining is available in many diagnostic laboratories. Virus isolation procedures are available in some laboratories.

12.2.6.3 Treatment and Prevention
Similarly to EEE, there is no effective treatment. Prevention and control are best achieved through reducing vector populations by management of the habitat that produces them. Experimentally, vaccination has been shown to be helpful in preventing clinical signs and death in some species of gamebirds such as ruffed grouse [20, 22].

12.2.7 Newcastle Disease

Newcastle disease (ND) is caused by infection with avian paramyxovirus serotype 1 (APMV-1) [25]. It is an RNA virus that causes an acute, rapidly spreading disease of birds of all ages. Although the details of clinical signs and diagnosis are given in Chapter 11, it is discussed here because infection of pheasants and quail is frequently associated with neurologic signs [26, 27].

12.2.7.1 Clinical Signs

The incubation period varies between 2 and 15 days and averages 5–6 days. In some cases, it may take 3–4 weeks for disease development. Infected pheasants may display nervous signs such as incoordination, depression, failure to feed, and head shaking [26]. Mortality is highly variable and has been reported from 3% up to 77% in natural outbreaks in captive reared pheasants [26]. In the late stages of the disease, infected birds may display greenish diarrhea, facial swelling, clonic spasms, and other neurologic signs.

12.2.7.2 Diagnosis

The microscopic findings in the brain are typical of a viral infection but not specific. There is perivascular cuffing by lymphocytes and gliosis in the brain [9, 10]. Definitive diagnosis requires detection of the virus. For this, swabs of trachea, pharynx/choanae, cloaca, or brain are collected. They can be used for the PCR assay or as inoculum for virus isolation in embryonated chicken eggs. The advantage of the PCR assay is that it potentially can be performed the same day whereas virus isolation can take a few days, depending on the availability of fertile eggs.

12.2.7.3 Treatment and Prevention

There is no treatment for the viral infection itself. Environmental conditions should be optimized to reduce additional stresses on the sick birds. Birds that survive the less virulent forms of ND are immune for a period of time, but this depends on the species involved. Killed and modified-live vaccines are available. Vaccination programs similar to those used in commercial poultry production are followed. More detail on vaccination is provided in Chapter 11.

12.2.8 Avian Encephalomyelitis

Avian encephalomyelitis (AE) is a viral disease that occurs in natural outbreaks in chickens, pheasants, coturnix quail, turkeys, and pigeons [3, 9, 28, 29]. It is caused by infection with a picornavirus and is the sole member of the genus *Tremorovirus*. The virus is transmitted by ingestion and is shed in droppings for several days. It is a durable virus in the environment and resistant to many disinfectants. Contaminated litter is an important source of infection. It can be easily spread on fomites or tracked on footwear. The infection spreads rapidly in a pen or house. It is more likely to occur in multiage operations than in flocks reared in isolation or as a single age group. The virus is also transmitted vertically, from an infected hen through the egg to the chick. Once hatched, the infected chick acts as a source of infection for other chicks in the group. The virus can also be transmitted in the incubator.

12.2.8.1 Clinical Signs

It is usually seen in flocks between 1 and 2 weeks of age. Some infected chicks may show signs at hatching if it has been transmitted from an infected hen. Affected chicks first appear dull. Gradually, ataxia and incoordination develop. Chicks tend to sit and are reluctant to move. They may walk on their hocks or shanks. Fine tremors of the head and neck become evident. Exciting or disturbing the chicks may bring on the tremors. Ataxia progresses and the chicks are unable to move, become prostrate, and die. Severely affected chicks are often trampled by their pen mates. Some chicks may survive and grow to maturity. The clinical signs in these birds may resolve completely. Survivors often are blind due to a bluish discoloration of the lens (cataracts). Chicks over 2–3 weeks of age are resistant to clinical signs. Infection of mature birds is associated with a drop in egg production. Mature birds do not develop neurologic signs.

12.2.8.2 Diagnosis

Except for cataracts, gross lesions are not commonly seen in pheasants [29]. Whitish streaks in the muscularis of the gizzard are seen in chickens but have not been reported in pheasants [28, 29]. The microscopic changes in the CNS are well described in chickens and are very suggestive [10]. Microscopic changes are minimal or nonexistent in both chickens and pheasants under 7 days of age despite the presence of severe clinical signs. In older chicks, the lesions are more apparent and include the presence of multiple and extensive infiltrations of lymphocytes and perivascular cuffing by lymphocytes [10]. Microgliosis is present in the cerebellum in the molecular layer. The central chromatolysis visible in motor neurons and Purkinje cells of chickens is not a prominent feature of the disease in pheasants. Peripheral nerves are not involved. The lymphoid infiltrations seen in the proventriculus, gizzard, pancreas, or myocardium of chickens are not seen in pheasants. The diagnosis can be confirmed by isolation of the virus, PCR assay, or by detecting a rise in antibody titer serologically. Antibody can be detected in gamebirds with the commercial ELISA tests.

12.2.8.3 Treatment and Prevention

There is no treatment. The morbidity varies from 40% to 60%. Mortality averages 25% and can exceed 50%. These rates are considerably lower if the chicks originate from immune breeders. Birds that survive infection are immune for life. Protection can also be achieved by vaccination of breeders during the growing phase. Vaccination at an older age can result in passage of the virus to the egg. Maternal antibody is protective of chicks during the first 3 weeks of age. The vaccine can be administered in the water, by aerosol, or by wing web stab. The virus is durable in the environment. It is susceptible to formaldehyde fumigation. Care should be taken to avoid introducing new stock during the breeding season, especially if the immune status of the resident hens is not known.

12.2.9 Aberrant Larval Migration

The larvae of the raccoon roundworm, *Baylisascaris procyonis*, may accidently be ingested by gamebirds and other animal species. After being ingested and hatching in the intestine of the normal host, the larvae migrate through the body harmlessly and eventually end up back in the intestine where they mature into adults. In the wrong host, however, the larvae hatch in the intestine and migrate aimlessly through the body, frequently ending up in the brain. The damage of their migration in the brain or spinal cord causes severe neurologic signs. The problem has been reported in partridges, emu, quail, and other birds [10].

12.2.9.1 Clinical Signs

Affected birds may show torticollis, ataxia, and depression.

12.2.9.2 Diagnosis

The distinctive tracts of aberrant larval migration in the brain or spinal cord are visible microscopically. Multiple serial sections may be required to find the larva itself. No gross lesions are usually visible.

12.2.9.3 Treatment and Prevention

No treatment is available for affected birds. The flock may be dewormed with the objective of removing the larvae from birds that are not yet affected. Control of exposure to the host raccoons is important. The eggs are passed in the feces of the raccoons. Contamination of the pens by the feces is the primary source of exposure. A possibility for consideration of control is to put out bait that contains a dewormer to treat the resident raccoon population. The problem with eradication of the resident population is that it allows new raccoons to move into the area, potentially bringing more of the parasite. Hopefully, maintenance of a dewormed local population will allow them to defend the territory against entrance of nonmedicated raccoons from outside the area.

12.2.10 Vitamin E/Selenium Deficiency in Chicks

Deficiency of vitamin E or selenium is associated with three different presentations: (i) softening of the cerebellum of the brain (encephalomalacia); (ii) subcutaneous edema (exudative diathesis); and (iii) muscle degeneration [9, 10]. Either nutrient can be inadvertently left out of the ration and cause the deficiency [10]. Vitamin E deficiency is more common than selenium deficiency because the vitamin can break down during storage, especially if there is a high level of fat or oil in the feed mix.

12.2.10.1 Clinical Signs

Encephalomalacia affects the cerebellum of young chicks. This is the hind portion of the brain that moderates movement. Damage to the cerebellum results in retractions or twisting of the head, incoordination, prostration, and death. The affected birds may sprawl on their breasts with legs back. This appearance may mimic the effects of ionophore toxicity. Exudative diathesis is characterized by accumulation of edema fluid in the subcutis. Muscle degeneration is not commonly seen in gamebirds and occurs when there is deficiency of vitamin E and sulfur-containing amino acids.

12.2.10.2 Diagnosis

In encephalomalacia, there is swelling and hemorrhage visible grossly in and limited to the cerebellum (Figure 12.4) [9]. The rest of the brain is spared. Microscopically, there are multiple coalescing areas of necrosis and hemorrhage in the cerebellar folia (Figure 12.5). The necrosis is caused by blockage of capillaries by fibrin thrombi in the affected areas [9]. The damage caused by the deficiency must be differentiated from that caused by a fungal infection. Detection of a fungus may require the use of a special stain such as PAS or GMS.

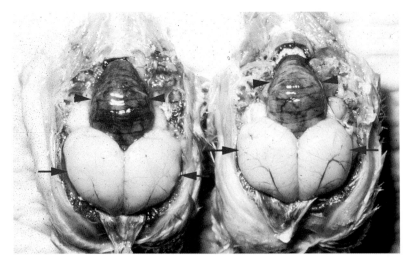

Figure 12.4 Encephalomalacia. The dorsal portion of the skull has been removed in each of the heads of the turkey poults. The cerebellums (arrowhead) are swollen and reddened. The cerebral hemispheres (arrows) are normal.

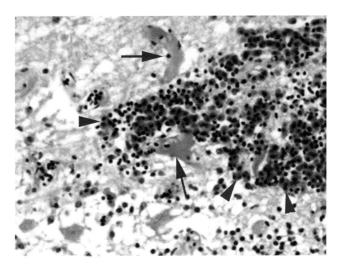

Figure 12.5   Encephalomalacia in cerebellum due to vitamin E deficiency. Necrosis and hemorrhage (arrowheads). Capillaries serving the affected area contain fibrin thrombi (arrows). (H&E stain, 40×).

In exudative diathesis, the viscous fluid that accumulates in the subcutaneous tissues has a green-blue tint [9, 10]. There may be weeping sores in the skin. Microscopic examination and bacterial culture can help confirm the diagnosis and rule out infectious causes of cellulitis.

With muscle degeneration, there are light-colored streaks in the breast muscle, heart, or gizzard. Microscopically, the muscle fibers have a hyaline appearance with loss of striations. The fibers may become disrupted and contain eosinophilic globules. Extravasation of proteinaceous fluid separates individual and groups of muscle fibers. The fluid often contains red blood cells and heterophils. Later in the course of disease, the reparative process produces proliferations of muscle cell nuclei and fibrous connective tissue. The pathologic changes induced by ionophore toxicity are very similar and must be differentiated from vitamin E/selenium deficiency [10]. The distinction may ultimately be based on whether the feed contained an ionophore coccidiostat. The presence of exudative diathesis in at least a few of the affected birds would bolster the likelihood of vitamin E deficiency rather than ionophore toxicity.

12.2.10.3   Treatment and Prevention

Supplementation with a water-soluble product that contains a high level of vitamin E will help prevent problems in the chicks that do not yet have cerebellar damage. It is difficult to reverse the damage in the cerebellums of affected chicks. Exudative diathesis and muscle degeneration can be treated by administering vitamin E orally in the feed or by giving vitamin E and selenium by injection. The presence of an adequate level of selenium in feed may have protective effects against deficiency of vitamin E in mature coturnix quail [30].

12.3   Generalized Disease

12.3.1   Botulism

Botulism, also referred to as limberneck, is caused by absorption of the botulism toxin produced by the bacterium *Clostridium botulinum* [31]. The organism is a spore-forming anaerobic bacterium

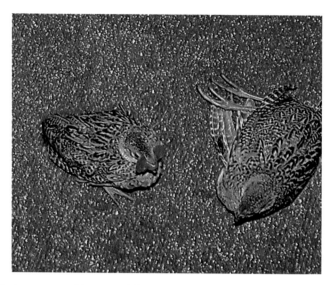

Figure 12.6 Weak pheasants unable to stand. Botulism would be the likely consideration if no lesions are found in the necropsy examination.

that is present in soil. It can survive in the soil in the spore stage for many years. *Clostridium* sp. are activated to grow when anaerobic conditions develop. *Clostridum botulinum* then produce the botulism toxin, which is released into the surrounding material. Once ingested by an animal, the toxin is absorbed and binds to the nerve endings of voluntary and autonomic nerves. All species of birds and mammals are susceptible. There is, however, variation between species in tolerance to the toxin.

12.3.1.1   Clinical Signs

Affected birds are weak and reluctant to move (Figure 12.6). They may appear lame when forced to move. There is flaccid paralysis of legs, wings, neck, and eyelids [31, 32]. The signs usually start in the legs and spread forward to the wings, neck, and eyelids. The birds may appear comatose or dead because of paralysis of the eyelids. Feathers may be ruffled and fall out with handling [33]. Death is due to heart and respiratory failure and occurs within hours.

12.3.1.2   Diagnosis

Clinical signs are very suggestive. Botulism does not induce any specific gross or microscopic changes in the tissues [32, 34]. The toxin does not affect insects and larval forms may carry enough toxin that, when eaten, can cause clinical signs in birds. Finding maggots in the crop or gizzard can be very suggestive if typical clinical signs are present in the host or other members of the flock. Confirmation of the diagnosis requires detection of the toxin or the organism.

The mouse bioassay is a sensitive and reliable method for detecting botulism toxin in serum. In this assay, groups of mice are inoculated with suspect serum samples. Other mice receive samples treated with type-specific antiserum. If toxin is present in the suspect serum, the mice develop signs and die within 48 hours. Mice that received the suspect serum treated with specific antitoxin will be protected. The mouse bioassay method is not offered at very many diagnostic laboratories because it is expensive and time-consuming to perform. A PCR assay is available that detects and identifies *C. botulinum* types A, B, and C toxin genes in vegetative cells after a culture enrichment step. The assay was originally offered at the Botulism Reference Center, PennVet-New

Bolton Center, but is now performed at the National Veterinary Services Laboratory, Diagnostic Bacteriology and Pathology Laboratory in Ames, Iowa (www.aphis.usda.gov/aphis/ourfocus/ animalhealth/lab-info-services/). Most cases of avian botulism are caused by *C. botulinum* type C or mosaic type C/D. Finding *C. botulinum* organisms or spores in a fecal or digestive tract sample or feed sample is strongly supportive of a diagnosis of botulism in birds exhibiting compatible clinical signs. Samples from normal birds are rarely positive.

12.3.1.3 Treatment and Prevention

The organism grows in the anaerobic conditions in dead or rotting organic material. There is also a form of the disease, called autointoxication, in which the organism colonizes the ceca and releases the toxin to be absorbed by the host bird. There is no direct treatment for the condition. Less severely affected birds may recover if given time and supportive care. Antibiotics may be administered to the flock if the autointoxication form of the disease is suspected. The antibiotic is expected to inhibit or kill the organism in the intestine. The disease occurs sporadically in different pens on an affected farm. Gamebirds are opportunistic in their foraging behavior so it is important to pick up dead birds and other rotting material in pens to reduce the chance of ingestion of contaminated materials. Insect larvae may ingest the toxin but are not affected by it. They can then serve as a source of toxicity when eaten by a gamebird.

References

1 Ferguson-Noel, N., Armour, N.K., Noormohammadi, A.H. et al. (2019). Mycoplasmosis. In: *Diseases of Poultry*, 14e (ed. D.E. Swayne, M. Boulianne, C. Logue, et al.), 907–965. Hoboken, NJ: Wiley.

2 Crespo, R. (2019). Developmental, metabolic, and other noninfectious disorders. In: *Diseases of Poultry*, 14e (ed. D.E. Swayne, M. Boulianne, C. Logue, et al.), 1286–1329. Hoboken, NJ: Wiley.

3 Greenacre, C.B. (2020). Musculoskeletal diseases. In: *Backyard Poultry Medicine and Surgery*, 2e (ed. C.B. Greenacre and T.Y. Morishita), 234–258. Hoboken, NJ: Wiley.

4 Nair, V., Gimeno, I., and Dunn, J. (2019). Marek's disease. In: *Diseases of Poultry*, 14e (ed. D.E. Swayne, M. Boulianne, C. Logue, et al.), 559–587. Hoboken: Wiley.

5 Schat, K.A. and Nair, V. (2013). Marek's disease. In: *Diseases of Poultry*, 13e (ed. D.E. Swayne, J. Glisson, L. McDougald, et al.), 515–552. Hoboken, NJ: Wiley-Blackwell.

6 Schock, A., Garcia-Rueda, C., Byas, R. et al. (2016). Severe outbreak of Marek's disease in crested partridges (*Rollulus rouloul*). *Vet. Rec.* 179 (17): 443–444.

7 Lin, J.A., Kitagawa, H., Ono, M. et al. (1990). Isolation of serotype 2 Marek's disease virus from birds belonging to the genus Gallus in Japan. *Avian Dis.* 34 (2): 336–344.

8 Pradham, H.K., Mohanty, G.C., and Mukit, A. (1985). Marek's disease in Japanese quails (Coturnix coturnix japonica): a study of natural cases. *Avian Dis.* 29 (3): 575–582.

9 Crespo, R., França, M.S., Fenton, H., and Shivaprasad, H.L. (2018). Galliformes and Columbiformes. In: *Pathology of Wildlife and Zoo Animals* (ed. K.A. Terio, D. McAloose and J. Leger St,), 747–773. St Louis, MO: Elsevier.

10 Fletcher, O.J. and Abdul-Aziz, T. (ed.) (2008). *Avian Histopathology*, 3e. WI: Omni Press: Madison.

11 Klasing, K.C. and Korver, D.R. (2019). Nutritional diseases. In: *Diseases of Poultry*, 14e (ed. D.E. Swayne, M. Boulianne, C. Logue, et al.), 1255–1285. Hoboken: Wiley.

12 Nolan, L.K., Vaillancourt, J.-P., Barbieri, N.L. et al. (2019). Colibacillosis. In: *Diseases of Poultry*, 14e (ed. D.E. Swayne, M. Boulianne, C. Logue, et al.), 770–830. Hoboken: Wiley.

13 Boulianne, M., Blackall, P.J., Hofacre, C.L. et al. (2019). Pasteurellosis and other respiratory bacterial infections. In: *Diseases of Poultry*, 14e (ed. D.E. Swayne, M. Boulianne, C. Logue, et al.), 831–889. Hoboken: Wiley.

14 Gast, R.K. and Porter, R.E. (2019). *Salmonella* infections. In: *Diseases of Poultry*, 14e (ed. D.E. Swayne, M. Boulianne, C. Logue, et al.), 719–753. Hoboken: Wiley.

15 Gu, Y., Liang, X., and Huang, Z. (2015). Outbreak of Listeria monocytogenes in pheasants. *Poult. Sci.* 94 (12): 2905–2908.

16 Arne, P. and Lee, M.D. (2019). Fungal infections. In: *Diseases of Poultry*, 14e (ed. D.E. Swayne, M. Boulianne, C. Logue, et al.), 1111–1133. Hoboken: Wiley.

17 Guy, J.S. (2019). Arbovirus infections. In: *Diseases of Poultry*, 14e (ed. D.E. Swayne, M. Boulianne, C. Logue, et al.), 507–516. Hoboken: Wiley.

18 McLean, R.G., Frier, G., Parham, G.L. et al. (1985). Investigations of the vertebrate hosts of eastern equine encephalitis during an epizootic in Michigan, 1980. *Am. J. Trop. Med. Hyg.* 34 (6): 1190–1202.

19 Steele, K.E., Linn, M.J., Schoepp, R.J. et al. (2000). Pathology of fatal West Nile virus infections in native and exotic birds during the 1999 outbreak in New York City, New York. *Vet. Pathol.* 37 (3): 208–224.

20 Clark, L., Hall, J., McLean, R. et al. (2006). Susceptibility of greater sage-grouse to experimental infection with West Nile virus. *J. Wildl. Dis.* 42 (1): 14–22.

21 Eckstrand, C.D., Woods, L.W., Diab, S.S. et al. (2015). Diagnostic exercise: high mortality in a flock of Chukar partridge chicks (*Alectoris chukar*) in California. *Vet. Pathol.* 52 (1): 189–192.

22 Nemeth, N.M., Bosco-Lauth, A.M., Williams, L.M. et al. (2017). West Nile virus infection in ruffed grouse (*Bonasa umbellus*): experimental infection and protective effects of vaccination. *Vet. Pathol.* 54 (6): 901–911.

23 Gamino, V., Escribano-Romero, E., Blázquez, A.-B. et al. (2016). Experimental North American West Nile virus infection in the red-legged partridge (*Alectoris rufa*). *Vet. Pathol.* 53 (3): 585–593.

24 Wünschmann, A. and Ziegler, A. (2006). West Nile virus-associated mortality events in domestic Chukar partridges (Alectoris chukar) and domestic Impeyan pheasants (Lophophorus impeyanus). *Avian Dis.* 50 (3): 456–459.

25 Miller, P.J. and Koch, G. (2020). Newcastle disease. In: *Diseases of Poultry*, 14e (ed. D.E. Swayne, M. Boulianne, C. Logue, et al.), 111–129. Hoboken: Wiley.

26 Aldous, E.W. and Alexander, D.J. (2008). Newcastle disease in pheasants (*Phasianus colchicus*): a review. *Vet. J.* 175 (2): 181–185.

27 Susta, L., Segovia, D., Olivier, T.L. et al. (2018). Newcastle disease virus infection in quail. *Vet. Pathol.* 55 (5): 682–692.

28 Suarez, D.L. (2019). Avian encephalomyelitis. In: *Diseases of Poultry*, 14e (ed. D.E. Swayne, M. Boulianne, C. Logue, et al.), 520–527. Hoboken: Wiley.

29 Welchman, D., Cox, W.J., Wood, A.M. et al. (2009). Avian encephalomyelitis in reared pheasants: a case study. *Avian Pathol.* 38 (3): 251–256.

30 Kling, L.J. and Soares, J.H. Jr., (1980). Vitamin E deficiency in the Japanese quail. *Poult. Sci.* 59 (10): 2352–2354.

31 Boulianne, M. and Uzal, F.A. (2020). Botulism. In: *Diseases of Poultry*, 14e (ed. D.E. Swayne, M. Boulianne, C. Logue, et al.), 976–980. Hoboken: Wiley.

32 Linares, J.A., Walker, R.L., Bickford, A.A. et al. (1994). An outbreak of type C botulism in pheasants and subsequent occurrence in chickens. *J. Vet. Diagn. Invest.* 6 (2): 272–273.

33 Vadlamudi, S., Lee, V.H., and Hanson, R.P. (1959). Case report – botulism type C outbreak on a pheasant game farm. *Avian Dis.* 3 (3): 344–350.

34 Shave, H.J. (1970). Progressive pathologic signs of botulism in pheasants. *J. Wildl. Dis.* 6 (4): 402–403.

13

Gamebird Skin Diseases and Multisystemic Diseases
Robert E. Porter, Jr and Teresa Y. Morishita

From a dermatology standpoint, conditions affecting either the skin or the feathers of gamebirds are often interrelated; therefore, no attempt will be made to differentiate these conditions based on anatomic site. These conditions will be presented based on the designation of infectious versus noninfectious conditions. Additionally, there are several infectious agents, some of them previously described in the text, that were associated with one particular body system when, in fact, they can have a multisystemic presentation. These multisystemic agents will be readdressed in this chapter. The topics addressed in this chapter are ones that the authors have encountered in captive gamebirds.

13.1 Infectious Agents of the Skin

13.1.1 Avipoxvirus

Avian pox is an infectious disease of domestic and wild birds, caused by the genus *Avipoxvirus* from the family Poxviridae. Avipoxviruses are large (250 × 350 nm), enveloped, oval-shaped viruses that contain linear, double-stranded DNA [1]. Avipoxvirus (APV) has been detected in 374 avian species in 23 orders, including pheasants [2, 3], partridges [4–6], quail [7–9], guineafowl [10], and peafowl [1].

Infected birds are the main reservoir for avipoxviruses. The most frequent route of infection is via biting insects – midges and mosquitoes – but pecking trauma to skin, objects contaminated with viable poxviruses, and inhalation or ingestion of dust, infected skin scabs and aerosols are other possible routes [11]. Mosquito-borne infections are considered to be the most common route of transmission [12]. In some instances, cutaneous or diphtheritic pox lesions can develop as a result of viremia rather than direct inoculation [13]. APV infections can be introduced to captive populations from wild birds, newly introduced captive birds, fomites or arthropod vectors. Infected carrier birds with no clinical signs have been shown to spread APV infection in aviaries after a 10-day quarantine [14]. Outbreaks of poxvirus are more commonly observed in warm, humid seasons (summer, fall) when the vector population is at the highest point [11]. Reported mortality in gamebirds affected by avipoxvirus is usually low [5]; however, mortality can vary depending on age, host, and strain of avipoxvirus [12]. In most reports of poxvirus in gamebirds, the infected birds are usually juveniles that have not developed full innate immunity or were not previously immunized from a virus exposure during the previous season [11, 14].

Gamebird Medicine and Management, First Edition. Edited by Teresa Y. Morishita and Robert E. Porter, Jr.
© 2023 John Wiley & Sons, Inc. Published 2023 by John Wiley & Sons, Inc.

The duration of infection in individual birds is poorly understood. It may vary according to virus strain and host. For example, poxvirus isolates from bobwhite quail were shown to cause temporary skin lesions when inoculated into the skin of chicks and poults, but were nonpathogenic for coturnix quail [12].

The varying susceptibility of birds to avipoxviruses depends on the presence of host-adapted strains and differences in virulence of the avipoxviruses [15]. Mosquito-borne transmission is the most important route of infection [12]. Avian pox can occur in two forms: the cutaneous (dry) form and the diphtheritic (wet) form. Both forms of the disease can occur in the same birds [16]. The cutaneous form is caused by virus entry into breaks in the nonfeathered skin over the cere, eyelids, head, legs, and feet. These lesions are usually self-limiting unless the extent of skin lesions is overwhelming and interfere with sight or prehension of feed. Eyelids can be sealed by the accumulation of dried exudate and secondary bacterial conjunctivitis [7]. The diphtheritic form develops on the mucous membrane of the oral cavity, nasal passage, and upper respiratory tract. The wet lesions are usually more severe than the cutaneous forms and can interfere with respiration as well as swallowing.

At a minimum, affected birds can be expected to show reduced activity and weight loss [17], but signs can be more severe if lesions are extensive. Pox infections can cause high mortality with both dry and wet forms in captive quail [9]. Brower et al. described severe beak necrosis and deformation in Hungarian partridges caused by avipoxvirus and likely exacerbated by the placement of beak bits [6]. In one report, peafowl chicks incurred high mortality from large scabs developing on the eyelids, nostrils, beak, and legs [18] which is typical for avipoxviral disease (Figure 13.1). Additionally, a poxvirus closely related to fowlpox virus caused high mortality from beak and periocular lesions in captive peafowl [19]. Kirmse showed that most cutaneous pox lesions disappear in 3–4 weeks, but some can remain for up to 10 weeks [15]. Davidson et al. also indicated that typical pox skin lesions regress spontaneously after 6–12 weeks [7].

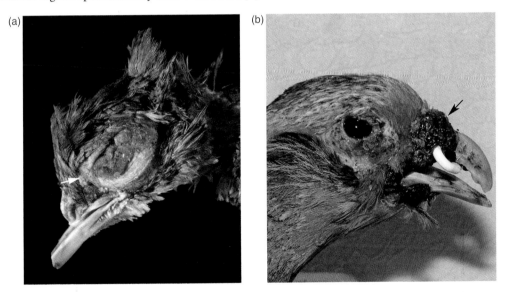

Figure 13.1 (a) A 5-week-old ring-necked pheasant with Avipoxvirus infection has proliferative dermatitis and scabs (arrow) on the eyelids, which have fused shut. The chick also has an upper beak defect that is unrelated to the pox infection. (b) A Hungarian partridge with Avipoxvirus infection has prominent proliferative dermatitis around the beak and cere (arrow).

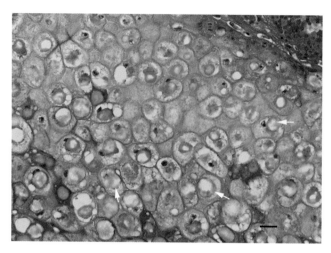

Figure 13.2 A histological section of skin from the pheasant in Figure 13.1 reveals marked hyperplasia and ballooning degeneration of epithelium. Epithelial cells contain round, eosinophilic intracyoplasmic inclusions (arrows) consistent with Avipoxvirus. H&E stain, bar = 20 μm.

Diagnosis is based on clinical signs, gross lesions, and a variety of tests that confirm the presence of poxvirus, including histopathology, immunohistochemistry, transmission electron microscopy, virus isolation, and PCR of affected tissue [16]. Histopathology of both cutaneous and diphtheritic lesions will reveal extensive epithelial hyperplasia with subepithelial fibrosis and infiltrates of heterophils and macrophages. The epithelial cells have ballooning degeneration with prominent eosinophilic intracytoplasmic inclusions (Bollinger bodies) [18] as shown in Figure 13.2. Inflammation and necrosis of the skin lesions caused by secondary bacterial infection is commonly observed in histologic sections.

The control of avipoxvirus infection is based on prevention rather than treatment. Poor husbandry conditions in the pen along with abundance of blood-sucking arthropods can trigger APV infection; hence, maintaining adequate air movement to reduce the amount of dust and dander in the house is important [20]. Increased bird activity, bright lights, and increased stocking density can increase bird-to-bird contact and exacerbate skin trauma. Effective insect control measures in the house or pen are also indicated.

Vaccination of commercial gamebirds is generally not practiced, but it might be effective in high-risk situations. Commercial poxvirus vaccines are generally administered by subcutaneous injection of the wing web. Commercial vaccines are not available for all specific strains of avipoxvirus that affect gamebirds; however, as an example, a commercial fowlpox vaccine was shown to protect bobwhite quail against the bobwhite quail strain of APV [12]. Additionally, a live commercial fowlpox vaccine has been used to control avipoxvirus infection in 16-week-old breeder bobwhite quail [21]. Fatunmbi et al. showed that chickens vaccinated with various avipoxvirus strains (multivalent vaccines) show the greatest resistance to challenge with fowlpox virus [22], and perhaps a similar use of multiple strains of avipoxvirus would be effective in gamebirds. However, one study indicated that administration of a combination of live pigeonpox and fowlpox vaccines in coturnix quail did not protect the birds from challenge with a quail strain of poxvirus [9]. Captive peafowl that were previously vaccinated with fowlpox virus still broke with cutaneous pox lesions affecting the beak and periocular skin, even though the field virus infecting the peafowl was shown to be nearly identical to fowlpox [19]. To effectively determine if a vaccine would be successful one should attempt to isolate and genetically characterize the field virus, then differentiate it from other avipoxvirus strains by cross-immunity and pathogenicity tests [3].

13.1.2 Staphylococcosis

Staphylococcal infection of the foot (pododermatitis) was addressed in Chapter 12, but this microorganism deserves further attention here because of the association with breast blisters, cellulitis, and omphalitis in gamebirds. The microorganisms are Gram-positive cocci (0.5–1.5 µm diameter) belonging to the family Staphylococcaceae and genus *Staphylococcus*. These microorganisms are often observed as pairs, tetrads or grape-like clusters, and are readily isolated on blood agar.

More than 50 species and subspecies have been described [23] but *Staphylococcus aureus* is the most important and common isolate from poultry. This microorganism is a common inhabitant of the skin and mucous membranes, but a break in the integrity of those tissues will allow this opportunistic bacterium to penetrate the skin or membrane, colonize the subcutis and, in some instances, progress to sepsis [24]. Skin that is chronically wet (high humidity, leaking drinkers, wet litter) is more pliable and subject to puncture wounds and lacerations. Common forms of *S. aureus* infection in poultry include omphalitis, necrotic dermatitis, tenosynovitis/arthritis, pododermatitis, and osteomyelitis in chickens and turkeys [25]. In terms of gamebirds, particularly pheasants, the authors have most often isolated *Staphylococcus* spp. (*S. aureus*, *S. hyicus*, *S. intermedius*), with or without coliforms (*Escherichia coli*), in cases of omphalitis (Figure 13.3), cellulitis and breast blisters. Raidal described staphylococcal dermatitis with crust formation on the beak, eyelids, and nares in captive-reared Japanese quail experiencing 8% mortality and a nutritional deficiency [26].

Reduction of staphylococcal infection is based on reducing trauma in the flock: mitigate cannibalism and feather picking, eliminate sharp objects, avoid crowding, avoid wet litter or leaking drinkers, and have adequate feeder space so that birds do not crowd or climb on each other when taking a meal. In general, flocks under conditions of high humidity, wet litter, and skin trauma can develop staphylococcal disease. Antibiotics might be effective in reducing lesions in problem flocks, but attention should be given to appropriate culture and antibiotic sensitivity testing [25].

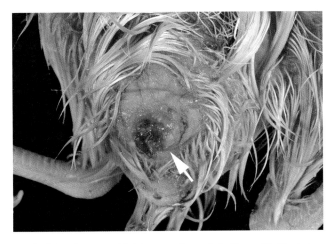

Figure 13.3 A 1-day-old white pheasant chick has a yolk sac infection with *Staphylococcus* sp. The omphalitis is characterized by a red, enlarged navel (arrow).

13.1.3 Lice (Phthiraptera)

Lice (Insecta: Phthiraptera) are wingless, dorsoventrally flattened insects that are divided into two groups: sucking lice and chewing lice (Mallophaga). Many chewing lice parasitize birds and, in fact, birds serve as hosts for only chewing lice [27]. The lice feed by ingesting host feathers, skin secretions and skin dander, using their broad mandibles to fragment the feather or dander into bite-size pieces. Different genera of lice usually colonize different areas of the body. Lice are small (350 µm to 10 mm long in adult stage) and normally rest on the feathers, but they quickly disperse from feathers onto skin if they are disturbed. Immature lice (nymphs) resemble the adults, but they are smaller and lack external genitalia. Immature lice increase in size after each nymphal molt. At least six species of chewing lice are found on domestic fowl, particularly chickens [27], and many lice have been described on pheasants, partridges, quail, guineafowl, and pea fowl (Table 13.1).

The life cycles of different avian lice can vary slightly but the wing louse (*Lipeurus caponis*) will be used here as an example of a typical life cycle. Eggs of the wing louse hatch 4–7 days after the female has cemented them to the base of a feather shaft. Each nymphal stage will each last 5–18 days and total generation time is 18–27 days [27]. Direct host contact (e.g., young in nest, copulation) is the primary route of transmission for lice; however, chewing lice can survive for days off the avian host [63]. Any time the lice spend off the host can promote transmission through contaminated nests, litter, cages, or truck beds.

The clinical signs observed with a louse infestation in a flock are hyperirritability, increased grooming, poor feathering or feather loss, weight loss, and reduced egg production. The gross lesions include red, irritated skin from the scratching activity of the lice and frayed feathers from mite chewing and excessive grooming. Large numbers of lice can debilitate the host. The lice are very active on the host, are larger than mites and are visible to the naked eye as they move about on the host (Figure 13.4a). Inspection of individual feathers can reveal the large masses of eggs (nits) glued to the feather shaft, generally toward the base (Figure 13.4b). Speciation of the lice is based on body morphology (Figure 13.5) [63, 64].

The approach to control and treatment of lice and mites is similar and will be addressed in the section on mites below.

13.1.4 Mites (Acari)

More than 250 species of mites are known to cause health-related issues in domestic animals and humans. Based on the classification schemes described by Zhang [65], mites or Acari consist of two major groups: the superorder Parasitiformes (Anactinotrichida) and the superorder Acariformes (Actinotrichida). These superorders are further divided into six orders. The orders of mites that are known to contain species of veterinary importance are Ixodida, Mesostigmata, Trombidiformes, and Sarcoptifomes. Most of the mites identified on gamebirds are feather and skin mites or environmental mites that migrate onto captive birds. The list of gamebird mites is likely incomplete and new species will be identified in future surveillance studies. *Knemidocoptes* sp. is the scaly leg mite and will be described later in the chapter. In most poultry, feather mites can cause discomfort and excessive grooming and promote weight loss, reduced egg production, or mortality in severe cases [50, 66]. For example, feather loss from mites can reduce marketing of quail [50].

The life cycle of mites consists of the egg, prelarva, protonymph, deutonumph, tritonymph, and adult. Mites typically have four pairs of legs as nymphs and adults, but larvae have only three pairs. Surveys of ectoparasites in many types of wild and captive gamebirds have identified a variety of mites, and *Ornithonyssus sylviarum*, the northern fowl mite, and *Dermanyssus gallinae*, the red roost mite, are cited most often; therefore, these two mites will be emphasized in this section.

Table 13.1 Louse species referenced in gamebirds, guineafowl, and peafowl.

Bird	Louse	References
Pheasant	*Amyrsidea megalosoma*	Emerson [28]
	Amyrsidea monostoecha	Goldova et al. [29]
	Amyrsidea perdicus	Hillgarth [30]
	Amyrsidea suabaequale	Weselmann [31]
	Cuculotogaster heterographus[a]	Lewin and Mahrt [32]
	Lagopoecus colchicus	Payne et al. [33]
	Lagopoecus sp. *(8 species)*	Sychra [34]
	Lipeurus caponis[b]	Arnold [35]
	Lipeurus maculosus	Ashraf et al. [36]
	Menacanthus stramineus[c]	Curland et al. [37]
	Menopon sp.	Chu et al. [38]
	Oxylipeurus colchicus	
	Goniodes capitatus	
	Goniodes colchici	
	Goniodes dissimilis	
	Goniocotes albidus	
	Goniocotes cervinicornis	
	Goniocotes chrysocephalus	
	Goniocotes gallinae[d]	
Partridge	*Amyrsidea perdicus*	Emerson [39]
	Brueelia coquimbana	Calvete et al. [40]
	Cuculotogaster heterographus	Millan et al. [41]
	Lypeurus caponis	Sychra [34]
	Lypeurus maculosus	Ali-Bawar and Saeed [42]
	Menacanthus pallidus	Khattak et al. [43]
	Menacanthus lyali	Gustafsson and Zou [44]
	Menacanthus numidae	
	Menacanthus stramineus	
	Menopon gallinae[e]	
	Menopon pallens	
	Myrsidea picae	
	Goniodes microthorax	
	Goniodes dispar	
	Goniocotes galli	
	Goniocotes obscurus	
	Gionocotes simillimus	
	Cuculotogaster heterographus	
	Cuculotogaster obscurior	

(continued)

Table 13.1 (Continued)

Bird	Louse	References
Quail	*Amyrsidea perdicus*	Hightower et al. [45]
	Amyrsidea saudiensis	Bergstrand and Klimstra [46]
	Brueelia illustris	Kellog and Doster [47]
	Colinicola numidana	Doster et al. [48]
	Cuculotogaster maculipes	Sychra [34]
	Goniocotes chrysocephalus	Askin [49]
	Goniodes colchici	El-Sharabasy and Hanafy [50]
	Goniodes gigas[f]	Adamu et al. [51]
	Goniodes mamillatus	Alahmed et al. [52]
	Goniodes ortygis	
	Lagopaecus colchicus	
	Lipeurus maculosus	
	Menacanthus pricei	
	Menacanthus stramineus	
	Oxylipeurus clavatus	
Peafowl	*Amyrsidea minutes*	Emerson [28]
	Amyrsidea perdicus	Hollamby et al. [53]
	Colpocephalum tausi	Millan et al. [41]
	Colpocephalum thoracicum	Corn et al. [54]
	Columbicola columbae	Kattach et al. [43]
	Goniocotes chrysocephalus	Khursheed et al. [55]
	Goniocotes mayuri	Ganjali et al. [56]
	Goniocotes parviceps	Nasser et al. [57]
	Goniocotes rectanulatus	Yadav et al. [58]
	Goniodes dissimilis	
	Goniodes gigas	
	Goniodes meinertzhageni	
	Goniodes pavonis	
	Menacanthus kaddoui	
	Menacanthus stramineus	
Guineafowl	*Amyrsidea powelli*	Emerson [39]
	Cuculotogaster occidentalis	Emerson [28]
	Goniodes gigas	Martin-Mateo et al. [59]
	Goniocotes gallinae	Ayeni et al. [60]
	Goniocotes maculatus	Fabiyi [61]
	Lipeurus caponis	Okaeme [62]
	Lipeurus tropicalis	Sychra [34]
	Menacanthus numidae	Gustafsson and Zou [44]
	Menacanthus stramineus	
	Menopon gallinae	
	Numidilipeurus tropicalis	

Common names: [a]Chicken head louse, [b]Wing louse, [c]Chicken body louse, [d]Fluff louse, [e]Shaft louse, [f]Large chicken louse.

(a)

(b)

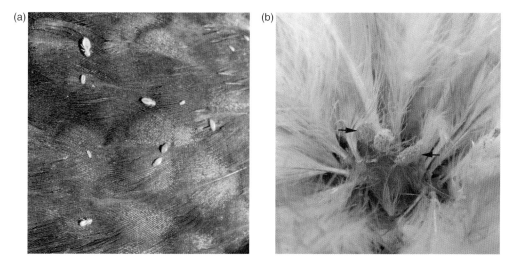

Figure 13.4 Lice. (a) In heavy infestations, chewing lice, which are larger than mites, are readily observed with the naked eye as they course across the feathers of the wing and neck. (b) Clusters of louse eggs (arrows) are glued onto the feather shaft and barbs.

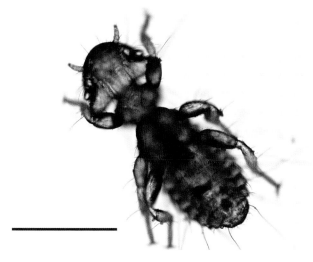

Figure 13.5 Lice. *Menacanthus* sp., the chicken body louse, has been described on a variety of game birds. Bar = 0.5 mm.

Feather and skin mites are usually identified by distribution on the host, by inspecting (usually with magnification) the entire feather and by scraping the feather exudate onto a glass slide with or without the use of mineral oil for microscopic examination (Figure 13.6) [66]. It should be noted that avian mites, particularly *O. sylviarum* and *D. gallinae*, are associated with "avian mite dermatitis" in humans. These blood-sucking mites can use humans as a short-term feeding host but will not reproduce on human hosts. Poultry workers and people residing close to bird nests are most often affected. Mite numbers in the surrounding environment are usually heavy if there are human infestations [67].

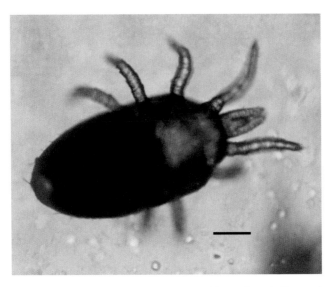

Figure 13.6   Mites. Scrapings of feather exudate can be placed into mineral oil on a glass slide to confirm the presence of mites, in this case an adult *Ornithonyssus sylviarum*. Bar = 100µm.

13.1.4.1   Northern Fowl Mite

Ornithonyssus sylviarum, a mite that spends its entire life on the avian host, is generally located on feathers of the tail, wing, and neck (Figure 13.7). Surveys have documented this this mite in at least 72 species of birds [68] and it can likely be spread to captive bird farms by wild birds [69]. The northern fowl mite is a blood feeder and has been documented in pheasants [29, 66], partridges [43], quail [47], and guineafowl [70]. Multiple surveys of ectoparasites in wild and captive peafowl failed to list feather mites [53, 54, 58]; however, because of the broad host range of the northern fowl mite and the red roost mite, it is likely that peafowl are susceptible to these mite species as well. Economic loss can result from discomfort, decreased egg production, reduced feed consumption,

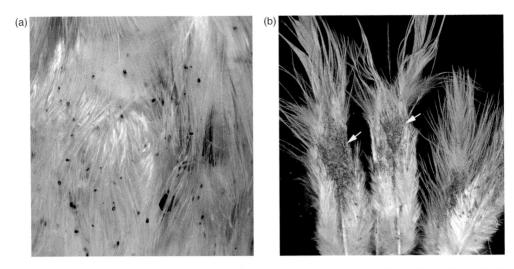

Figure 13.7   (a) Mites of the northern fowl mite, *Ornithonyssus sylviarum*, are visible on the feathers. (b) The feathers from the vent region are often discolored and coated with mite feces, mite debris, and eggs (arrows).

and reduced weight gain. Male birds tend to be more heavily infested than hens and the mites are readily spread between genders while breeding [30].

The entire life cycle is completed in 5 days and in most instances the mite remains on the host bird for the entire life cycle and at all times of the day. The infestation and disease caused by the northern fowl mite are worse during cold months of the year because of the close contact of birds during these periods.

13.1.4.2 Red Roost Mite

Dermanyssus gallinae is found on feathers of the tail, wing, and neck, and has been described in pheasants [29, 66], partridges [40, 43], quail [50], and guineafowl [62]. This mite feeds on blood and is primarily active at night (night feeder), while during the day it will leave the host to reside in nest boxes and 2 mm cracks and crevices of perches and slats in the poultry house. Red mites survive well in cage-free, open-housing units if there are sheltered areas or nests where the birds rest at night [69]. *Dermanyssus* mites can live off the host for 5 months under laboratory conditions [67]. The mites are most often observed on young birds and cause rough, scaly skin and dark, stained feathers over the entire body, but most often on the feathers of the vent. The dark staining of the vent feathers is caused by accumulation of mite eggs, scabs, and fecal material. The mites will feed on blood, and heavy mite infestations can cause anemia. Decreased egg production can occur. Multiple birds should be checked for ectoparasites and associated lesions because not all birds may be infected at one time.

13.1.4.3 Tropical Fowl Mite

Ornithonyssus bursa infests domestic and wild birds throughout the warmer regions of world. The mite eggs that are laid in nesting material will hatch in 2–3 days and after 6–8 days become adults that cause skin irritation during blood feeds. The mite can survive off the host for 10 days [69]. The tropical feather mite, *Bdellonysus bursa*, has been described in guineafowl raised in Nigeria [61].

13.1.4.4 Fowl Cyst Mite

Laminosioptes cysticola occurs on a variety of domestic birds and, in particular, has been described in pheasants and pigeons, thus wild pigeons should be considered as a potential vector for captive gamebirds. The mites can invade the skin to form small yellow subcutaneous nodules [66].

13.1.4.5 Miscellaneous Feather Mites

Over 2000 species of mites that live on or in the feathers of many orders of birds have been identified. These mites vary in which portion of the feather they prefer to inhabit or consume – the barbules or the shaft. The feather mites *Meginia cubitalis* or *Meginia* sp. and *Pterolichus* sp. have been described in gamebird health surveys. *Megninia* sp. has been identified in pheasants [33] and quail [46, 48] while *Pterolichus* sp. has also been described in quail [46, 48]. Shaft mites, such as *Apionacarua wilsoni* and *Colinophlius wilsoni*, have been described in surveys of captive quail [48, 66]. These mites live inside the base of the feather (calamus) to feed on the feather tissue or penetrate the shaft to absorb host fluids. Infestation with the shaft mite is generally not economically important.

A variety of mites are occasionally referred to as feather mites, but the term "skin mite" is more accurate because these ectoparasites can live on the skin surface or in feather follicles, eating scale and crust. They can cause irritation, scaly skin, and dermatitis. *Microlichus* sp. and *Rivoltasia* sp. have been described in quail [48], while *Rivoltasia* sp. have also been described in ectoparasite surveys of pheasants [33] and guineafowl [61]. *Epidermoptes phasianus* is a skin mite described in pheasants [33, 71].

13.1.4.6 Trombiculoid Mites (Chiggers)

Domestic animals, birds, and humans can be short-term atypical hosts for chiggers, resulting in pruritus and dermatitis. Chiggers or red bugs are members of the family Trombiculidae, and the larval stage is the only parasitic stage of the trombicuoid life cycle. They are most numerous in areas with moist grasslands, brush, and thickets, with the preferred environment varying between species. The deutonymph stage is a free-living predator that feeds on small arthropods [66]. *Neoschoengastria americana* of quail [47], *Neotrombicula autumnalis* of pheasants, partridges [66] and quail [48], and *Eutrombicula alfreddugesi* of pheasants [33] and quail [47] have been identified in field surveys.

A variety of environmental mites that live in litter or feed can be identified on poultry. For example, *Tyroglyphus* sp. is the flour and grain mite but can also contaminate cheese. Under conditions of probable feed contamination, this mite has been found on the feathers of partridges [43] and quail [50]; however, the clinical effects are minimal.

13.1.5 *Knemidocoptes* Infection (Scaly Leg Mites)

Scaly leg disease is a condition caused by *Knemidocoptes* mites that burrow into the nonfeathered skin of the feet and legs, resulting in hyperkeratosis and grossly thickened skin with disfigurement and loss of function in severe cases. There are a variety of burrowing mite species described in birds, and *Knemidocoptes mutans* is the major mite described in poultry. The primary Knemokoptinae described in gallinaceous birds are *K. mutans* and *Neocnemidocoptes gallinae*. *Knemidocoptes jamaicensis* is described in the green peafowl, while *K. mutans* has been described in the helmeted guineafowl [72]. Among gamebirds, *K. mutans* is most often reported in pheasants [29, 36]. Wild birds can serve as a source of knemidocoptic infection for confined poultry.

Mites are transmitted directly from bird to bird through contact. The mites spend their entire 3-week life cycle on their bird hosts. Female mites are viviparous, producing nymphal offspring with three pairs of legs. There are two nymphal stages before adult mites develop with four pairs of legs, and then burrow into feather follicles and the epidermal stratum corneum of the nonfeathered feet, shanks, eyelids, and beak. The burrowing of adult mites causes increased hyperkeratosis and in extreme cases can cause discomfort and reduced function of the affected appendage. Severe hyperkeratosis of the affected skin can impair blood supply to result in eventual loss of digits or entire feet (Figure 13.8). *Neocnemidocoptes gallinae*, the depluming itch mite, burrows into the feather shafts of the head, neck, back, abdomen, and upper legs of gallinaceous birds to cause irritation, feather picking, and feather loss. The affected skin underneath the feathers can be hyperkeratotic and thickened, but hyperkeratosis of the legs, feet or face is not observed [66, 73].

The primary lesions described in pheasants are prominent hyperkeratosis of the skin of the legs causing discomfort and associated plucking of feathers, weight loss, and reduced egg production [36]. The hyperkeratotic skin lesions, if focal, can resemble poxvirus infection and should be differentiated by histopathology of extruded crust. In histologic sections, the round, short-legged mites are embedded in pockets within keratin and range in size from 350–450 μm × 280–380 μm for females and 200–240 μm × 145–160 μm for males [74]. Diagnosis can also be made by cytologic examination of skin scrapings. In individual birds, ivermectin, as off-label medication, has been administered orally at 200 μg/kg given three times, 2 weeks apart, to effectively reduce the lesions in peafowl and other poultry [75, 76]. Prevention should focus on preventing entry of wild birds into the pen, reducing stocking density and practicing routine pen hygiene of the ground, equipment, and feeders/drinkers.

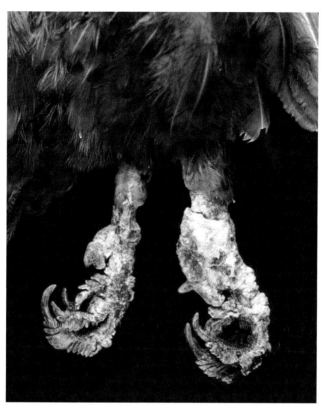

Figure 13.8 Scaly leg. An adult pheasant has thickened scales along the nonfeathered skin of the shanks and feet (hyperkeratosis) resulting from infection with *Knemidocoptes mutans*, the scaly leg mite.

13.1.6 Treatment and Prevention of Ectoparasites

Preventing the introduction of lice and mites onto a premises is most important because eradication can be difficult, medications are not readily available, and the use of insecticides may pose a risk to both human and bird health. Biosecurity should focus on insect control, rigid sanitation, regular removal of dead birds, and restricting movement of people and equipment from pen to pen or premise to premise. Litter should be thoroughly removed between flocks and dry cleaning and disinfection are essential [69, 77]. Wild birds and rodents that can serve as vectors for mites should be excluded. This can be difficult in a flight cage arrangement.

   The authors have never encountered heavy mite loads on farmed gamebirds, but in instances of heavy infestation, one can consider chemical insecticide sprays, for which veterinary supervision is strongly recommended. The insecticides are available as wettable powders, emusifiable concentrates, soluble concentrates, granular and microencapsulated products. The spray must be at high enough pressure (100–125 psi with 1 gallon of water per 100 birds) to penetrate the feathers of the vent region. Commercial acaricides include pyrethroids (e.g., permethrin) and organophosphates such as tetrachlorviphos (Rabon® or Ravap®) often contain wetting agents to help the active chemical penetrate to the feathers [78]. Commercial insecticide sprays should have a Material Safety Data Sheet (MSDS) with directions that should be carefully followed. Birds raised in cages should receive the spray from beneath the cage to increase access to the vent region. Because the red roost mite commonly spends time off the bird by day, these infestations require that, in addition to bird treatment, the nests and cracks/crevices of the housing structure should be sprayed or dusted with insecticide. Other products available for mites include a spinosad compound (Elector®), which can be sprayed onto the birds.

Alternative measures for small gamebird flocks include preparing one or more dust boxes that contain a variety of inert materials, such as kaolin (clay), diatomaceous earth (DE), and elemental sulfur [69]. Recent studies have shown that sulfur either in a dust bath or suspended in dust bags is effective in controlling northern fowl mites [79].

13.2   Miscellaneous Skin Conditions

13.2.1   Sternal Bursitis (Breast Blister)

The sternal bursa is a subcutaneous, narrow, elongated synovium-lined sac oriented along the keel of the sternum. The bursa is attached to the fascia of the underlying keel bone as well as to the aponeurosis (connective tissue sheath) of the superficial pectoral muscle. The subcutaneous bursa is covered by a linear tract of nonfeathered skin (sternal apteryium). The width of the sternal bursal cavity varies between species of birds and the cavity is traversed by connective tissue bundles [80]. The bursa is barely discernible at hatch and becomes more elongated and deeper as the bird ages. In turkeys, the sternal bursa is not observed histologically until 4–12 weeks of age [81].

Under a variety of conditions, the bursa can progressively enlarge and become fluid filled (cystic); this is a result of chronic irritation and subsequent inflammation of the bursal wall. This condition has long been recognized in meat-type chickens and turkeys, upon which much of the research is based. The authors have observed this condition in both mature pheasant breeders and market-age pheasants. The sternal bursa in heavy meat-type birds can become quite large, cystic, and infected with bacteria, resulting in substantial carcass downgrades at the processing plant; the downgrades can be exacerbated further by ulcerative dermatitis (breast buttons) over the enlarged sternal bursae [82]. Similar conditions occur in meat-type pheasants graded at processing plants (author observation).

There are genetic, environmental, physical (conformation), and infectious factors that have been shown to influence the development of sternal bursitis [82]. The condition is observed more often in older, heavier birds with prominent keel bones and occurs more often when there is poor feathering along the skin of the keel. Body weight and gender are significant factors as the condition is observed more often in male, heavy meat-type birds [83]. Physical irritation of the sternal bursa is considered as the initiating factor [81, 84], and this is generally enhanced by coarse litter, wire flooring, increased litter moisture, and crowding. The early brooding environment does not affect development of this condition; in one study, newly hatched turkey poults placed on wet or coarse litter did not have an increased incidence of breast blisters as poults [85]. It has been shown that older turkeys (juvenile or adult) are much more prone to developing breast blisters, compared to young poults, when exposed to bursal trauma [86]; sternal bursitis is a condition of the grow-out rather than the brooder environment. Additionally, infections with *Staphylococcus*, *E. coli*, *Mycoplasma gallisepticum*, and *Mycoplasma synoviae* can be associated with sternal bursitis [83].

Because the condition does not hinder bird activity, it is usually observed at the processing plant on scalded, defeathered carcasses. The enlarged, cystic sternal bursa will have an inflamed, fibrous wall with varying amounts of clear to turbid fluid or blood, depending on the degree of secondary bacterial infection (Figure 13.9). Practices to reduce this condition have been described in chickens and turkeys [87], and should be effective for pheasant as well.

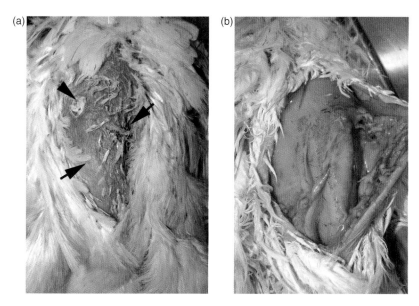

Figure 13.9   Ten-month-old white pheasant. (a) The sternal bursa is enlarged (arrows) and there is a solitary skin ulcer (arrowhead). (b) The sternal bursa (open) has a fibrous cyst wall and the cavity contains fibrin and clear fluid.

Prevention should focus on controlling bird weights, avoiding wet and coarse litter, maximizing breast feathering, and reducing stocking density. The presence of underlying systemic or localized bacterial infections should also be reduced.

13.2.2   Cannibalism

Cannibalism is defined as damage to the feathers and skin of birds by pecking aggression from other birds. It has long been recognized as a production issue in domestic poultry as well as gamebirds such as pheasants [88–90], partridge [91], and quail [92, 93]. The aggressive behavior can begin as feather pecking, but then progress to skin damage. If feather pecking starts at a young age, the small feathers on the back, wings, vent, and tail are easily accessible. Soft quill feathers that are filled with blood will attract aggressive birds [88]. Toe, beak, and feather picking are more commonly observed in chicks while trauma from vent, wing and head picking is observed more often in older birds [94]. Feather pecking can progress to cannibalism, particularly if the birds develop a taste for skin and blood as a learned behavior. Repetitive pecking or picking can open wounds and eventually result in loss of toes. Birds will often repeatedly peck at open, bleeding wounds on others and will keep on attacking until the affected bird is fatally wounded (Figure 13.10).

Cannibalism is a particular gamebird issue during the brooding and growing period, but it can also increase during the mating and egg-laying period in captive breeder pheasants, for example [89]. It is most economical for the grower to take husbandry measures to minimize cannibalism before it occurs. Common causes for cannibalism are high stocking density, bright ambient light, inadequate feed or water space, extremes of heat or cold, and the general cannibalistic nature of wild birds placed in confinement [94]. Suggested methods to reduce cannibalism include the following.

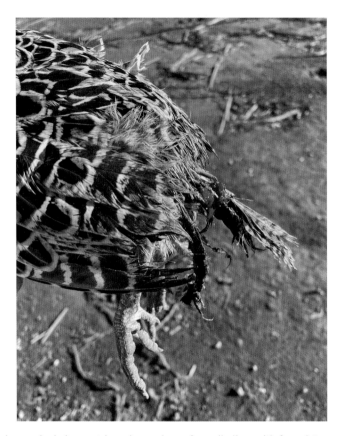

Figure 13.10   A ring-necked pheasant hen shows signs of cannibalism with frayed, truncated tail feathers and bleeding from both skin and damaged pin feathers.

1. Reduce light intensity to less than 1.0 fc in the brooding house. The birds should be able to find feed and water [93]. The use of red bulbs has also been suggested [95].
2. Provide adequate feed and water space for all birds.
3. Maintain adequate floor space per bird as per documented recommendations for the various species or based on your growing experience. For example, a stocking density of no more than 10 birds per square foot has been recommended for bobwhite quail [93].
4. Feed the birds a balanced ration that meets recommended requirements. For example, dietary deficiencies of arginine or crude protein have been associated with cannibalistic behavior in pheasants and partridges [89, 91, 96].
5. Provide disposable cover or barriers (e.g., straw bales, crates, cornstalks, switch grass) in pens that allow birds to hide from more aggressive penmates.
6. Regularly monitor birds for ectoparasites, such as lice and mites, that can promote pecking behavior.
7. Maintain flock uniformity in terms of size and weight.
8. Remove dead birds or cull dying birds quickly from the flock.
9. Place spectacles (Figure 13.11a) that alter forward vision or bits (Figure 13.11b) that prevent full closure of the beak to reduce trauma from aggressive behavior [93, 94]. Spectacles and bits have been shown to reduce feather pecking and skin trauma and improve feather quality in both pheasants and partridges [97–99].

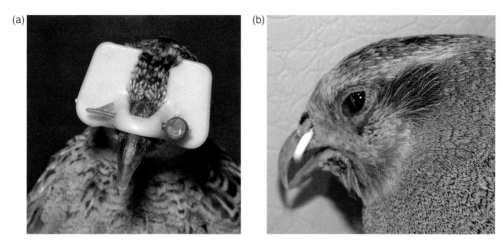

Figure 13.11 (a) The ring-necked pheasant has spectacle blinders. (b) The Hungarian partridge has a curved bit applied through the nares and mouth.

10. Beak trim the flock to reduce the pecking ability of aggressive birds [92]. For example, this has been practiced on bobwhite quail around 6 weeks of age [93] and has been used in pheasants as an alternative to spectacles [99]. There are animal welfare issues to consider, and the practice of beak trimming should be conducted safely and aseptically.

13.3 Gamebird Multisystemic Infections

13.3.1 Marble Spleen Disease (MSD)

Marble spleen disease (MSD) is a fatal disease of commercial pheasants that are over 3 months of age, and is caused by a siadenovirus (nonenveloped, icosahedral DNA virus) that is closely related to hemorrhagic enteritis virus (HEV) of turkeys (turkey adenovirus 3, TAdV-3). Together, the MSD and HEV viruses, along with avian adenovirus splenomegaly (AAS) virus of broiler chickens, are classified as turkey adenovirus A, previously listed as Group II adenovirus [100, 101]. Additionally, siadenoviruses have distinct genomic and ultrastructural differences from aviadenoviruses [100]. It has been shown experimentally that the virus causing MSD in pheasants can infect turkeys and that HEV from turkeys can infect pheasants, but this does not generally occur under natural conditions [102, 103]. The virus is spread through contaminated feces and direct bird-to-bird contact [102].

Infection commonly occurs in pheasants and is characterized by sudden death caused by respiratory distress and suffocation. The infection has occasionally been observed in chukar partridges and guineafowl. The infection is promoted by captive rearing and high stocking density that enhance viral transmission, which likely explains why captive-reared ring-necked pheasants are largely affected and why antibodies to MSD and HEV have not been found in serologic surveys of wild birds, including the wild turkey [104, 105]. It has been shown that captive-bred wild turkeys experimentally infected with MSD virus can develop clinical disease with associated lesions [106]. There is usually peracute or acute death of pheasants that are of reproductive age. Some birds are in respiratory distress just prior to death. Pheasants infected with MSD virus have enlarged, pale, mottled spleens as a hallmark lesion (Figure 13.12). The lungs of dead birds are dark red and wet (edema). Pulmonary edema is often the cause of death [107]. Histology of spleens from affected

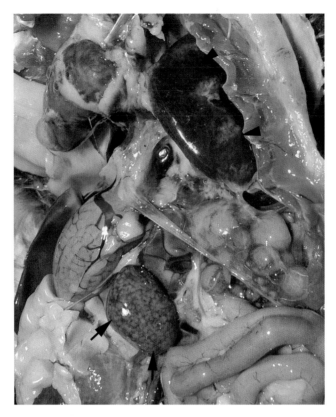

Figure 13.12 One-year-old ring-necked pheasant with marble spleen disease. Note the enlarged and mottled spleen (arrows) and marked pulmonary edema and hemorrhage (arrowheads).

birds often reveals splenic necrosis, lymphoid depletion and histiocytic hyperplasia. Macrophages have enlarged nuclei with marginated chromatin and single, colorless to basophilic intranuclear inclusions. Similar inclusions can occasionally be observed in lung and liver.

Diagnosis can be based on the clinical history, distinctive gross lesions, and the characteristic intranuclear inclusion bodies in spleen (Figure 13.13). The virus can be grown on cell culture and the MDV viral antigen can be detected by polymerase chain reaction. There is no specific treatment for MSD aside from immediate culling of sick and dead birds and use of antibiotics to prevent a secondary bacterial infection. Historically, commercial HEV vaccine marketed for turkeys has effectively been used to vaccinate pheasant flocks [103, 108].

13.3.2 *Escherichia coli* Infection (Colibacillosis)

Colibacillosis is a disease caused by strains of avian pathogenic *E. coli* (APEC). *E. coli* is a normal inhabitant of the avian digestive tract and most strains do not cause disease. *E. coli* is a member of the Enterobacteriaceae family, and is Gram negative and motile, possessing both flagella and fimbriae. Somatic (O), flagellar (H), and capsular (C) antigens have classically been used to differentiate *E. coli* serotypes. The most common serotypes in poultry are 01, 02, and 078, but a large variety have been identified [109]. More recently, it has been recognized that *E. coli* isolates from poultry share various virulence genes such as those associated with adherence, multiplication, and cytotoxicity. These virulence genes are used to characterize APEC which, by definition, are

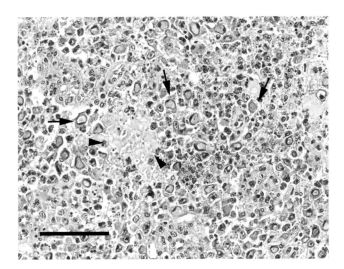

Figure 13.13 Photomicrograph of spleen from 1-year-old ring-necked pheasant with marble spleen disease. Islands of necrosis and fibrin exudation (arrowheads) are bordered by macrophages that contain angular, clear to basophilic intranuclear inclusions (arrows) consistent with adenovirus. H&E stain; bar = 60μm.

associated with diseases in poultry. Although most studies on APEC have been conducted in chickens and turkeys and similar reports in gamebirds are limited, APEC virulence-associated genes have also been identified in pheasants, quail, partridges, guineafowl, and peafowl [110–112].

The factors of captive rearing may play a role in propagating avian infections. Diaz-Sanchez et al. demonstrated that *E. coli* was commonly present in the intestine of farmed partridges (45–50% of flocks), but was practically absent from wild partridges [110]. *E. coli* infections in poultry are manifested as systemic or localized lesions. The authors have observed most of these lesions in farmed gamebirds as well. These lesions include omphalitis/yolk sac infection, cellulitis, salpingitis, peritonitis, and colisepticemia (Figure 13.14). Creitz and Small described *E. coli* septicemia in a flock of 4-month-old pheasants with mortality and either weakness or no premonitory signs. Gross findings included mild lung congestion, but were otherwise unremarkable [113]. In another report, pheasants with systemic *E. coli* infection incurred high mortality and there were gross findings of fibrinous pericarditis, perihepatitis, peritonitis, and hepatosplenomegaly [90]. Ragione et al. described high mortality in red-legged partridges with lethargy and yellow diarrhea; gross lesions were unremarkable [114]. Diaz-Sanchez isolated *E. coli*, characterized with APEC virulence genes, from 1-day-old partridge chicks with weight loss, yellow diarrhea, and 50% mortality. The chicks had enlarged, friable livers and multifocal hepatic necrosis was observed microscopically [111]. Roy et al. observed high mortality in 3–4-week-old farmed Japanese quail with fibrinous perihepatitis, hepatocyte necrosis, and intrahepatic granulomas containing *E. coli* [115]. In another report, *E. coli* cellulitis in 35-day-old quail resulted in high condemnations at the processing plant [116]. Coligranuloma, characterized by tan to yellow, granulomatous nodules on all internal viscera, caused 15% mortality and an 85% drop in egg production in 8–12 month-old breeder quail [117]. Arenas et al. reported on Japanese quail with septicemic colibacillosis (colisepticemia) [118]. The birds were depressed with high mortality; gross necropsy revealed mild splenomegaly with generalized organ congestion.

In another report, *E. coli* with APEC virulence genes was isolated from adult peafowl that died after showing depression, anorexia, and green diarrhea. These birds had a variety of classic *E. coli*

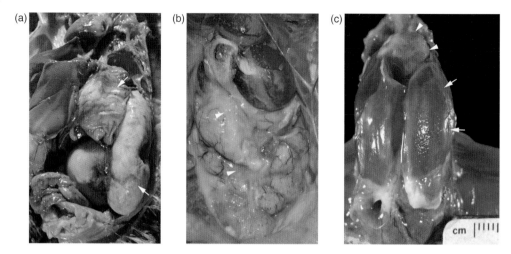

Figure 13.14 Examples of *Escherichia coli* infection in ring-necked pheasants. (a) An adult hen has an oviduct (arrows) distended with exudate (salpingitis). (b) An adult hen has free fibrin (arrowheads) within the coelomic cavity (peritonitis). (c) A pheasant chick with perihepatitis and pericarditis; there is prominent fibrin coating of the enlarged liver (arrows) and heart (arrowheads).

lesions, including fibrinous peritonitis, pneumonia, airsacculitis, and pericarditis [119]. Finally, APECs were readily detected in cloacal swabs of healthy guineafowl with no clinical signs [120].

The diagnosis of colibacillosis is primarily based on clinical signs, gross lesions and culture of *E. coli* from internal organs, particularly liver, spleen, heart, lung or predominant lesions. Diaz-Sanchez et al. demonstrated that APEC isolated from farmed and restocked partridges can develop resistance to frequently used antimicrobials [120]. The authors of this chapter have observed a general resistance of avian *E. coli* isolates to the traditional veterinary antibiotics and these findings are supported by recent surveys [121].

Prevention of *E. coli* infection can be a challenge, but efforts should be made to reduce overall coliform contamination in the poultry environment. Additionally, there is a paucity of antibiotics that are readily available for treatment of bacterial infections in poultry. Therefore, preventive biosecurity is of the utmost importance. Biosecurity procedures include changing clothing and shoes when entering pens, maintaining adequate floor space (minimize crowding), and providing quality ventilation and adequate feeder and water space to reduce stress. Pest and wild bird control is essential. Feed, rodent manure, and contaminated well water can be sources of pathogenic *E. coli* [109], so minimizing pest and fecal contamination of these sources is essential. Probiotics have been added to feed or drinking water in an effort to reduce fecal shedding of APEC into the environment [122].

Vaccines are of uncertain efficacy for reducing *E. coli* in gamebirds because of the diversity of APEC strains and because vaccination programs in gamebirds are not standard practice. The use of commercial *E. coli* vaccines might be helpful in large-scale gamebird production where colibacillosis is a recurring issue. For example, one option would be to isolate the predominant APEC from breeders or growing birds and create a killed autogenous bacterin to administer to the adults prior to breeding season. Passive antibodies from the hens could provide a degree of protection for the chicks for 2–3 weeks post hatch [122]. Additionally, the use of live *E. coli* vaccines can be considered. For example, commercial live *E. coli* vaccines administered to broiler chicks by spray or eyedrop had no deleterious effect, and both clinical signs and *E. coli*-associated lesions in vaccinated/challenged broilers were reduced when compared to nonvaccinated/challenged controls [123]. Similar effects might be achievable in gamebird farms with a history of *E. coli* infection.

13.3.3   *Pasteurella multocida* Infection (Fowl Cholera)

The species *Pasteurella multocida* is divided into four subspecies: *multocida*, *gallicida*, *septica* and *tigris*. *P. multocida* subsp. *multocida* is the primary agent of concern and is generally referred to as *P. multocida*. This agent is classified into serogroups A, B, C, D, E, and F based on capsule antigen and into 16 somatic serotypes (1–16) based on lipopolysaccharide antigen [124]. All capsular and somatic serotypes (except 8 and 13) have been isolated from birds [125]. Although the capsule is considered the major virulence factor for avian *P. multocida*, other bacterial factors that can influence virulence are endotoxin, outer membrane proteins, heat shock proteins, neuraminidase, and iron binding proteins [126]. *P. multocida* is a common pathogen in cattle, pigs, sheep, and rabbits and is often referred to as "fowl cholera" or "avian cholera" in birds, particularly poultry and gamebirds. The bacterial infection is common in domestic chickens, turkeys, and waterfowl, and has been described in pheasants [127–129], partridges [130], quail [131–133], peafowl [134], and guineafowl [135]. Quail are reported to be more susceptible to *P. multocida* infection than other gamebirds [134]; however, in the Midwest US, the authors observe this condition most often in pheasants. Because the strains of *P. multocida* are similar across poultry species, infected turkeys and chickens can pose a risk to domestic gamebirds and vice versa.

The bacterial agent is usually transmitted through the mucosal membranes of the respiratory tract. It has been shown that *P. multocida* inoculated into the skin can result in localized skin infection or progress to septicemia [126, 136]. High population density can be a predisposing factor to infection, along with adverse weather such as rain or sudden change from hot to cold temperatures [130]. In domestic poultry, a major source of *P. multocida* infection is chronic carrier birds that have recovered from previous infection or had subclinical infections [127]. Additionally, aside from the bacterial strain, the virulence of *P. multocida* can vary depending on the host species, age of birds, nutrition, climate, and crowding. Predators (skunk, racoon, fox) entering the pen can introduce *P. multocida* into the flock. Acute infections usually result in septicemia and sudden death as the most common clinical sign, but septicemia with lethargy, ruffled feathers, diarrhea, respiratory distress, and oculonasal discharge can be observed. In birds that survive acute infection, bacteria can localize in wattle or footpad, leg joints, brain, and lung. Confined pheasants may be less likely to develop a carrier state compared to chickens and turkeys [127].

In the authors' experience, pheasants can often die rapidly in high numbers without gross lesions; mortality as high as 9.5% within 24 hours has been recorded [128]. If gamebirds are observed closely, aside from rapid mortality, ruffled feathers, decreased feed consumption, lethargy, and weakness might be observed in a small percentage of the flock [127, 131]. Dead birds may have no gross lesions or mild hepatosplenomegaly with pinpoint necrosis (Figure 13.15) and systemic hemorrhages, but these lesions are usually not as extreme as those observed in chickens and turkeys.

Diagnosis is based on isolation of the organism from infected internal organs (lung, liver, and spleen) and should include antibiotic sensitivity for treatment. *P. multocida* isolates can be further characterized by serotyping, DNA fingerprinting (restriction endonuclease analysis), and whole-genome sequencing. These analyses are useful for tracking the epidemiology of flock infection and have been used to select isolates for autogenous bacterin preparation [137, 138].

In terms of treatment, outbreaks in pheasants and quail were effectively reduced with the use of chlortetracycline in the feed; this antibiotic is now off-label in the US [127, 131]. Birds with subclinical infections can spread the agent through oral secretions and aerosols. To detect subclinical

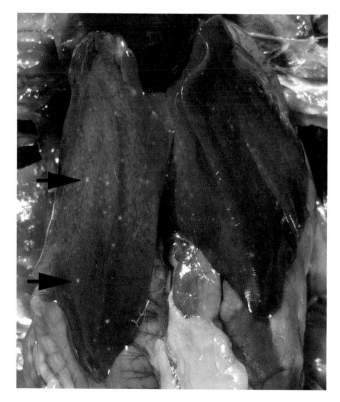

Figure 13.15   An adult ring-necked pheasant hen with *Pasteurella multocida* infection has an enlarged liver with scattered pale, necrotic foci (arrows).

infections, one should focus on culturing visible lesions on the skin of the head, conjunctival sac, infraorbital sinus, and swollen joints on the wing or leg. If assessing valuable breeding stock for individual carrier birds, one can collect oropharyngeal swabs for PCR or mouse inoculation [139].

Confinement and biosecurity are probably the most effective ways to prevent introduction of *P. multocida*. This includes rodent and insect control, regular disinfection of drinkers and feeders, all-in, all-out husbandry, and vaccination [131]. Vaccination is a common practice and can be the most effective control measure in confinement-reared poultry systems. Most commercial vaccines in domestic poultry contain *P. multocida* serotypes Al, A3, and A4 that are emulsified in oil adjuvant or aluminum hydroxide [126]. Killed vaccines with adjuvant can adulterate skin, subcutis, and muscle. The live attenuated vaccines marketed in North America are the Clemson University and M-9 strains, which are serotype A3,4; however, these strains have occasionally been implicated in causing active *P. multocida* infection in domestic poultry [140, 141]. The use of these live vaccines in gamebirds is poorly documented.

13.3.4   *Erysipelothrix rhusiopathiae* Infection (Erysipelas)

Erysipelothrix rhusiopathiae is a slightly curved, nonspore-forming, Gram-positive rod (facultative anaerobe) that can survive for long periods in dead animal tissue, soil, and organic matter [142]. The microorganism has a wide host range and can infect humans as well.

Erysipelas is usually septicemic bacterial disease with the greatest economic impact in swine and turkeys and has been described in most commercial poultry [143, 144]. Infected birds can readily contaminate the environment and serve as a source of infection, either directly or through fomites. Infected ducks and sheep can also serve as a source of infection [145]. Historically in poultry, this infection is described most often in domestic turkeys raised in outdoor ranges or pasture, and disease outbreaks have been significantly reduced by modern indoor confinement practices. The infection has also been reported in a variety of domestic birds including pheasants [146–149], quail [150–152], partridge [153], peafowl [142], and guineafowl [154, 155].

Human exposure to *E. rhusiopathiae* is a significant occupational hazard, and can occur through contact with sick animals, viscera, blood, or contaminated soil/bedding. Three forms of human disease that have been described are a localized cutaneous lesion form, termed "erysipeloid," a generalized cutaneous form, and a septicemic form that is often associated with endocarditis [142].

Infections with *E. rhusiopathiae* occur through inoculation of damaged skin or mucous membranes, by ingesting the agent in contaminated soil or through cannibalism of infected carcasses [145]. Infected birds can transmit the bacterium in feces, saliva, and nasal secretions. Older birds tend to be more sensitive to the infection, which is why the diagnosis is most often made in young adults or mature breeder birds. Birds raised with outdoor access will have greater exposure to infection through contact with contaminated soil and carriers such as wild birds, rodents, and insects [156]. Additionally, artificially inseminated (AI) turkey hens can be infected through contaminated semen and a similar mode of spread might be possible in specialized gamebird breeder flocks in which AI is practiced. Skin damage caused by fighting or pecking (cannibalism) is a common mode of spread in turkeys, and this likely also occurs in gamebirds such as pheasants. Exposure will be greatest in gamebirds raised in outdoor flight pens on soil floors. Gamebirds raised in indoor confinement are less likely to contract the infection, but the agent can be brought inside by pests.

Erysipelas in domestic poultry usually has an acute course with sudden onset and the resulting flock mortality can be large. An outbreak in chukar partridges resulted in 55% mortality in the flock [157]. One might observe weakness or ataxia, ruffled feathers, or decreased feed consumption prior to death, but rapid death with no premonitory signs is often the only sign at 2–3 days after infection. Infection in quail often causes death without premonitory signs, but may also be preceded by watery diarrhea [150]. The disease can persist for 2–3 weeks in infected poultry flocks [143].

Diagnosis is based upon flock history, clinical signs, and observed lesions. Hallmark lesions in turkeys are cutaneous and systemic hemorrhages, hepatosplenomegaly, swollen joints on legs or wings (septic arthritis), and possibly valvular endocarditis; however, lesions in gamebirds are usually more subtle. Birds are often well fleshed because of the rapid sepsis and mortality. The primary lesions described in pheasants range from none to pale kidney and spleen with enlarged mottled livers [148, 149]. Lesions described in coturnix quail include myocardial, muscular, ovarian, and hepatic hemorrhages as well as enlarged liver, spleen, and kidney [150, 152]. Hepatosplenomegaly and pinpoint hemorrhages (Figure 13.16) have been described in chukar partridges [153, 157]. A guineafowl flock demonstrated 10% mortality with lesions of splenomegaly and pinpoint, white, necrotic splenic foci [155].

Histologic lesions of *E. rhusiopathiae* in birds usually consist of acute septicemia- generalized vascular thrombi of bacteria and fibrin with necrosis or hemorrhage in many organs, particularly liver, spleen, and lung [144]. Blood vessels usually contain clusters of small, curved Gram-positive bacterial rods. Definitive diagnosis of the causative agent can be made by bacterial culture, immunohistochemistry or PCR analysis of organs [149]. The mouse protection test has also been used to confirm the presence of *E. rhusiopathiae* [145].

Penicillin is generally the drug of choice to treat *E. rhusiopathiae* infection in turkeys [142]. Other measures to reduce exposure during an outbreak include immediate removal of dead and sick birds,

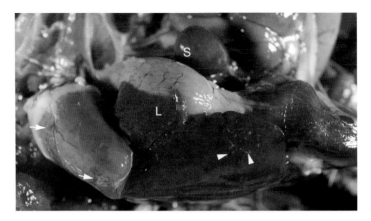

Figure 13.16 An adult chukar partridge with *Erysipelothrix rhusiopathiae* septicemia has hepatosplenomegaly with petechiae (hemorrhages) in the heart (arrows), and pinpoint necrotic foci (arrowheads) in the liver and spleen. L, liver; S, spleen.

thorough cleaning and disinfection of the pen, feeders, drinkers, and equipment. The numbers of possible vectors such as rodents and insects should be reduced in the house. Vaccination for erysipelas has been an effective control measure in commercial poultry. Inoculation of turkeys and chickens with either killed bacterin or live attenuated vaccine has been effective in reducing infection; however, these products have received little attention in gamebirds [158, 159]. Commercial vaccines prepared for swine and turkeys have been shown to be efficacious in emus and geese [143]. One might consider the use of such products in large, high-risk gamebird breeder flocks that have incurred repeated outbreaks.

References

1 Weli, S. and Tryland, M. (2011). Avipoxviruses: infection biology and their use as vaccine vectors. *Virol. J.* 8 (1): 49.

2 Crawford, J.A., Oates, R.M., and Helper, D.H. (1979). Avian pox in California quail from Oregon. *J. Wildl. Dis.* 15 (3): 447–449.

3 Al-Ani, M.O.A. (1986). An outbreak of pox among pheasants in Iraq. *Avian Pathol.* 15 (4): 795–796.

4 Gortazar, C., Millan, J., Hofle, U. et al. (2002). Pathology of avian pox in wild red-legged partridges (*Alectoris rufa*) in Spain. *N. Y. Acad. Sci.* 969 (1): 354–357.

5 Buenestado, F., Gortazar, C., Milan, J. et al. (2004). Descriptive study of an avian pox. *Epidemiol. Infect.* 132 (2): 369–374.

6 Brower, A.I., Cigel, F., Radi, C. et al. (2010). Beak necrosis in Hungarian partridges (*Perdix perdix*) associated with beak-bits and avian poxvirus infection. *Avian Pathol.* 39 (3): 223–225.

7 Davidson, W.R., Kellog, F.E., and Doster, G.L. (1980). An epornitic of avian pox in wild bobwhite quail. *J. Wildl. Dis.* 16 (2): 293–296.

8 Crawford, J.A. (1986). Differential prevalence of avian pox in adult and immature California quail. *J. Wildl. Dis.* 22 (4): 564–566.

9 Gulbahar, Y.M., Cabalar, M., and Boynukara, B. (2005). Avipoxvirus infection in quails. *Turk. J. Vet. Anim. Sci.* 29 (2): 449–454.

10 Bolte, A.L., Meurer, J., and Kaleta, E.F. (1999). Avian host spectrum of avipoxviruses. *Avian Pathol.* 25 (5): 415–432.

11 Williams, R.A., Truchado, D.A., and Benitez, L. (2021). A review on the prevalence of poxvirus disease in free-living and captive wild birds. *Microbiol. Res.* 12 (2): 403–418.

12 Davidson, W.R., Kellog, F.E., and Doster, G.L. (1982). Avian pox infections in southeastern bobwhites: historical and recent information. *Natl. Quail Symp. Proc.* 2 (11): 64–68.

13 Tanizaki, E., Kotani, T., Odagiri, Y. et al. (1989). *Avian Dis.* 33 (2): 333–339.

14 Giddens, W.E. Jr., Swango, L.J., Henderson, J.D. Jr., et al. (1971). Canary pox in sparrows and canaried (Fringillidae) and in weavers (Ploceidae). *Vet. Pathol.* 8 (3): 1971.

15 Kirmse, P. (1969). Host specificity and pathogenicity of pox viruses from wild birds. *Bull. Wildl. Dis. Assoc.* 5 (4): 376–386.

16 Beytuti, E. and Haliguri, M. (2007). Pathological, immunohistochemical, and electron microscopic findings in the respiratory tract and skin of chickens naturally infected with avipoxvirus. *Turk. J. Vet. Anim. Res.* 31 (5): 311–317.

17 Pages-Mante, A., Majo, N., March, R. et al. (2004). Pathology and experimental prophylaxis of avian poxvirus in red-legged partridges (*Alectoris rufa*). *Vet. Rec.* 153 (10): 307–308.

18 Khan, A., Yousaf, A., Khan, Z. et al. (2009). Cutaneous form of pox infection among captive peafowl (Pavo cristatus) chicks. *Avian Pathol.* 38 (1): 65–70.

19 Falluji, A., Tantawi, M.M., Albana, A. et al. (1979). Pox infection among captive peacocks. *J. Wildl. Dis.* 16 (4): 597–600.

20 Tsai, S.S., Chang, T.C., and Yang, S.F. (1997). Unusual lesions associated with avian poxvirus infection in rosy-faced lovebirds (*Agapornis orseicollis*). *Avian Pathol.* 26 (1): 75–82.

21 Poonacha, K.B. and Wilson, M.S. (1981). Avian pox in pen-raised bobwhite quail. *J. Am. Vet. Med. Assoc.* 179 (11): 1264–1265.

22 Fatunmbi, O.O., Reed, W.M., and Olufemi, O.O. (1993). Evaluation of commercial modified live virus fowl pox vaccine for the control of 'variant' fowl poxvirus infections. *Avian Dis.* 40 (3): 582–587.

23 Hermans, K., Devriese, L.A., and Haesebrouck, F. (2010). Staphylococcus. In: *Pathogenesis of Bacterial Infections in Animals*, 4e (ed. C.L. Gyles), 75–89. Danvers, MA: Wiley.

24 Harris, L.G., Foster, S.J., and Richards, R.G. (2002). An introduction to *Staphylococcus aureus* and techniques for identifying and quantifying *S. aureus* adhesins in relation to adhesion to biomaterials: review. *Eur. Cell. Mater.* 4. 39–60.

25 Lorenzoni, G. (2020). Staphylococcosis in chickens. Penn State Extension https://extension.psu.edu (accessed February 2022).

26 Raidal, S.R. (1995). Staphylococcal dermatitis in quail with a parakeratotic hyperkeratotic dermatosis suggestive of pantothenic acid deficiency. *Avian Pathol.* 24 (3): 579–583.

27 Durden, L.A. (2019). Lice (Phthiraptera). In: *Medical and Veterinary Entomology*, 3e (ed. G.R. Mullen and L.A. Durden), 79–105. San Diego, CA: Elsevier.

28 Emerson, K.C. (1962). Mallophaga (chewing lice) occurring on the Turkey. *J. Kansas Ent. Soc.* 35 (1): 196–201.

29 Goldova, M., Palus, V., Letkova, V. et al. (2006). Parasitoloses in pheasants (*Phasianus colchicus*) in confined systems. *Vet. Archiv.* 76 (suppl): 83–89.

30 Hillgarth, N. (1966). Ectoparasite transfer during mating in ring-necked pheasants *Phasianus colchicus*. *J. Avian Biol.* 27 (3): 260–262.

31 Weselmann, R.J. (1968). Population density of Mallophaga on the *Phasianus colchicus*. Masters thesis. Drake University. http://hdl.handle.net/2092/1238 (accessed February 2022).

32 Lewin, V. and Mahrt, J.L. (1983). Parasites of Kalij pheasant (Lophura leucomelana) on the island of Hawaii. *Pac. Sci.* 37 (1): 81–83.

33 Payne, W.R., Oates, D.W., and Dappen, G.E. (1990). Ectoparasites of ring-necked pheasants in Nebraska. *J. Wildl. Dis.* 26 (3): 407–409.

34 Sychra, O. (2005). Chewing lice (Phthiraptera: Amblycera, Ischnocera) from chukars (Alectoris chukar) from a pheasant farm in Jinacovixce (Czech Republic). *Vet. Med. Czech.* 50 (5): 213–218.

35 Arnold, D.C. (2008). The pheasant group of the genus Lagopoecus (Phthiraptera: Ischoncera: Philopteridae). *J. Kansas Entomol. Soc.* 81 (2): 153–160.

36 Ashraf, S., Javid, A., Akram, M. et al. (2015). Studies on the parasitic prevalence in ring necked pheasants (*Phasianus colchicus*) in captivity. *J. Anim. Plant Sci.* 25 (3): 359–364.

37 Curland, N., Gethoffer, F., van Neer, A. et al. (2018). Investigation into diseases in free-ranging ring-necked pheasants (*Phasianus colchicus*) in northwestern Germany during population decline with special reference to infectious pathogens. *Eur. J. Wildl. Res.* 64 (2): 12.

38 Chu, X., Dik, B., Gustafsson, D.R. et al. (2019). The influence of host body size and good guild on prevalence and mean intensity of chewing lice (Phthiraptera) on birds in southern China. *J. Parasitol.* 105 (2): 334–344.

39 Emerson, K.C. (1956). Mallophaga (chewing lice) occurring on the domestic chicken. *J. Kansas Ent. Soc.* 30 (1): 9–10.

40 Calvete, C., Estrada, R., Lucientes, J. et al. (2003). Ectoparasite ticks and chewing lice of red-legged partridge, *Alecorus rufa*, in Spain. *Med. Vet. J.* 17 (1): 33–37.

41 Millan, J., Gortazar, C., Martin-Mateo, M.P. et al. (2004). Comparative survey of the ectoparasites fauna of wild and farm-reared red-legged partridges (*Alectoris rufa*), with an ecological study in wild populations. *Parasitol. Res.* 93 (1): 79–85.

42 Al-Bawar, S. and Saeed, I. (2012). Parasitoses of the chukar partridge, *Alectoris* chukar in North Iraq. *Turk. Parazitol. Derg.* 36 (4): 240–246.

43 Khattak, R.M., Ali, S., Jahangir, M. et al. (2012). Prelaence of exctoparasites in wild and domesticated grey (*Francolinus pondicerianus*) and black partirdges (*Francolinus francolinus*) from Khyber Pakhtoonkhwa province of Pakistan. *Pak. J. Zool.* 44 (5): 1239–1244.

44 Gustafsson, D.R. and Zou, G. (2020). Gallancyra gen. nov. (Phthiraptera: Ischnocera), with an overview of the geographical distribution of chewing lice parasitizing chicken. *Eur. J. Taxon.* 686 (1): 1–36.

45 Hightower, B.G., Lehman, V.W., and Eads, R.B. (1953). Ectoparasites from mammals and birds on a quail preserve. *J. Mammal.* 34 (2): 268–271.

46 Bergstrand, J.L. and Klimstra, W.D. (1964). Ectoparasites of the bobwhite quail in southern Illinois. *Am. Midl. Nat.* 72 (2): 490–498.

47 Kellog, F.E. and Doster, G.L. (1972). Diseases and parasites of the bobwhite. *Natl. Quail Symp. Proc.* 1: 233–267.

48 Doster, G.L., Wilson, N., and Kellog, F.E. (1980). Ectoparasites collected from bobwhite quail in the southeastern United States. *J. Wildl. Dis.* 16 (4): 515–520.

49 Askin, N. (2010). The presence of chewing lice (Insects: Phthiraptera) species on wild quails (*Coturnix coturnix*). *J. Anim. Vet Adv.* 9 (9): 1377–1379.

50 El-Sharabasy, H.M. and Hanafy, A.M. (2014). Ectoparasitic and predaceous mites inhabiting litters of the Japanese quail, coturnix japonica in Ismailia Governorate, Egypt. *Egypt. J. Biol. Pest Control* 24 (2): 359–362.

51 Adamu, Y.A., Alayande, M.O., Bello, A. et al. (2015). Lice infestation on Japanese quail (*Coturnix coturnix japonica*) Temminck & Schlegel 1849 in Sokoto metropolis, Nigeria. *Net J. Agric. Sci.* 3 (1): 32–34.

52 Alahmed, A., Aldryhim, Y., Shobruck, M. et al. (2017). A new species of the genus Amyrsidea (Phthirapter: Amblycera: Menoponidae) parasitizing domestic chickens in Saudi Arabia. *Zootaxa* 4238 (2): 253–257.

53 Hollamby, S.H., Sikarskie, J.G., and Stuht, J. (2003). Survey of peafowl (*Pavo cristatus*) for potential pathogens at three Michigan zoos. *J. Zoo Wildl. Med.* 34 (4): 375–379.

54 Corn, J.L., Berger, P., and Mertens, J.W. (2009). Surveys for ectoparasites on wildlife associated with *Amblyomma variegatum* (Acari: Ixodidae)-infected livestock in St. Croix, U.S. Virgin Islands. *J. Med. Entomol.* 46 (6): 1483–1489.

55 Khursheed, A., Sial, N., Malik, S. et al. (2014). Parasitic infestation in peafowl of Bahawalpur Zoo, Punjab, Pakistan. *Stand. Sci. Res. Essays* 2 (9): 401–405.

56 Ganjali, M., Keighobadi, M., and Hajopour, N. (2015). First report of new species of Goniodes Pavonis (the chewing lice) from Indian peacock in Iran. *J. New Biol. Rep.* 4 (1): 76–78.

57 Nasser, M., Al-Ahmed, A., Schobrak, M. et al. (2015). Identification key for chewing lice (Phthiraptera: Amblycera: Ischnocera) infesting peafowl (Pavo cristatus) with one new country record and new host record for Saudi Arabia. *Turk. J. Zool.* 39 (1): 88–94.

58 Yadav, S.K., Sarkar, S., Sarkar, S. et al. (2021). Prevalence of endoparasites and ectoparasites of captive peafowl farm. *Adv. Anim. Vet. Sci.* 9 (3): 442–445.

59 Martin-Mateo, M.P., Albala, F., and Sanchez, A.C. (1980). Malofagos ectoparasites de aves de la provincial de Zaragoza. *Graellsia, Revista de Entomologos Ibericos* 34 (1): 121–145.

60 Ayeni, J.S.O., Dipeolu, O.O., and Okaeme, A.N. (1983). Parasitic infections in the grey-helmeted guinea fowl. *Vet. Parasitol.* 12 (1): 59–63.

61 Fabiyi, J.P. (1986). Exclusion in Nigeria of chickens and guinea-fowl from the host range of *Menacanthus stramineus* (Mallophaga: Insecta). *Rev. Elev. Med. Vet. Pays Trop.* 39 (3–4): 377–379.

62 Okaeme, A.N. (1988). Ectoparasites of guinea fowl (*Numida meleagris glaeata pallas*) and local domestic chicken (*Gallus gallus*) in southern Guinea savanna, Nigeria. *Vet. Res. Commun.* 12 (4–5): 277–280.

63 Clayton, D.H. and Drown, D.M. (2001). Critical evaluation of five methods for quantifying chewing lice (Insecta: Phthiraptera). *J. Parasitol.* 87 (6): 1291–1300.

64 Ramli, R., Cusack, M., Curry, G.B. et al. (2000). Morphological variation of chewing lice (Insecta: Phthiraptera) from different skua taxa. *Biol. J. Linnean Soc.* 71 (1): 91–101.

65 Zhang, Z.-Q. (2011). Animal biodiversity: an outline of higher level classification and survey of taxonomic richness. *Zootaxa* 3148: 1–237.

66 Mullen, G.R. and OConnor, B.M. (2019). Mites (Acari). In: *Medical and Veterinary Entomology*, 3e (ed. G.A. Mullen, L.A. Durden and J.G. King), 533–602. Cambridge, MA: Elsevier.

67 Orton, D.I., Warren, L.J., and Wilkinson, J.D. (2000). Avian mite dermatitis. *Clin. Exp. Dermatol.* 25 (2): 129–131.

68 Knee, W. and Proctor, H. (2007). Host records for *Ornithonyssus sylviarum* (Mesostigmata: Macronyssidae) from birds of North America (Canada, United States, and Mexico). *J. Med. Entomol.* 44 (4): 709–713.

69 Mullens, B.A. and Murillo, A.C. (2018). The future of poultry pest management. In: *Advances in Poultry Welfare* (ed. J.A. Mench), 295–321. Cambridge, MA: Elsevier/Woodhead Publishing.

70 Ogada, S., Lichoti, J., Oyier, P.A. et al. (2016). A survey on disease prevalence, ectoparasite infestation and chick mortality in poultry popoulations of Kenya. *Livestock Res. Rural Dev.* 28 (12): 1–13.

71 McDaniel, B. and Parikh, G.C. (1969). A new species of *Epidermoptes* from a South Dakota Pheasant (Acarina: Epidermoptidae). *J. Kansas Entomol. Soc.* 42 (1): 34–38.

72 Lawal, M.D., Mohammad, L., Bello, A. et al. (2016). Seasonal incidence of scaly leg mite (Cnemidiokoptes mutans) on guinea fowls (Numida meleagrisgaleata) from Sokoto, north western Nigeria. *Schol. J. Biotechnol.* 3 (1): 1–3.

73 Jackson, B., Heath, A., Harvey, C. et al. (2015). Knemidokoptinid (epidermoptidae: knemidokoptinae) mite infestation in wild red-crowned parakeets (*Cyanoramphus novaezelandiae*): correlations between macroscopic and microscopic findings. *J. Wildl. Dis.* 51 (3): 651–651.

74 Kirmse, P. (1966). Cnemidocoptic mite infestations in wild birds. *Bull. Wildl. Dis. Assoc.* 2 (4): 86–99.

75 Morishita, T.Y., Johnson, G., Johnson, G. et al. (2005). Scaly-leg mite infestation associated with digit necrosis in bantam chickens (Gallus domesticus). *J. Avian. Med. Surg.* 19 (3): 230–233.

76 Siti Aminah, Y., Donny, Y., Zubaidah, K. et al. (2016). A case report of scaly leg mite in green peafowl (*Pavo muticus*). *Malaysian J. Vet. Res.* 7 (1): 77–80.

77 Ruff, M.D. (1999). Important parasites in poultry production systems. *Vet. Parasitol.* 84 (3–4): 3437–3447.

78 Sato, Y. (2019). Poultry external parasite and pest control. Iowa State University Extension and Outreach. www.abe.iastate.edu/extension-and-outreach (accessed February 2022).

79 Murillio, A.C. and Mullen, B.A. (2016). Sulfur dust bag: a novel technique for ectoparasite control in poultry systems. *J. Econ. Entomol.* 109 (5): 2229–2233.

80 Lucas, A.M. and Stettenheim, P.R. (1972). *Avian Anatomy – Integument Part II. Agricultural Handbook 362*. Washington, D.C.: U.S. Government Printing Office.

81 Miner, M.L. and Smart, R.A. (1975). Causes of enlarged sternal bursas (breast blisters). *Avian Dis.* 19 (2): 246–256.

82 Wisman, E.L. and Beane, W.L. (1964). Effect of some management factors on the incidence of breast blisters in heavy broilers. *Poult. Sci.* 44 (3): 737–741.

83 Pass, D.A. (1989). The pathology of the avian integument: a review. *Avian Pathol.* 18 (1): 1–72.

84 McCune, E.L. and Dellman, H.D. (1968). Developmental origin and structural characters of "breast blisters" in chickens. *Poult. Sci.* 47 (3): 852–858.

85 Muller, H.D. (1968). Juvenile initiation of keel bursa enlargement in tom turkeys. *Poult. Sci.* 47 (6): 1897–1901.

86 Adams, A.W., Carlson, C.W., Kahrs, A.J. et al. (1967). Relationship of several environmental factors to the incidence of breast blisters in large type male market turkeys. *Poult. Sci.* 46 (3): 569–577.

87 Kamyab, A. (2001). Enlarged sternal bursa and focal ulcerative dermatitis in male turkeys. *World Poult. Sci. J.* 57 (1): 5012.

88 Wilson, W.O. (1949). Cannibalism in poultry. *California Agric.* 3 (6): 13–14.

89 Pulliainen, E. (1965). Cannibalism in the pheasant (Phasianus colchicus L.) during the egg-laying period. *Ann. Zool. Fennici* 2 (3): 208–214.

90 Pennycott, T.W. (2000). Causes of mortality and culling in adult pheasants. *Vet. Rec.* 146 (10): 273–278.

91 Madsen, H. (1966). On feather picking and cannibalism in pheasant and partridge chicks, particulary in relation to the amino acid arginine. *Acta Vet. Scand.* 7 (2): 272–287.

92 Walker, W. and Smith, T.W. (2005). Raising bobwhite quail for commercial use. Cooperative Extension Service, Mississippi State University. http://extension.msstate.edu (accessed February 2022).

93 Dozier, W.A., Bramwell, K., Hatkin, J. et al. (2010). Bobwhite quail production and management guide. University of Georgia Cooperative Extension. Bulletin 1215. https://extension.uga.edu (accessed February 2022).

94 Ernst, R.A., Woodard, A.E., and Vohra, P. (2007). Raising game birds. University of California Division of Agriculture and Natural Resources. Publication 8155. http://anrcatalog.ucdavis.edu (accessed February 2022).

95 Clauer, P.J. (2016). Poultry cannibalism: prevention and treatment. Penn State Extension. https://extension.psu.edu/poultry-cannibalism-prevention-and-treatment (accessed February 2022).

96 Blake, J.P., Hess, J.B., and Berry, W.D. (2013). Effect of 2 protein regimens and 2 lighting intensities on performance of the Hungarian partridge (*Perdix perdix*). *J. Appl. Poultry Res.* 22 (3): 365–369.

97 Butler, D.A. and Davis, C. (2010). Effects of plastic bits on the condition and behavior of captive-reared pheasants. *Vet. Rec.* 166 (13): 398–401.

98 Butler, D.A. and Davis, C. (2014). Effects of plastic spectacles on the condition and behavior of pheasants. *Vet. Rec.* 174 (8): 198.

99 Nicol, C.J., Bouwsema, J., Caplan, G. et al. (2017). Guinea fowl, pigeons, partridges, quail, and pheasants. In: *Farmed Bird Welfare Science Review, October 2017.*, 215–235. Melbourne, Australia: Department of Economic Development, Jobs, Transport and Resources.

100 Hess, M. (2000). Detection and differentiation of avian adenoviruses: a review. *Avian Pathol.* 29 (3): 195–206.

101 McFerran, J.B. and Smyth, J.A. (2000). Avian adenoviruses. *Rev. Sci. Tech.* 19 (2): 589–601.

102 Iltis, J.P., Jakowski, R.M., and Wyand, D.S. (1975). Transmission of marble spleen disease in turkeys and pheasants. *Am. J. Vet. Res.* 36 (1): 97–101.

103 Fadly, A.M., Cowen, B.S., and Nazerian, K. (1988). Some observations on the response of ring-necked pheasants to inoculation with various strains of cell-culture-propagated type II avian adenovirus. *Avian Dis.* 32 (3): 548–552.

104 Domermuth, C.H., Forrester, D.J., Trainer, D.O. et al. (1977). Serologic examination of wild birds for hemorrhagic enteritis of Turkey and marble spleen disease of pheasants. *J. Wildl. Dis.* 13 (4): 405–408.

105 Hopkins, B.A., Skeeles, J.K., Houghton, G.E. et al. (1990). A survey of infectious diseases in wild turkeys (Meleagris gallopavo silvestris) from Arkansas. *J. Wildl. Dis.* 26 (4): 468–472.

106 Iltis, J.P., Jakowski, R.M., and Wyand, D.S. (1975). Experimentally transmitted marble spleen disease in pen-raised wild turkeys. *J. Wildl. Dis.* 11 (4): 484–485.

107 Fitzgerald, S.D. and Reed, W.M. (1989). A review of marble spleen disease of ring-necked pheasants. *J. Wildl. Dis.* 25 (4): 455–461.

108 Domermuth, C.H., Douglass, C.S., DuBose, R.T. et al. (1979). Vaccination of ring-necked pheasant for marble spleen disease. *Avian Dis.* 23 (1): 30–38.

109 Panth, Y. (2019). Colibacillosis in poultry: a review. *J. Agric. Nat. Resour.* 2 (1): 301–311.

110 Diaz-Sanchez, S., Moriones, A.M., Casas, F. et al. (2012). Prevalence of *Escherichia coli*, *Salmonella sp.* and *Campylobacter sp.* in the intestinal flora of farm-reared, restocked and wild red-legged partridges (*Alectoris rufa*): is restocking using farm-reared birds a risk? *Eur. J. Wildl. Res.* 58 (1): 99–105.

111 Diaz-Sanchez, S., Lopez, A., Gamino, V. et al. (2013). A colibacillosis outbreak in farmed red-legged partridges (*Alectoris rufa*). *Avian Dis.* 57 (1): 143–146.

112 Borzi, M.M., Cardozo, M.V., de Oliveira, E.S. et al. (2018). Characterization of avian pathogenic *Escherichia coli* isolated from free-range helmeted guineafowl. *Braz. J. Microbiol.* 49S (suppl. 1): 107–112.

113 Creitz, J.R. and Small, N.N. (1967). Escherichia coli septicemia in pheasants. *Bull. Wildl. Dis. Assoc.* 3 (2): 68–69.

114 La Ragione, R.M., Cooley, W.A., Parmar, D.D.G. et al. (2004). Attaching and effacing *Escherichia coli* 0103:K+:H- in red-legged partridges. *Vet. Rec.* 155 (3): 397–398.

115 Roy, P., Hemalatha, S., and Purushothaman, V. (2013). Unusual coligranuloma very young Japanese quail chicks. *Pak. J. Biol. Sci.* 16 (24): 2020–2072.

116 Burns, K.A., Otalora, R., Glisson, J.R., and Hofacre, C.L. (2003). Cellulitis in Japanese quail (Coturnix coturnix japonica). *Avian Dis.* 47 (1): 211–214.

117 Da Silva, P.L., Coelho, H.E., de Almeida Ribeiro, S.C., and de Oliveira, R. (1989). Occurrence of coligranulomatosis in coturnix quail in Uberlandia, Minas Gerais, Brazil. *Avian Dis.* 33 (3): 590–593.

118 Arenas, A., Vicente, S., Luque, I. et al. (1999). Outbreak of septicaemic colibacillosis in Japanese quail (*Coturnix coturnix japonica*). *J. Vet. Med.* 46 (6): 399–404.

119 Barbieri, N.L., Tejkowski, T.M., de Oliveira, A.L. et al. (2102). Characterization of extraintestinal *Escherichia coli* isolated from a peacock (*Pavo cristatus*) with colicepticemia. *Avian Dis.* 56 (2): 436–440.

120 Diaz-Sanchez, S., Sanchez, S., Ewers, C. et al. (2012). Occurrence of avian pathogenic *Escherichia coli* and antimicrobial resistant E. coli in red-legged partridges (*Alectoris rufa*): sanitary concerns of farming. *Avian Pathol.* 41 (4): 337–344.

121 Agunos, A., Carson, C., and Leger, D. (2013). Antimicrobial therapy of selected diseases in turkeys, laying hens and minor poultry species. *Can. Vet. J.* 54 (11): 1041–1052.

122 Kabir, S.M.L. (2010). Avian colibacillosis and salmonellosis: a closer look at epidemiology, pathogenesis, diagnosis, control and public health concerns. *Int. J. Environ. Res. Public Health* 7 (1): 89–114.

123 Assad, H.M., Amen, O., Elazeem, M.A. et al. (2019). Comparative study on commercial vaccines against E. coli in broiler chickens. *Assiut Vet. Med. J.* 65 (161): 22–29.

124 Harper, M., Boyce, J.D., and Adler, B. (2006). *Pasteurella multocida* pathogenesis: 125 years after Pasteur. *FEMS Microbiol. Lett.* 265 (1): 1–10.

125 Chaves Hernandez, A.J. (2014). Poultry and avian diseases. In: *Encyclopedia of Agriculture and Food Systems* (ed. N.K. van Alfen), 504–520. St Louis, MO: Elsevier.

126 Christensen, J.P. and Bisgaard, M. (2000). Fowl cholera. *Rev. Sci. Tech.* 19 (2): 626–637.

127 Brown, J.D., Dunn, P., Wallner-Pendleton, E. et al. (2016). Pheasants (*Phasianus cholchicus*) after an avian cholera and after an outbreak of avian cholera and apparently successful antibiotic treatment. *Avian Dis.* 60 (1): 87–89.

128 Popova, T.P. and Tzvetkov, Y.M. (2002). Fowl cholera in pheasants (*Phasianus colchicus*) – etiological investigation and effect of therapy with thiamphenicol. *Bulg. J. Vet. Med.* 5 (1): 23–28.

129 Sakuri, K., Kurihara, T., Matsuoka, Y. et al. (1986). An outbreak of fowl cholera in green pheasants (Phasianus cholchicus) in Japan (1986). *Nihon Juigaku Zasschi* 48 (4): 711–717.

130 Pedersen, K., Dietz, H.H., Jorgensen, J.C. et al. (2003). Pasteurella multocida from outbreaks of avian cholera in wild and captive birds in Denmark. *J. Wildl. Dis.* 39 (4): 808–816.

131 Glisson, J.R., Cheng, I.N., Rowland, G.N. et al. (1989). *Pasteurella multocida* infection in Japanese quail (Coturnix conturnix japonica). *Avian Dis.* 33 (4): 820–822.

132 Goto, Y., Nakura, R., Nasu, T. et al. (2001). Isolation of Pasteurella multocida during an outbreak of infectious septicemia in Japanese quail (Coturnix coturnix japonica). *J. Vet. Med. Sci.* 63 (9): 1055–1056.

133 Panigrahy, B. and Glass, S.G. (1982). Outbreaks of fowl cholera in quail. *Avian Dis.* 26 (1): 200–203.

134 Christensen, J.P. and Bisgaard, M. (1997). Avian pasteurellosis: taxonomy of the organisms involved and aspects of pathogenesis. *Avian Pathol.* 26 (3): 461–483.

135 Sellyei, B., Thuma, A., Volokhov, D. et al. (2017). Comparative analysis of Pasteurella multocida isolates from acute and chronic fowl cholera cases in Hungary during the period 2005 through 2010. *Avian Dis.* 61 (4): 457–465.

136 Frame, D.D., Clark, F.D., and Smart, R.A. (1994). Recurrent outbreaks of a cutaneous form of *Pasteurella multocida* infection in turkeys. *Avian Dis.* 38 (2): 390–392.

137 Blackall, P.J., Miflin, J.K., and Miflin, J.K. (2000). Identification and typing of Pasteurella multocida: a review. *Avian Pathol.* 29 (4): 271–287.

138 Dziva, F., Muhairwa, A.P., Bisgaard, M. et al. (2008). Diagnostic and typing options for investigating diseases associated with Pasteurella multocida. *Vet. Microbiol.* 128 (1): 1–22.

139 Muhairwa, A.P., Christensen, J.P., and Bisgaard, M. (2000). Investigations on the carrier rate of Pasteurella multocida in healthy commercial poultry flocks and flocks affected by fowl cholera. *Avian Pathol.* 29 (1): 133–142.

140 Hofacre, C.L. and Glisson, J.R. (1986). A serotypic survey of *Pasteurella multocida* isolated from poultry. *Avian Dis.* 30 (3): 632–633.

141 Snipes, K.P., Hirsch, D.C., Kasten, R.W. et al. (1990). Differentiation of field isolates of *Pasteurella multocida* serotype 3,4 from liver vaccine strain by genotypic characterization. *Avian Dis.* 34 (3): 419–424.

142 Wang, Q., Chang, B.J., and Riley, T.V. (2010). *Erysipelothrix rhusiopathiae*. *Vet. Microbiol.* 140 (3): 405–417.

143 Bobrek, K., Gawel, A., and Masurkiewicz, M. (2013). Infections with *Erysipelothrix rhusiopathiae* in poultry flocks. *Worlds Poult. Sci. J.* 69 (4): 803–811.

144 Silva, A.P., Cooper, G., Blakey, J. et al. (2020). Retrospective summary of *Erysipelothrix rhusiopathiae* diagnosed in avian species in California (2000–19). *Avian Dis.* 64 (4): 499–506.

145 Ugochukwu, I.C.I., Samuel, F., Orapoghenor, O. et al. (2019). Erysipelas, the opportunistic zoonotic disease: history, epidemiology, pathology, and diagnosis – a review. *Comp. Clin. Pathol.* 28 (3): 853–859.

146 Raines, T.V. and Winkel, F.H. (1956). Erysipelas in pheasants. *J. Am. Vet. Med. Assoc.* 129 (1): 399–400.

147 Bygrave, A.C. (1971). An outbreak of erysipelas in pheasant poults (Phasianus cholchicus). *Vet. Rec.* 89 (10): 279–280.

148 Milne, E.M., Windsor, R.S., Rogerson, F. et al. (1997). Concurrent infection with enteric protozoa and *Erysipelothrix rhusiopathiae* in chicken and pheasant flocks. *Vet. Rec.* 141 (13): 340–341.

149 Henning, G.E., Goebel, H.D., and Fabis, J.J. (2002). Diagnosis by polymerase chain reaction of Erysipelas septicemia in a flock of ring-necked pheasants. *Avian Dis.* 46 (2): 509–514.

150 Panigrahy, B. and Hall, C.F. (1977). An outbreak of erysipelas in Coturnix quails. *Avian Dis.* 21 (4): 708–710.

151 Githkopoulos, P.R. and Xenos, G.X. (1984). Erysipelas in quails (Coturnix Coturnix Japonica). *J. Hell. Vet. Med. Soc.* 35 (1): L53–L58.

152 Mutalib, A., Keirs, R., and Austin, F. (1995). Erysipelas in quail and suspected erysipeloid in processing plant employees. *Avian Dis.* 39 (1): 191–193.

153 Pettit, J.R., Gough, A.W., and Truscott, R.B. (1976). *Erysipelothrix rhusiopathiae* infection in chukar partridge (Alectorus graeca). *J. Wildl. Dis.* 12 (2): 254–255.

154 Baker, K.B. and Westwood, A. (1971). Erysipelas in the guinea fowl. *Vet. Rec.* 88 (4): 108–109.

155 Campbell, G.W., Taylor, J.D., and Harrower, B.J. (1992). Erysipelothrix rhusiopathiae infection of guinea fowl (*Numida meleagris*). *Aust. Vet. J.* 69 (1): 13.

156 Mazaheri, A., Philipp, H.C., Bonsack, H. et al. (2006). Investigations of the vertical transmission of Erysipelothrix rhusiopathiae in laying hens. *Avian Dis.* 50 (2): 306–308.

157 Butcher, G. and Panigrahy, B. (1985). An outbreak of erysipelas in chukars. *Avian Dis.* 29 (3): 843–845.

158 Bricker, J. and Saif, Y. (1988). Use of live oral vaccine to immunize turkeys against erysipelas. *Avian Dis.* 32 (4): 668–673.

159 Opriessnig, T., Forde, T., and Shimoji, Y. (2020). *Erysipelothrix* Spp.: past, present, and future directions in vaccine research. *Front. Vet. Sci.* 7: 174–192.

14

Gamebird Toxicologic Diseases
Richard M. Fulton

There are very few literature citations of toxicologic diseases of gamebirds (pheasants, quail, partridges). Only lead and selenium have been cited as naturally occurring in quail and pheasants respectively [1, 2]. After reviewing those reports, the remainder of this chapter will be focused on toxicants to which gamebirds might be exposed.

14.1   Lead

Lead toxicosis has historically been a problem with the poisoning of waterfowl, which prompted the change from the use of lead shot for hunting to that of steel and other compounds used for shot [3].

The typical gross findings of lead poisoning are those of cachexia, anemia, paresis, paralysis, proventricular impaction, and ventricular erosion with a bile-stained lining. While relatively common in waterfowl, lead toxicosis is rare in upland gamebirds. In quail, inability to fly and paralysis have been reported with lead toxicosis. The lesions found grossly in quail were emaciation, impacted proventriculus, and lesions affecting the ventriculus (gizzard). The ventriculus lining was stained green/brown, had two partially dissolved pellets, and had many erosions.

Diagnosis of lead toxicosis is based on clinical signs, both gross and microscopic lesions, lead shot in the ventriculus as well as finding a toxic lead level in blood and/or liver [1]. Prevention is accomplished by excluding gamebirds from soils heavily contaminated with lead shot. These areas are where there has been heavy hunting pressure using lead shot.

14.2   Selenium

Selenium toxicosis has occurred naturally in ducks and other waterbirds eating plants in areas with high soil selenium levels due to human activity [4]. In pheasants, and possibly in other gamebirds, selenium toxicosis has occurred due to a feed mixing error. Clinical manifestations were those of decreased egg production, increased mortality, and aggressive behavior [2]. Gross lesions were those of accumulation of fluid within the pericardial sac and a friable, normal size and color liver. Histologically, lesions were those of a degenerative cardiomyopathy and liver lesions associated with heart failure.

Gamebird Medicine and Management, First Edition. Edited by Teresa Y. Morishita and Robert E. Porter, Jr.
© 2023 John Wiley & Sons, Inc. Published 2023 by John Wiley & Sons, Inc.

Diagnosis is made by selenium analysis of suspect feed, liver, and kidney of affected birds with comparison to normal selenium levels of unaffected animals.

14.3 Other Toxicants

The following toxicants are those to which gamebirds may be exposed but as yet have not been reported in the current literature.

Sulfonamides are a class of antibiotics that have caused toxicity in avian species. Sulfaquinoxaline, sulfadimethoxine, and sulfamethazine are the specific sulfonamides used most commonly. Sulfonamides are used to treat many bacterial infections. The toxic level for these antibiotics is close to the therapeutic level. Published manuscripts on sulfonamide toxicity in poultry are rare. A 20-week-old leghorn flock of pullets experienced toxicosis with sulfaquinoxaline when it was administered through feed [5]. A large mortality had occurred and lesions were those of hemorrhage and bone marrow pallor. Experiments were then performed to duplicate the clinical case. Lesions in the experiment paralleled those of the clinical case. Levels of sulfaquinoxaline in the liver and kidneys were 1.6 ppm for the experimental toxicosis. Diagnosis of sulfonamide toxicity is made by a history of treatment with this antibiotic, gross and microscopic lesions as well as sulfonamide levels within the liver and kidneys.

Although monensin, an ionophore and a commonly used coccidiostat, has caused toxicosis in poultry, there is no citation of it occurring naturally or accidentally in gamebirds. In an attempt to illustrate what would happen if it occurred in gamebirds, a feed mixing error occurred in a broiler breeder flock which may serve as a good example [6]. A broiler breeder flock was fed feed with seven times the approved level of the ionophore monensin. Clinical presentation was that of increased mortality, feed refusal, decreased water consumption, inability to move, and paralysis. There were no gross lesions. Microscopically, the heart and skeletal muscle had degeneration with expansion of the interstitium by edema and inflammatory cells. In numerous cases of monensin toxicosis in turkeys, clinical signs have consisted of a dramatic increased mortality and birds that walk with the aid of their wings. There were few if any gross lesions except for pallor of the sternotrachealis muscle and an occasional heart with petechiae. Microscopic lesions are those that have been reported previously. Diagnosis of ionophore toxicosis is made by clinical signs, lesions, and elevated ionophore levels within the feed that caused the illness.

Another feed error-related toxicosis is salt (sodium chloride) poisoning. The sequelae of salt toxicosis vary with the age at which the birds are exposed. For young birds whose kidneys are developing, pulmonary hypertension and ascites result [7]. In older birds, clinical signs consist of wet droppings, increased water consumption with decreased feed consumption. Diagnosis of salt toxicosis is made by clinical signs, history of a recent feed change, and sodium analysis of feed being consumed during the illness. Often, tasting of the feed can detect increased levels of salt. Normally, poultry feed should be bland to the human taste while if it is salty, at the level of commercially available potato chips, the feed has too much salt.

Coal tar toxicosis could occur in areas where trap or skeet shooting existed for a prolonged period of time. It used to be that clay pigeons, used for these sports, were made of coal tar which was extremely toxic to swine [8]. In an attempt to produce more environmentally friendly clay pigeons, manufacturers have moved to using more nontoxic components and those which are biodegradable [9]. When ducklings were fed different levels of ground clay pigeons, toxicity developed at week 3 with hydropericardium, ascites, and fibrin around the spleen and liver. Microscopically, there was proliferation of bile duct epithelium and necrotic hepatocytes. Although not mentioned in the publication, mortality rate would have increased [8]. Diagnosis of coal tar toxicosis is made by a history of exposure, increased mortality, and gross and microscopic lesions.

Ammonia toxicosis, although not cited in the literature, could occur naturally in gamebirds. Based on gamebird management, this toxicosis would most likely occur in closed buildings, typically considered to be the brooder, where ventilation may be at low levels. Avian manure contains nitrogenous waste material from the digestive tract and uric acid excreted from the kidney. With the addition of litter moisture and litter bacteria, uric acid breaks down into ammonia [10]. Ammonia gas, when it dissolves in the moisture of mucous membranes, becomes ammonium hydroxide which is caustic to tissues. If ammonia gas is in high concentrations, birds could be blinded due to ulceration of the cornea. Birds will sit with their eyes closed and not move. If they cannot find food or water, they will die. If they can find food and water, like birds that are kept in cages, they can eventually survive, and the corneal ulcers will heal if ammonia levels are controlled. Also, if ammonia concentrations are high enough, it can cause paralysis of the cilia lining the trachea and may predispose the birds to respiratory infections [10]. Diagnosis of ammonia toxicity is made based on clinical history of ammonia exposure and gross lesions. No treatments are available other than removing the ammonia gas and keeping birds close to feed and water.

Aflatoxicosis is caused by aflatoxin which is produced by the fungi *Aspergillus favus* and *A. parasiticus*. Exposure to aflatoxins may result in immunosuppression, anemia, hemorrhage, liver damage with bile duct hyperplasia, and increased mortality [11]. There is a variation in species susceptibility: ducklings, goslings, and turkey poults are the most susceptible to aflatoxicosis [12]. Diagnosis of aflatoxicosis is made by clinical signs, gross and microscopic lesions and finding the appropriate mycotoxin in the feed that caused the illness. Often, the feed that caused the illness had been consumed before clinical signs appear. Therefore, it is wise to reserve at least 2 lb of feed from all feed batches or deliveries. Then, if issues arise, samples of previous feed batches can be analyzed. There is no treatment for aflatoxicosis except to remove the offending feed and provide new feed. There are ingredients that can be added to feed in an attempt to reduce or control aflatoxin in feeds. The reader is referred to Chapter 8 of this book for a discussion on mycotoxin control in feed.

There are many other toxicants that have caused illness in poultry. The purpose of this chapter is not to discuss all of those items. The reader is referred to the Toxins and Poisons chapter in the latest edition of the Avian Diseases text [13].

References

1 Lewis, L.A. and Schweitzer, S.H. (2000). Lead poisoning in a norther bobwhite in Georgia. *J. Wildl. Dis.* 36 (1): 180–183.

2 Latshaw, J.D., Morishita, T.Y., Sarver, C.F. et al. (2004). Selenium toxicity in breeding ring-necked pheasants (*Phasianus colchicus*). *Avian Dis.* 48 (4): 935–939.

3 Wheeler, W.E. and Gates, R.J. (1999). Spatial and temporal variation in lead levels related to body condition in Mississippi valley population of Canada geese. *J. Wildl. Dis.* 35 (2): 178–186.

4 Hoffman, D.J. (2002). Role of selenium toxicity and oxidative stress in aquatic birds. *Aquatic Toxicol.* 57 (1–2): 11–26.

5 Daft, B.M., Bickford, A.A., and Hammarlund, M.A. (1989). Experimental and field sulfaquinoxaline toxicosis in leghorn chickens. *Avian Dis.* 33 (1): 30–34.

6 Guillermo, Z., Anderson, D.A., Davis, J.F. et al. (2011). Acute monensin toxicosis in broiler breeder chickens. *Avian Dis.* 55 (3): 516–521.

7 Julian, R.J., Caston, L.J., and Leeson, S. (1992). The effect of dietary sodium on right ventricular failure-induced ascites, gain and fat deposition in meat-type chickens. *Can. Vet. J. Sci. Res.* 56 (3): 214–219.

8 Carlton, W.W. (1966). Experimental coal tar poisoning in white Pekin duck. *Avian Dis.* 10 (4): 484–502.

9 Buckenmeyer, J. (2011). Composition of clay pigeons. www.sportsrec.com/composition-clay-pigeons-8283200.html (accessed February 2022).

10 Carlile, F.S. (1984). Ammonia in poultry houses: a literature review. *Worlds Poult. Sci. J.* 40 (2): 99–113.

11 Diaz, G.J., Calabrese, E., and Blain, R. (2008). Aflatoxicosis in chickens (*Gallus gallus*): an example of hormesis? *Poult. Sci.* 87 (4): 727–732.

12 Dalvi, R.R. (1986). An overview of aflatoxicosis of poultry: its characteristics, prevention, and reduction. *Vet. Res. Commun.* 10 (6): 429–443.

13 Fulton, R.M. (2020). Toxins and poisons. In: *Diseases of Poultry* (ed. D.E. Swayne), 1349–1382. Hoboken, NJ: Wiley.

15

Gamebird Necropsy Procedures
Robert E. Porter, Jr

Necropsy of birds in a flock is a standard procedure for gauging overall flock health or accurately identifying the cause of a disease or underlying conditions that could affect production. Selection of birds for this purpose is very important and will affect the necropsy findings. The most obvious reason to conduct necropsies is to determine the cause of death in a flock with high mortality. Alternatively, when investigating respiratory, musculoskeletal or neurologic disease in a flock, one can select live birds with those signs and include birds that have died while showing those clinical signs. One should avoid selecting birds that are culled because of injury, poor feathering, undersized or other miscellaneous conditions because in most instances those birds will not provide information on the primary disease in the flock.

Dead birds should be necropsied within 24 hours or less of death because of carcass decomposition at ambient temperature; however, the condition of the carcass may be prolonged if the birds die during cooler temperatures or are refrigerated at 35–38 °F (4 °C) shortly after death.

This chapter will introduce the novice to the steps for opening a carcass and locating the various body systems. Although the necropsy follows a specific order, it is up to the prosector to develop an orderly, stepwise pattern of dissection so that a particular body system or organ is not missed in the process.

15.1 Equipment

A standard set of necropsy tools is shown in Figure 15.1. These tools should be used only for necropsy and the hardware should be disinfected and authoclaved on a regular basis. The prosector should work on a smooth, waterproof surface, preferably a stainless steel table, with adjacent sink and faucet that can be washed and disinfected before and after each use.

Gamebird Medicine and Management, First Edition. Edited by Teresa Y. Morishita and Robert E. Porter, Jr.
© 2023 John Wiley & Sons, Inc. Published 2023 by John Wiley & Sons, Inc.

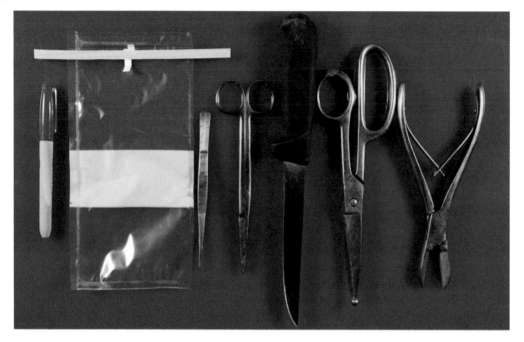

Figure 15.1 The recommended tools for necropsy include water-resistant marker or pen, sterile, sealable sample bags, scissors, forceps, necropsy knife, poultry shears, and bone rongeur.

15.2 Necropsy Procedure

1. Birds may need to be euthanized prior to necropsy. The procedures approved for humane euthanasia of poultry include cervical dislocation, carbon dioxide asphyxiation, intravenous barbiturate injection, and intracranial captive bolt for very large birds. However, barbiturates should not be used for on-farm necropsy or during dressing of hunted birds, or any birds entering the human/pet food chain.

2. Carefully examine the external features of the carcass prior to necropsy. Any abnormal findings arising from external examination of the carcass provide vital clues that the prosector can investigate further.

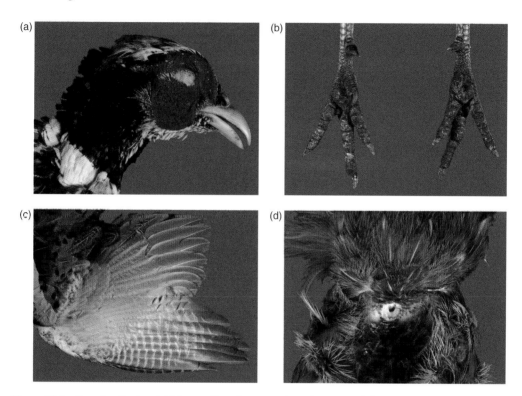

Figure 15.2 Examine the head (a) for swollen sinuses and exudate around the eyelids, nares or mouth. The feet (b) should be clean with symmetric digits and no plantar ulcers. Wing feathers (c) should be assessed for frayed feathers, ectoparasites, and exudate. The vent and adjacent feathers (d) should not have pecking injuries, blood or pasted feces.

3. In a laboratory setting, it is useful to drench the carcass with soap by grasping the neck and immersing the body in soapy water, such as mild dishwashing liquid.

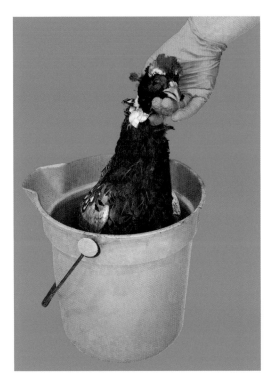

Figure 15.3 A detergent will wet down the feathers and make it easier to cut the skin and expose the body cavity. Do not use a bactericidal detergent, which could interfere with pathogen isolation. Avoid getting detergent into the eyes, mouth or nares of the carcass.

4. Lay the carcass on its dorsum on the dissection table and extend both the legs and neck.

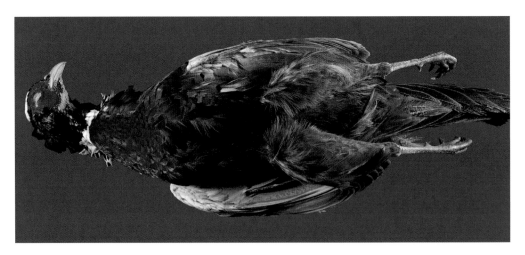

Figure 15.4 The carcass is placed on its back with the neck and legs extended.

5. Make the first skin incision between the legs and body.

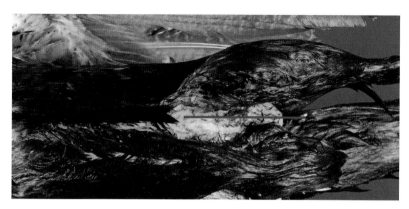

Figure 15.5   Incise the skin between the keel bone/breast muscle and the femur (upper legs) on both sides by following the line shown in red.

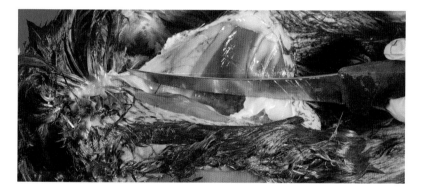

Figure 15.6   After the skin is incised, the thigh and leg muscles will be exposed.

6. Fold the legs laterally to expose the heads of the right and left femurs.

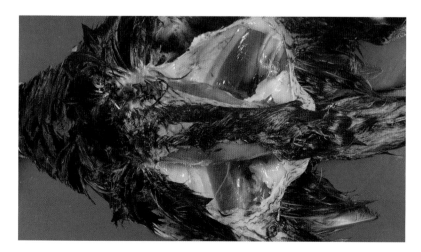

Figure 15.7   Fold the legs laterally (away from the body) to separate (dislocate) the coxofemoral (hip) joints. This will stabilize the carcass on the table and expose the femoral heads and the thigh muscles on the medial aspect of either leg.

7. Remove the skin from the breast muscle.

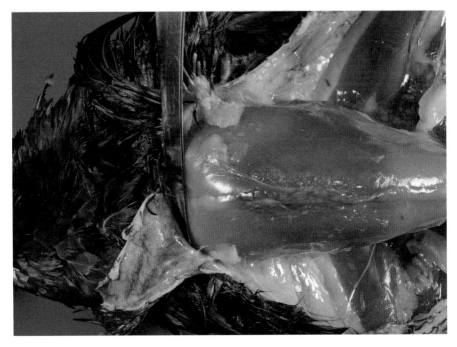

Figure 15.8 Tent the skin near the caudal edge (tip) of the keel bone and peel or cut that skin off the breast muscle, moving toward the neck. Note whether the breast muscle is normal sized or if there is decreased muscle mass. Note the presence or absence of subcutaneous fat.

8. Remove the skin along the neck up to the mandible or jaw to expose the trachea, esophagus and crop.

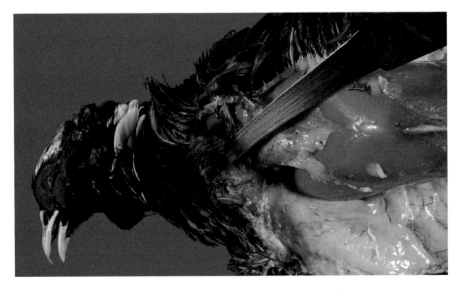

Figure 15.9 Continue to cut skin along the base of the neck up to the mandible or jaw.

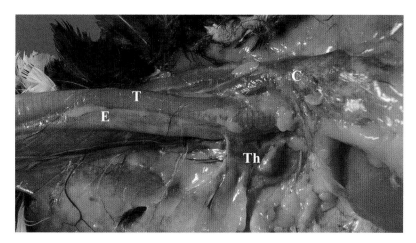

Figure 15.10   The cut along the neck will expose the trachea (T), esophagus (E), crop (C) and, in sexually immature birds (<20 weeks), the thymus (Th).

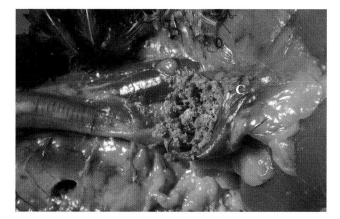

Figure 15.11   Open the crop and note the contents. The crop (C) of a clinically healthy bird will usually contain feed and have a glistening pink surface (mucosa).

9. Incise the body wall along the caudal border of the keel bone. Emaciated birds will have reduced or absent coelomic and subcutaneous fat. If the liver is enlarged, it will extend past the caudal edge of the keel bone. There should not be free fluid or blood in the coelom.

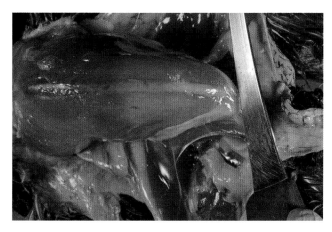

Figure 15.12   Incise the body wall along the caudal border of the keel bone to expose the liver and gizzard.

10. Starting at the caudal edge of the keel bone, cut the mid-aspect of the ribs, moving cranially toward the shoulder joint. This allows one to remove the keel bone and expose the underlying viscera.

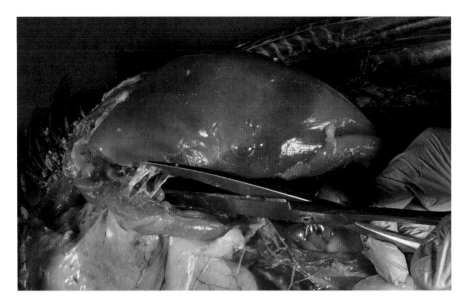

Figure 15.13 Cut across the ribs and breast muscle on both sides and reach the scapulohumeral joints ("armpit").

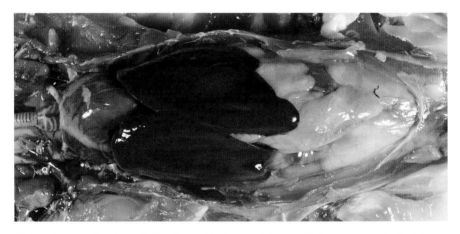

Figure 15.14 After cutting through the ribs and both scapulohumeral joints, remove the keel bone and breast muscle from the carcass to expose the internal viscera.

11. Examine the body (coelomic) cavity after the keel bone is removed. Identify each organ and note the color and shape to establish whether there are any lesions.

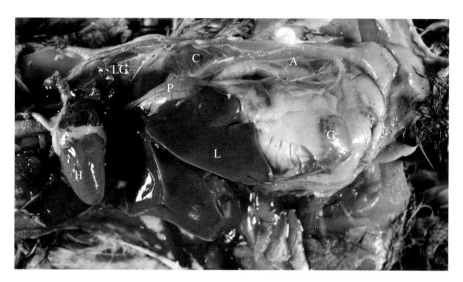

Figure 15.15   In the caudal coelom, observe the abdominal (A) air sacs, which should be clear and free of exudate. The liver (L), proventriculus (P), cecum, and gizzard (G) can be easily viewed at this point of the necropsy. Similarly, in the cranial coelom, observe the caudal thoracic (C) air sacs, heart (H) with pericardial sac, and lung (LG).

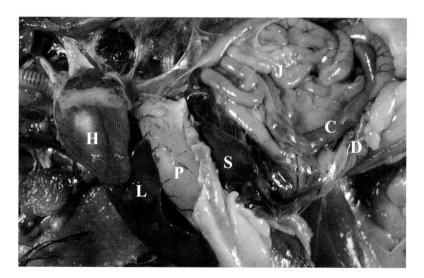

Figure 15.16   Bluntly dissect through the air sacs, grasp the gizzard and exteriorize it toward the bird's right side. This will reveal the ovoid spleen (S). A normal spleen is about one-third the length of the proventriculus (P). The liver (L), heart (H), duodenum (D), jejunum (J), and cecum (C) can now be viewed more extensively.

12. The entire digestive tract can be exteriorized by bluntly dissecting the mesenteric attachments. It is recommended to identify the various segments of the digestive tract using Figure 15.17 as a guide.

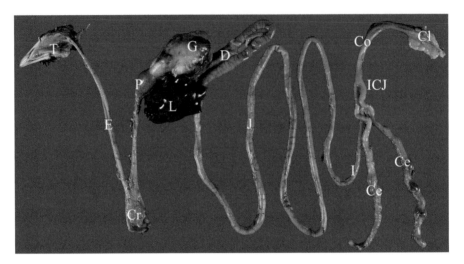

Figure 15.17   Identify the various segments of the digestive tract. (T) Tongue, (E) Esophagus, (Cr) Crop, (P) Proventriculus, (G) Gizzard, (L) Liver, (D) Duodenal loop with pancreas, (J) Jejunum: occupies most of the small intestine and contains the Meckel's diverticulum, (I) Ileum, (ICJ) Ileocecal junction and adjacent cecal tonsils (lymphoid nodules: swellings in proximal ceca that can be observed in young animals), (Ce) Paired ceca, (Co) Colon, (Cl) Cloaca: internal end of digestive tract.

13. Identify the proventriculus (secretory stomach) and gizzard (ventriculus). Open these organs to view the lining and contents.

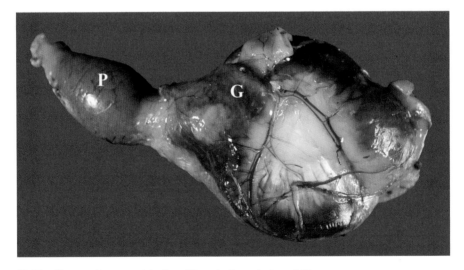

Figure 15.18   Observe the proventriculcus (P) and adjacent gizzard (G).

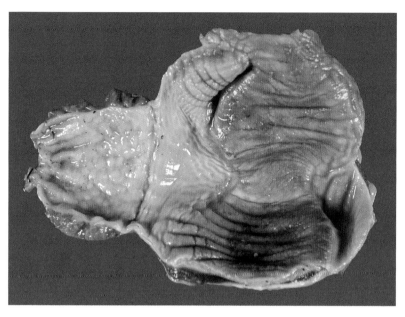

Figure 15.19   Open the proventriculus to observe the pale, nodular mucosal glands. The open gizzard will usually contain feed, plant fibers, and grit in healthy birds. When the digestive contents are removed from the gizzard, one can observe koilin, the thickened, rugose, protective protein-polysaccharide that coats the mucosal surface.

14. Open several sites along the small intestine to observe the contents and the color and character of the intestinal mucosa (walls). One might observe blood, foreign bodies, or nematode (worms) and/or cestode parasites. The mucosal lining can either be scraped for cytologic evaluation or intestinal contents can be collected to examine for nematode ova or coccidial oocysts by fecal flotation.

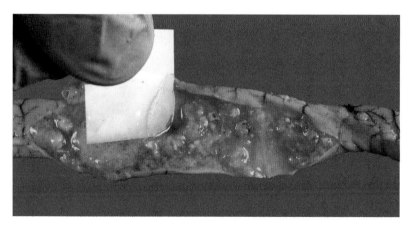

Figure 15.20   In several birds, use glass microscope coverslips to separately scrape the mucosa of three segments of the intestinal tract: duodenum, jejunum, and cecum.

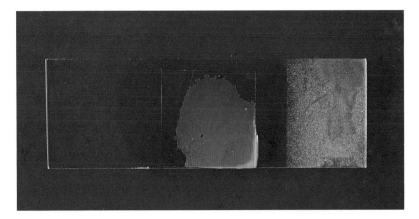

Figure 15.21 Place each coverslip with mucosal scrapings on a glass slide. Examine the slides microscopically on low-power magnification for the presence of blood, protozoa or nematode ova.

15. Cranial coelom ("chest"): Note the four-chambered heart which will be covered by a pericardial sac. Remove the heart and cut off the pericardial sac. The heart can be opened to observe the left and right ventricles.

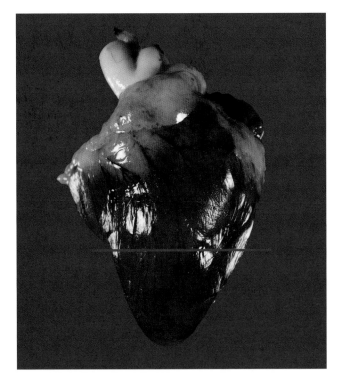

Figure 15.22 The heart has four chambers. Cut transversely across left and right ventricles as shown by the red line.

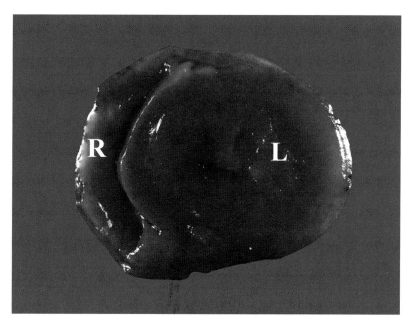

Figure 15.23   A transverse section of the heart shows the thin wall of the right ventricle (R), compared to the thick wall of the left ventricle (L).

16. After removing the liver and digestive tract from the coelom, one can observe the gonads and the paired and trilobed kidneys. Observe the organs for swelling or atrophy.

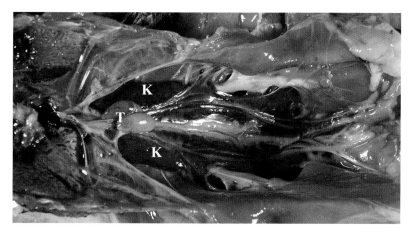

Figure 15.24   The kidneys (K) are partially nestled within the bone of the lumbosacral spine. In the carcass of this male pheasant, the paired testes (T) are present along the cranial aspect of the kidney.

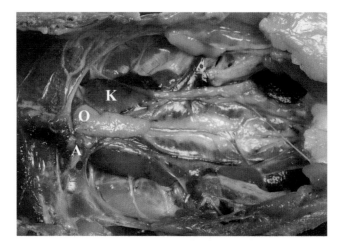

Figure 15.25 Coelomic cavity of a female pheasant. The ovary (O) is unilateral, located at the cranial pole of the left kidney (K), adjacent to the bilateral adrenal glands (A).

17. Using the blunt end of forceps or your finger, gently dissect the lungs from the ribs. A segment of lung can be collected aseptically for microbiological testing.

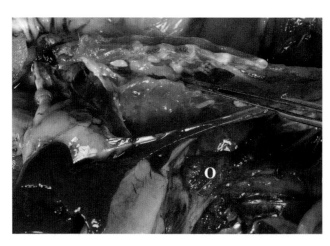

Figure 15.26 Coelomic cavity of a female pheasant. One can detach the lungs for full examination by inserting a forceps between the lungs and ribs. Note the ovary (O) in the female.

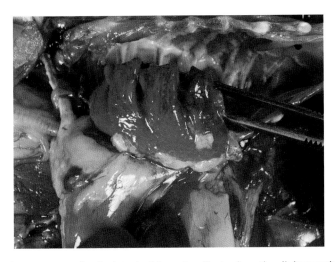

Figure 15.27   The lungs are completely detached from the ribs to show the rib impressions. Normal lungs are pinkish red, dry and spongy.

18. The mouth can be opened by cutting the jaw through the temporomandibular joint. This will expose the tongue, choana, glottis, and trachea. The trachea is an excellent location to collect swabs for bacterial culture, virus isolation, and molecular diagnostics (e.g., avian influenza and Newcastle disease virus testing).

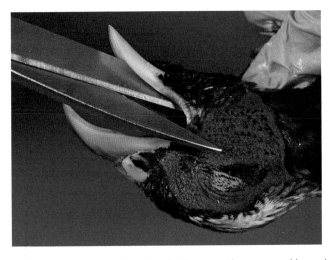

Figure 15.28   Cut through the temporomandibular joint between the upper and lower beak to expose the oral cavity and trachea.

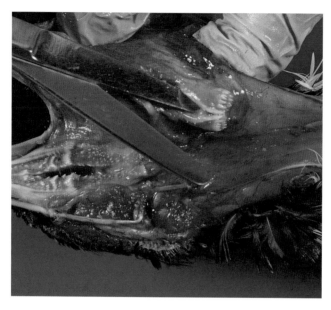

Figure 15.29 The oropharynx has been exposed. Note the tongue, choana (slit on the roof of the mouth that is the channel between the oral and nasal cavities), and the glottis, the opening of the trachea, which has the tip of the scissors inserted into it.

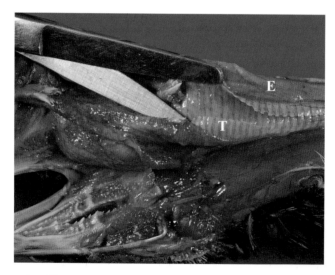

Figure 15.30 The trachea (T) can be opened by cutting through the glottis with scissors. A normal trachea will have a relatively dry, glistening, white lining (mucosa). Note the adjacent esophagus (E).

19. To examine the nasal cavity and infraorbital sinuses (upper respiratory tract), cut transversely across the beak, just caudal to the nares. These spaces should be free of fluid or exudate and can be sampled with swabs for bacterial culture, virus isolation, and molecular diagnostics.

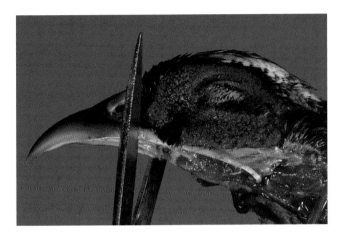

Figure 15.31 Place the shears across the beak and caudal to the nares to make a transverse cut, which will expose the nasal cavity.

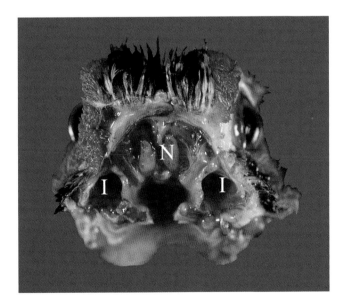

Figure 15.32 The transverse cut of the beak has been completed to reveal the nasal cavity (N) and paired infraorbital sinuses (I). The nasal cavity contains coiled turbinates of bone and cartilage, while the infraorbital sinuses course beneath the globes of the eye. The choanal slit, the connection between the nasal and oral cavities, runs between the infraorbital sinuses.

20. Observe the stifle and hock (intertarsal) joints for any swelling. Excise these joints to expose the joint spaces. Observe the articular cartilage and monitor for exudate, blood or an increased volume of synovial fluid in the joint space.

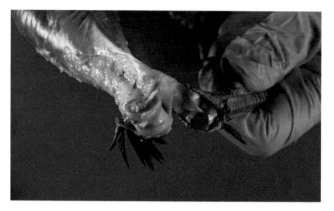

Figure 15.33 Excised intertarsal joint. The joint articular cartilage should be white and glistening and the joint space should not contain blood or other exudate.

21. In some instances, such as in neurologic cases, it will be necessary to examine the brain by removing it from the skull. Using sturdy shears or bone rongeurs, make a series of five skull bone incisions to remove the dorsal aspect of the calvarium (skull cap) and expose the brain as shown in Figures 15.34–15.39. The brain can be used for microbiologic and toxicologic testing, and a portion of the brain can be placed in formalin for microscopic examination.

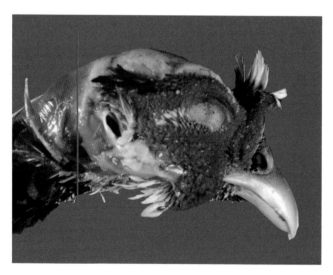

Figure 15.34 The skull can be disarticulated by cutting across the region where the caudal aspect of the skull meets the first cervical vertebrae (red line).

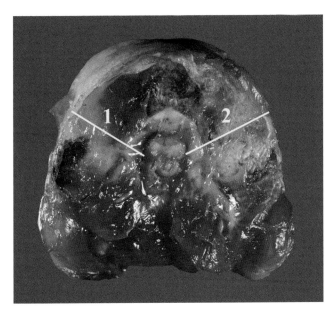

Figure 15.35 Once the skull is disarticulated, remove the skin and skeletal muscle that cover the caudal and dorsal aspects to expose the occipital and parietal bones. Make two angled cuts (yellow lines 1 and 2) from the foramen magnum along the occipital bone to extend to the dorsal parietal bone of the skull.

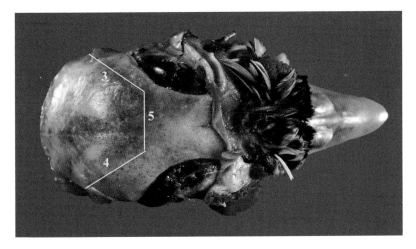

Figure 15.36 Dorsum of pheasant skull with skin removed. Make two caudorostral cuts (yellow lines 3 and 4) in the bone and connect these cuts with a final lateromedial cut (yellow line 5) running along the frontal bone at the rostral aspect of the skull.

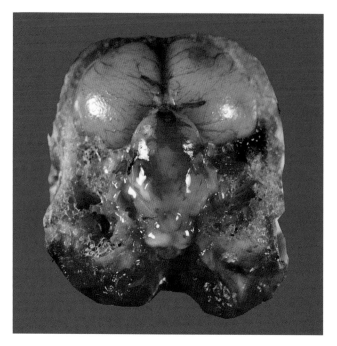

Figure 15.37 Caudal view of pheasant skull with bone removed. Making a series of five cuts to the skull bone creates a boney cap that can be carefully dissected and lifted off to expose the brain.

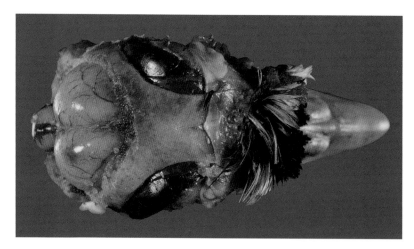

Figure 15.38 Dorsal view of pheasant skull, which has bone removed to expose the brain.

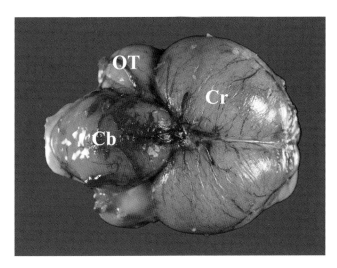

Figure 15.39   Dorsal view of pheasant brain after removal from the skull. The brain can be gently dissected from the base of the skull by incising the cranial nerves and dura mater, then lifting the brain out of the brain case. This view of the dorsal aspect of the exteriorized brain shows the cerebrum (Cr), cerebellum (Cb), and optic tectum (OT).

16

Gamebird Medication Regulations
Lisa A. Tell, Krysta L. Martin, and Tara Marmulak

16.1   Introduction and Overview

Medicating gamebirds is a worldwide practice since they are commercially raised as an alternative avian meat source. Medication use in gamebirds has both rewards and challenges. It prevents or treats illness, thus producing healthier animals and increasing production. However, consumers, regulators, and legislators are increasingly concerned about direct and indirect hazards of drug use and potential impacts on public health. For example, when medications are administered to gamebirds, drug residues can be present within edible products if an insufficient drug withdrawal time (WDT) is not observed. In order to minimize drug residues in food products from gamebirds, it is important that all veterinarians are educated and inform their clients about how to minimize drug residues in the human food chain.

   This chapter provides veterinarians with information that will help them navigate the legal and logistical hoops of medication use in gamebirds, provide resources for finding WDTs for drugs approved for gamebirds, provide guidance for estimating withdrawal intervals when drugs are used in an extra-label manner, and highlight guidance recommendations regarding prudent use of antibiotics. The information presented in this chapter is the authors' interpretation of the legislation, guidelines, and literature; however, the regulatory agencies have the ultimate authority and should be contacted with any questions. For most of the chapter, the resources and legislative/legal information are focused on the United States, but information relative to other worldwide geographic areas is briefly highlighted.

16.2   Definition of a Gamebird

The United States Food and Drug Administration (FDA) has defined gamebirds as "minor species." "Minor species" are all animals, other than humans, that are not one of the major species (horses, dogs, cats, cattle, pigs, turkeys, and chickens) [1]. The United States Department of Agriculture (USDA) considers gamebird species to include wild turkeys, wild geese, wild ducks, grouse, quail, pheasant, and other nondomesticated species of fowl [2]. For the purposes of this chapter, "gamebird" is deemed to refer to those avian species outlined by the USDA that have the potential for their meat, eggs, offal (entrails and internal organs of an animal used as food), byproducts (i.e., feathers), or manure to directly or indirectly enter or influence any portion of the human food chain.

16.3   Drug Administration, On-Label and Extra-Label Drug Use in Gamebirds

Medications can be administered to an individual bird or an entire flock depending on the number of birds needing treatment, disease, and/or overall management practices. The types of medications commonly administered to gamebirds include anticoccidials, anthelmintics, and antibiotics. Similar to any other animal species that are in need of medications, administration routes can be oral or parenteral. Since they require lower labor efforts, oral routes of drug administration for gamebirds commonly include medicated water or feed.

When medicating birds, practitioners should consider their unique gastrointestinal anatomy, physiology, and drug elimination processes that differ from those of mammals [3]. Practitioners treating gamebirds in the US can use FDA-approved veterinary products according to the label or in an extra-label manner. Use of medications according to the label directions is termed "on-label drug use," meaning that all of the drug label specifications (animal species and class, administration route, dose, dosing frequency/interval, indication, limitations) are fulfilled and the FDA-approved WDT is observed. The FDA-approved WDT is the amount of time that must be observed after the last dose is administered before the meat, eggs, or offal intended for human consumption can enter the food chain.

In contrast to on-label drug use, medications for gamebirds in the US can also be prescribed by a veterinarian for "extra-label drug use." Extra-label drug use (ELDU) occurs when the animal species/class, administration route, dose, dosing frequency/interval, duration of treatment, or indication differs from the FDA-approved label (veterinary or human). In the United States, ELDU was legalized with the passage of the Animal Medicinal Drug Use Clarification Act (AMDUCA) of 1994. When FDA-approved products are used in an extra-label manner, a withdrawal "interval" must be estimated based on scientific evidence and must be extended beyond the FDA-approved WDT regardless of the dose, route, or indication. It should be mentioned that the use of prohibited drugs or prohibited extra-label use of specified drug classes (such as fluoroquinolones) is illegal ELDU, unless there is an exception (such as for cephalosporins).

More details on the prohibition of certain drugs and drug classes in food-producing species will be discussed later in this chapter.

16.4   Definition of Residues

The word "residue" is defined in many ways by the literature and worldwide regulatory agencies. For the purposes of this chapter, a residue is deemed to be either the parent compound or metabolite of a parent compound that may accumulate, deposit, or otherwise be stored within the cells, tissues, organs, or edible products (e.g., milk, eggs) of an animal following its use to prevent, control, or treat animal disease or to enhance production [4].

According to the FDA, a residue is any compound that is present in edible tissues of the target animal that results from the use of the sponsored compound, including the sponsored compound, its metabolites, and any other substances formed in or on food because of the sponsored compound's use [5]. The main focus of this chapter is on drug residues; however, residues can also originate from pesticides [6], biotoxins, heavy metals, radionuclides, and so on. In general, residues that accumulate in food products can be problematic from a human health standpoint and should be considered when estimating how long to withhold meat, eggs, and/or offal before they enter the human food chain.

16.4.1 Human Health Hazards of Drug Residues

The human health hazards of drug residues can be classified as direct or indirect impacts [7]. Direct impacts are those that result more immediately and include toxic reactions that impact consumers directly, such as the clenbuterol exposure of 135 people in Spain in 1990 and similarly, 15 people in Italy in 1997 who consumed contaminated beef [8, 9]. Other examples of direct impacts include allergic/hypersensitivity reactions or bone marrow toxicity. Indirect impacts usually have negative effects over a longer time period and include carcinogenicity, mutagenicity, reproductive disorders, immunopathologic effects, and transfer of antibiotic-resistant bacteria to the human population. The US FDA Center for Veterinary Medicine (CVM) assesses the risks of veterinary drugs on public health prior to granting approval [10–13]. However, when drugs are used in an extra-label manner, these risk assessments have not been performed by a regulatory agency. A review of how risk assessment principles can be applied to evaluate the human health risks posed by different classes of drugs used in extra-label manner has been published [11].

16.4.2 Regulatory Monitoring of Drug Residues in Animal Products

Monitoring of drug residues in food-producing animals has been previously described [14]. In addition, regulatory systems for Europe, Australia, Canada, and Japan have also been reviewed [15].

In the United States, the primary mission of the National Residue Program (NRP) is to verify control of animal drug residues, pesticides, environmental contaminants, and any other chemical hazards in or on meat, poultry, or egg products. The principal agencies that work together to achieve the mission of the NRP include the Food Safety and Inspection Service (FSIS), the Environmental Protection Agency (EPA), and the FDA. Through the Federal Food, Drug and Cosmetic Act, the FDA is given the authority to establish drug tolerances (maximum permissible concentrations) that are published in Title 21 of the Code of Federal Regulations (CFR). Title 21 also contains tolerances set by the FDA for heavy metals, industrial chemicals, and pesticides that are no longer approved for use. The EPA is provided a similar responsibility for pesticide tolerances under the Federal Insecticide, Fungicide and Rodenticide Act (FIFRA). The tolerances for pesticides are published in Title 40 of the CFR.

The USDA oversees the FSIS, an agency that is responsible for the analytical testing program for residues in domestic and imported meat, poultry, and egg products. In particular, the NRP Sampling Plan, known as the Blue Book, is developed yearly and made publicly available, whereas the Red Book contains NRP drug residue testing results from previous years. Both the Blue and Red Books are available online by linking to their URLs, which are listed in Table 16.1.

Game animals are classified as nonamenable species and undergo voluntary inspection by the FSIS in accordance with the Agriculture Marketing Act [2]. While the NRP Sampling Plan is targeted toward major food-producing species, it can be used as a guide for potential residue testing of edible products derived from gamebirds. An inspector may sample products that, according to their professional judgment, warrant testing and include analysis for approved and unapproved drugs, pesticides, hormones, and environmental contaminants.

In contrast to federally inspected large-scale commercial operations are the mid-size, smaller scale, and individual producers that are involved with local sales. To the authors' knowledge, there is minimal regulatory oversight for these operations; therefore, it is critical that the advising veterinarians take responsibility and educate their clients regarding best practices for avoiding drug residues.

Table 16.1 Web links for online resources that provide veterinary drug and/or gamebird-specific information.

Website	Description	Website address
Drugs @ FDA	FDA's searchable database of approved human drugs	www.accessdata.fda.gov/scripts/cder/daf
Animal Drugs @ FDA	FDA's searchable database of approved animal drugs and tolerances	https://animaldrugsatfda.fda.gov/adafda/views/#/search
Vetgram	FARAD's searchable drug database for food animal drugs and tolerances	www.farad.org/vetgram
Bayer Animal Health[a]	Searchable US compendium of veterinary products database; use charts tab for summarized label and WDT information	https://bayerall.cvpservice.com
Canadian Compendium of Veterinary Products presented by Bio Agri Mix Total Solutions	Searchable Canadian compendium of veterinary products database; use charts tab for summarized label and WDT information	www.bioagrimix.com/compendium
Drugs.com	Searchable database of veterinary drugs; can search by animal groups; also lists Canadian veterinary drugs	www.drugs.com/vet
CABI's Animal Health and Production Compendium	List of international animal drug databases	www.cabi.org/ahpc/more-resources/drug-databases
Australian Pesticides and Veterinary Medicines Authority	Pubcris is a searchable database of registered pesticides and veterinary drugs	https://portal.apvma.gov.au/pubcris
National Office of Animal Health	UK site with searchable drug compendium of approved drugs	www.noahcompendium.co.uk/Compendium/Overview
Health Products Regulatory Authority	Searchable compendium of approved drugs in Ireland	www.hpra.ie
European Medicines Agency Database	Public database providing online access to information about human and veterinary medicines registered in different Member States of the European Union	www.eudrapharm.eu/eudrapharm
USDA Foreign Agricultural Service	Veterinary drug and pesticide tolerance and MRL searchable database	www.fas.usda.gov/maximum-residue-limits-mrl-database
FAO/WHO Food Standards Codex Alimentarius	Definitions of terms used in discussing veterinary drug residues in food animals	www.fao.org/fao-who-codexalimentarius/codex-texts/dbs/vetdrugs/glossary/en

(Continued)

Table 16.1 (Continued)

Website	Description	Website address
Joint FAO/WHO Expert Committee on Food Additives (JECFA)	Description of JECFA and links to publications	www.fao.org/food/food-safety-qualityscientific-advice/jecfa/en/
JECFA "Residues of some veterinary drugs in foods and animals"	Searchable database of maximum residue levels for veterinary drugs as recommended by JECFA that includes pharmacokinetic data summaries	www.fao.org/food/food-safety-quality/scientific-advice/jecfa/jecfa-vetdrugs/en
Codex Alimentarius international food standards	Homepage for Codex Alimentarius	www.fao.org/fao-who-codexalimentarius/about-codex/en
European Medicines Agency European Public MRL Assessment Report	Summary report on the established MRL and the data supporting the MRL	www.ema.europa.eu/ema/index.jsp?curl=pages/medicines/landing/vet_mrl_search.jsp&mid=WC0b01ac058008d7ad
USDA/FSIS science chemistry page	Includes FSIS sampling plan (Blue Book) and results (Red Book)	www.fsis.usda.gov/wps/portal/fsis/topics/data-collection-and-reports/chemistry/residue-chemistry
USDA Food Safety and Inspection Service (FSIS)	Homepage with contact information and links to resources	www.fsis.usda.gov
FDA Center for Veterinary Medicine	Homepage with contact information and links to resources	www.fda.gov/about-fda/fda-organization/center-veterinary-medicine
AVMA: Animal Medicinal Drug Use Clarification Act (AMDUCA)	Reviews components of AMDUCA and includes list of prohibited drugs	www.avma.org/KB/Resources/Reference/Pages/AMDUCA.aspx
AVMA: VCPR Reference Guide	AVMA's definition of a valid VCPR	www.avma.org/KB/Resources/Reference/Pages/VCPR.aspx
FDA-CVM Compliance Policy Guide	Extra-label use of medicated feeds for minor species	www.fda.gov/regulatory-information/search-fda-guidance-documents/cpg-sec-615115-extralabel-use-medicated-feeds-minor-species
FARAD	Restricted and prohibited drugs in food animals	www.farad.org/prohibited-and-restricted-drugs.html
FARAD regulatory information	Details of the published law on compounding and AMDUCA	www.farad.org/amduca-law.html
FARAD species and topics pages	FARAD website pages that cover species related information and topics related to drug use in food animals.	www.usfarad.org
FARAD	Site where ELDU withdrawal requests may be made online and other resources for food animal veterinarians	http://farad.org

Resource	Description	URL
Canadian gFARAD	Canadian program providing withdrawal recommendations following extra-label drug use	https://cgfarad.usask.ca/index.php
National Pesticide Information Center	NPIC provides objective, science-based information about pesticides and pesticide-related topics	http://npic.orst.edu
US Environmental Protection Agency (EPA)	Home page for EPA; pesticide information	www.epa.gov
Centers for Disease Control and Prevention	CDC's Food Safety Program	www.cdc.gov/vitalsigns/food-safety.html
Minor Use Animal Drug Program (MUADP)	Searchable database for drugs approved in minor food animal species. MUADP project requests can be submitted via this website	www.nrsp7.org
American Association of Veterinary Laboratory Diagnosticians	Listing of AAVLD labs in USA by state	www.aavld.org/accredited-labs
US Food and Drug Administration: Animal & Veterinary. *CVM Guidance for Industry #152*	Appendix A identifies antibiotics deemed medically important by FDA and affected by Guidance #213	www.fda.gov/downloads/AnimalVeterinary/GuidanceComplianceEnforcement/GuidanceforIndustry/UCM052519.pdf
Australian Pesticides and Veterinary Medicines Authority Food safety studies for veterinary drugs used in food-producing animals	Guideline describing the food safety study design to determine maximum residue limits and withholding periods; contains sections specific to poultry	https://apvma.gov.au/node/746
FARAD Digests	FARAD digests are publications providing guidance specific to drug use in food-producing animals. A digest on drug use in wildlife, including game birds, is available through this URL	www.farad.org/publications/digests.asp

a) An account is required to access this database.

16.5 Legislation, Regulations, and Programs Related to Drug Use and Drug Residues

16.5.1 Minor Use/Minor Species (MUMs) Animal Health Act

The MUMs Animal Health Act was passed in 2004. This legislation added new options for approving limited-use drugs and provided a new mechanism to legally market some unapproved products. The intention of this legislation was to increase the number of FDA approvals for minor food animal species, such as gamebirds, and to provide sponsors with incentives to seek label claims for veterinary products that would have "minor uses" in major species of animals. "Minor use" is determined by frequency of use and geography. More specifically, minor use means that a drug can be used in a major species for an indication that occurs infrequently and in a small number of animals, or in a limited geographical area and in only a small number of animals annually.

The MUMs Animal Health Act modifies the Federal Food, Drug and Cosmetic Act to include conditional approval, designation, and indexing for veterinary drugs used in minor animal species [16]. Conditional approval and designation provide incentives to drug sponsors with the ultimate goal of drug approval. Drugs that are conditionally approved have shown a reasonable expectation of effectiveness, but the sponsor is granted up to 5 years to provide all the necessary data proving effectiveness. Conditionally approved drugs cannot be used in an extra-label manner. Designation provides incentives for approvals, including grants to support the studies required for approval, and up to 7 years' exclusive marketing rights by the sponsor. MUMs legislation also allows for medications to be categorized as "indexed" drugs. Indexed drugs have not undergone a formal drug approval process, but the designation allows drug companies to market and sell these medications for selected populations. Indexing is intended for drug treatment of diagnosed conditions in minor nonfood-producing animal species, specifically targeting laboratory animals and zoological collection specimens. The purpose of indexing is to make products available that cannot meet requirements of the drug approval process as a result of a limited animal population and a wide variety of species. Indexed drugs may not be legally used in an extra-label manner in food-producing animals. More details regarding MUMS legislation have been previously described [17].

16.5.2 Animal Medicinal Drug Use Clarification Act (AMDUCA) 1994

The AMDUCA 1994 made ELDU of FDA-approved medications by veterinarians in the United States legal. "Extra-label use" is defined in the CFR as: "Actual use or intended use of a drug in an animal in a manner that is not in accordance with the approved labeling. This includes, but is not limited to, use in species not listed in the labeling, use for indications (disease and other conditions) not listed in the labeling, use at dosage levels, frequencies, or routes of administration other than those stated in the labeling, and deviation from labeled withdrawal time based on these different uses" [18].

The requirements of the AMDUCA are listed in Table 16.2. Key points within the AMDUCA include the following. (i) ELDU can only occur on the order of a veterinarian within the context of a veterinarian–client–patient relationship (VCPR); (ii) ELDU must be limited to a therapeutic purpose to treat a sick or dying animal; (iii) ELDU in food-producing animals requires that no violative residues occur; (iv) certain compounds are prohibited from ELDU. The American Veterinary Medical Association (AVMA) has defined what constitutes a legal VCPR and the website address for this definition is included in Table 16.1. The AMDUCA stipulates that ELDU only

Table 16.2   Requirements of the Animal Medicinal Drug Use Clarification Act (AMDUCA) 1994.

Requirement	Explanation
Therapeutic purpose	Extra-label drug use can only occur for therapeutic purposes when an animal's health is suffering or threatened. Extra-label drug use for reproductive purposes, growth promotion, and efficiency is not allowable under AMDUCA
No effective labeled drugs	ELDU should not occur unless FDA-approved drugs as labeled are clinically ineffective for their intended use
VCPR	A valid veterinarian–client–patient relationship (VCPR) must exist. Table 16.1 includes the website address for AVMA's definition of a valid VCPR
Veterinarian' supervision	ELDU is permitted only under the supervision of a veterinarian. This includes the extra-label use of over-the-counter medications. Also, any over-the-counter product that is compounded in veterinary medicine is deemed a prescription drug and may only be used under veterinarian supervision
FDA-approved drugs	ELDU is permitted using only FDA-approved animal and human drugs. When using medications extra-label, medications approved for other food animal species should be used before medications approved only for nonfood animal species which should be used preferentially over drugs approved for humans only. Using bulk chemical or active pharmaceutical ingredient (API) is not allowed as they are not FDA approved
Not in feed	Extra-label use of an approved animal drug or human drug or feed additive in or on an animal feed is prohibited. Also, using combinations of medicated feed or feed additives not approved to be used together is not considered AMDUCA compliant. Extra-label drug use in water is permitted
No residues	ELDU must not result in violative residues
Additional food animal requirements	Make a careful diagnosis and evaluation of the conditions for which the drug is to be used. Establish a substantially extended withdrawal period supported by scientific information. Institute procedures to assure that the identity of the treated animal or animals is carefully maintained. If the individual animal cannot be identified for the extended withdrawal interval, then the extended withdrawal interval must be applied to the entire group. Take appropriate measures to assure that assigned timeframes for withdrawal are met and no illegal drug residues occur in any food-producing animal subjected to extra-label treatment

Source: Based on [18].

applies to FDA-approved human and veterinary medications. It does not legalize the extra-label use of EPA-regulated pesticides or USDA-regulated biologics.

As all FDA-approved veterinary products are assigned either a new animal drug application (NADA) or an abbreviated new animal drug applications (ANADA) number, if a veterinary product does not have a NADA or ANADA number, its use is most likely not AMDUCA compliant in an extra-label manner. In addition, drugs that are approved for humans have new drug application (NDA) numbers for pioneer drugs or abbreviated new drug application (ANDA) numbers for generic medications. Approval status of both animal and human drugs can be found on the FDA-CVM and FDA websites respectively. The website URLs are included in Table 16.1.

16.5.3 Compliance Policy Guide (CPG) 615.115 Extra-Label Use of Medicated Feeds for Minor Species

Extra-label use of medicated feed or drugs used extra-label in or on feed are prohibited by the AMD-UCA. However, for some minor food-producing species, medicating via the feed might be essential. Therefore, the CPG 615.115 was created to allow veterinarians to prescribe FDA-approved medicated feeds to be fed to minor food-producing animals in an extra-label manner. In 2016, the CPG was updated to include specifics on veterinary feed directives (VFDs) and to allow the nutritional content to be adjusted [19]. For the "minor" poultry species, such as pheasants and quail, medicated feeds that are approved for major species (turkeys or chickens) can be used under the supervision of a veterinarian. The CPG does not make it legal to use medicated feed for these minor poultry species. However, it does give field investigators "regulatory discretion," and if all the CPG requirements are followed correctly, field investigators do not have to take any action against the producer or veterinarian.

When medicated feeds are being used under the auspices of the CPG, the other requirements of the AMDUCA need to be met. Additional stipulations for the ELDU of medicated feed in minor species include the following.

1. A written recommendation that includes the medical rationale and dated within 3 months prior to use is required. The producer and veterinarian must keep copies of the written recommendation that must be available in the case of a FDA inspection.
2. A medicated feed to be used in a minor food-producing species must be approved in a similar food-producing species. Only medicated feeds approved for use in avian species can be used extra-label in a minor poultry species.
3. Extra-label use is limited to farmed or confined minor species. Treatment of unconfined wildlife is not permitted under the CPG.

16.6 Prohibited Drugs

In order to protect public health, the FDA has established a list of drugs or drug classes that are either completely prohibited or prohibited from ELDU in food-producing animals. Other countries have their own lists of drugs of high regulatory concern. Table 16.3 lists the veterinary products that the FDA-CVM prohibits from use in avian food-producing animals or drug classes that the FDA-CVM prohibits from extra-label use in the United States. A complete listing of the FDA-CVM prohibited drugs for all food-producing animal species can be found at website links referenced in Table 16.1. It is advised that the FDA-prohibited drug list be checked on a regular basis for updates as it is subject to change. If any of these prohibited drugs are mistakenly used, then the affected animal and its byproducts (i.e., eggs or poultry litter used as feed for other food-producing animals) are not allowed to enter the human food chain.

16.6.1 Prohibition of Extra-Label Drug Use of Cephalosporins in Major Food-Producing Animals

On 5 April 2012, prohibition of the extra-label use of cephalosporins in major food-producing animal species, including turkeys, took effect. The FDA enacted this prohibition because of concerns for increasing bacterial resistance to cephalosporins, many of which are used for treating humans. At the time that this chapter was written, there was only one cephalosporin

Table 16.3   FDA-Center for Veterinary Medicine prohibited drugs that have relevance to avian food-producing species; many have reported adverse reaction(s) in humans.

Prohibited drug	Adverse reaction(s) reported in humans
Chloramphenicol	Idiosyncratic, nondose-dependent, irreversible, aplastic anemia
Clenbuterol	B-adrenergic toxicities
Diethylstilbestrol (DES)	Reproductive tract abnormalities and tumors in female offspring, infertility
Nitroimidazoles such as metronidazole	Potential for carcinogenesis
Nitrofurans, including topical applications	Potential for carcinogenesis
Fluoroquinolones	Potential to cause development of resistant human pathogens
Glycopeptides such as vancomycin	Potential to cause development of resistant human pathogens
Gentian violet – prohibited from use in feed	Human food safety has not been assessed
Antivirals (adamantine and neuramidase inhibitors) in chickens, turkeys, and ducks	Potential to cause development of resistant human pathogens
Cephalosporins, not including cephapirin, must be used on-label in cattle, swine, chickens, and turkeys. They may be used extra-label only in the above species to treat a disease indication not labeled	Potential to cause development of resistant human pathogens

Source: Based on [20].

that was approved for poultry, ceftiofur sodium. Ceftiofur sodium is labeled for use in day-old chicks and turkey poults for control of early mortality associated with *Escherichia coli* infections. From a legal standpoint, ceftiofur sodium can only be used in an extra-label manner in the aforementioned species/class for a different indication. In other words, the label dose, administration route, treatment duration, and species (in this case, day-old chicks and turkey poults) must all be on-label. In ovo administration would be deemed prohibited. When this chapter was written, the minor food-producing poultry species (ducks, geese, etc.) were excluded from this ban; thus cephalosporins may continue to be used responsibly in an extra-label manner.

16.6.2   Prohibition of Fluoroquinolones

In the early 1990s, there was a rapid increase in fluoroquinolone-resistant *Campylobacter* spp., a known contributor to foodborne illness in humans, that was associated with increased use of fluoroquinolones in poultry [21]. As a result, the extra-label use of fluoroquinolones was banned in the United States in 1997. At that time, sarafloxacin and enrofloxacin were approved for use in poultry. Even with this prohibition, increased fluoroquinolone-resistant *Campylobacter* spp. in poultry were linked with resistant infections in humans, leading to the voluntary withdrawal of sarafloxacin products in 2001. In 2005, the FDA approval for enrofloxacin was withdrawn [22]. At the time this chapter was written, the use of any fluoroquinolones in US poultry and food-producing gamebird species is prohibited.

16.6.3 Prohibition of Specific Antiviral Medications

In 1999, avian influenza entered the limelight in the United States as a deadly zoonotic disease on a global scale. Given the serious nature of avian influenza infection, the antivirals rimantadine, amantadine, oseltamivir, and zanamivir were prohibited from use in chickens, turkeys, and ducks in the US in order to preserve their effectiveness for treatment of human beings. It has been reported that countries that have previously allowed the use of these medications in poultry have observed development of drug resistance [23, 24].

16.7 Compounding of Medications

Compounding is the term used for combining, mixing, or altering ingredients to create a medication that is tailored to the needs of an individual patient. It involves making a new drug for which safety and efficacy have not been demonstrated with the kind of data that FDA requires for new drug approval. In virtually all cases, the FDA regards compounded drugs as unapproved new drugs [25].

According to the CFR, a veterinarian may consider using a compounded product "when there is no approved new animal or approved new human drug that, when used as labeled or in conformity with criteria established in this part, will, in the available dosage form and concentration, appropriately treat the condition diagnosed" [26].

Given that gamebirds may be deemed food-producing animals, there are specific requirements for legal use of a compounded product [26]. These requirements are listed in Table 16.4.

Using compounded medications is deemed to be ELDU of an approved animal or human drug. As compounding falls under the AMDUCA, the requirements for ELDU are listed in Table 16.2 and compounded medications under the AMDUCA are listed in Table 16.4.

Often, bulk chemicals or active pharmaceutical ingredients (API) are used in commercial compounding. This is not deemed legal under the AMDUCA for food animal species because this chemical is not an FDA-approved drug. Defined in 21 CFR 207.3, "Bulk drug substance means any substance that is represented for use in a drug and that, when used in the manufacturing, processing, or packaging of a drug, becomes an active ingredient or a finished dosage form of the drug, but the term does not include intermediates used in the synthesis of such substances." In other words, by bulk chemical, we mean the drug in powdered chemical form, which is often used for

Table 16.4 Requirements for legal use of compounded products in food-producing animals.

- All requirements for ELDU under AMDUCA are met
- An approved animal drug should be used for compounding before a human drug
- Compounding is performed by the veterinarian or pharmacist within their scope of practice
- Adequate procedures are followed to ensure the safety and effectiveness of the compounded product
- Scale of compounding is in line with the need for the product and is for a particular patient. Compounding in anticipation of receiving prescriptions, except in limited quantities, is illegal. The compounding of large quantities can fall under "manufacturing" and thus the compounded product would be deemed a drug in need of FDA approval. Also, compounding for third parties to resell or selling it at wholesale to another individual or entity for resale is illegal
- All state laws relating to compounding are followed

Table 16.5   Required information to be included in the patient's medical record with extra-label drug use or compounded medication use.

- Identity of the animals, either as individuals or a group
- Animal species
- Number of animals treated
- Condition being treated
- Established name of the drug and active ingredient
- Dosage prescribed or used
- Duration of treatment
- Specified withdrawal, withholding, or discard time(s), if applicable, for meat, eggs, or animal-derived food

Table 16.6   Information to be included on the prescription label with extra-label drug use or compounded medication use.

- Name and address of the prescribing veterinarian
- Established name of the drug or each ingredient
- Any specified directions for use including the class/species or identification of the animal or herd, flock, pen, lot, or other group; dose, frequency, and route of administration; and the duration of therapy
- Any cautionary statements
- The veterinarian's specified withdrawal, withholding, or discard time for meat, eggs, or any other food that might be derived from the treated animal or animals

research purposes and may not be of pharmaceutical grade. Compounding with bulk chemicals can be less expensive than using an FDA-approved medication. However, according to the AMDUCA, ELDU (in this case compounding) is legal for therapeutic purposes only; therefore, cost is not an acceptable reason for compounding.

In order to be AMDUCA compliant, when compounded products or medications are used in an extra-label manner, the information listed in Tables 16.5 and 16.6 needs to be documented in the patient's medical records and on the prescription label respectively. These records must be kept for 2 years and be accessible to FDA inspectors, so that they can estimate the risk to public health.

There can be some liability associated with the use of compounded medications, as they generally do not undergo the same quality assurance testing as commercially manufactured medications. In addition, the AMDUCA requires that there be sufficient scientific data to estimate a withdrawal interval. In general, scientific pharmacokinetic data for compounded medication use in food-producing animals is limited, so estimating a withdrawal interval can be difficult. Recommending a withdrawal interval to the client is the legal responsibility of the veterinarian. It is particularly important that the veterinarian be aware of this, especially if a pharmacy is performing the drug compounding, as the pharmacy may not be aware of all the legal ramifications. If there is insufficient data to estimate a withdrawal interval, then the veterinarian must assure that the animal and its products never enter the human food chain.

It is also important to remember that medications can only be compounded for an individual patient with whom the veterinarian has a valid VCPR.

Overall, the compounding of medications for poultry and other food-producing animals should be rarely used. When treating an animal whose tissues or products have the potential to enter the human food chain, it is important to remember that food safety and public health come first. Additional resources regarding compounding and a link to the AVMA's brochure on veterinary compounding and choosing a compounding pharmacy are listed in Table 16.1.

16.8 FDA-CVM Guidance Documents

In April 2012, the FDA-CVM released the final version of Guidance for Industry (GFI) #209, "The judicious use of medically important antimicrobial drugs in food-producing animals" [27]. This document summarizes the agency's findings which have suggested that food-producing animals that have been treated with antimicrobials affect the bacterial populations of humans who consume them. Based on the interpretations of these findings, the FDA determined that use of antimicrobials that are important for therapeutic use in humans in food-producing animals should be limited to therapies necessary to maintain animal health only. In addition, the FDA determined that there should be veterinary oversight for any use of medically important antimicrobials in food-producing animals to ensure the judicious use of these important medications. Medically important antimicrobial drugs as identified by the FDA are listed in Appendix A of FDA-CVM's Guidance For Industry #152. The web URL for GFI #152 can be found in Table 16.1 of this chapter.

Implemented in 2017, the Guidance for Industry #213, "New animal drugs and new animal drug combination products, administered in or on medicated feed or drinking water of food-producing animals: recommendations for drug sponsors for voluntarily aligning product use conditions with GFI #209" goes further [28]. This document outlines changes that involved the withdrawal of marketed feed or water antibiotics, deemed medically important in the treatment of humans, that were labeled for production purposes, including weight gain and feed efficiency. Any remaining over-the-counter medicated feed or water treatments that contain medically important antimicrobials with therapeutic indications, including treatment, control, and prevention of specific diseases, were reclassified as VFD or prescription drugs. The guidance outlines the steps involved for manufacturers of previously over-the-counter medicated feeds or drinking water products to gain approval for therapeutic claims, making them VFDs or prescription drugs.

A VFD is a written statement issued by a veterinarian with a valid VCPR for the use of a VFD drug or VFD combination drug in or on animal feed. A list of drugs and approved VFD drug combinations can be found on the FARAD website (www.farad.org/vfd-drug-combinations.html). In order for a veterinarian to write for a VFD drug, they must be licensed to practice in the state the animals reside in, have a valid VCPR, and issue the VFD in compliance with the drug's approved labeling and conditions. Extra-label use of VFD drugs is prohibited, with the exception of minor species under CPG 615.115.

In the state of California, Senate Bill 27 (SB 27), which became effective on January 1, 2018, was created to address antimicrobial resistance. It is similar to the federal regulations on judicious use of medically important antimicrobials (MIA) but it extends veterinary oversite of MIA further. For animals being treated in California, all forms of MIA, including oral, injectable, topical, and intramammary, require a prescription from a veterinarian. This means that MIA formulations that are designated as OTC at the federal level are designated as Rx in the state of California. Prescription status for medications impacted by SB27 can be found on VetGram on the FARAD website.

16.9 Considerations for Avoiding Residues in Gamebird Products Intended for Human Consumption

16.9.1 General Recommendations

Some general recommendations to help avoid residues include the following.

- All waterers should be thoroughly rinsed and cleaned once the course of medication is complete.
- All equipment used for mixing and storing medicated feed and feeders should be cleaned once treatment is complete.
- If the label WDT requires it, all birds should be switched to a nonmedicated feed to allow residues to deplete prior to slaughter. Medicated feeds are a common source of drug residues if the proper WDT is not observed.
- Calculations of dosages for medicated water and feeds should be carefully performed and even double-checked by a second party in cases where large numbers of birds are to be treated. A list of conversions commonly used has been previously published [29].
- Bedding litter should be changed after completing treatment as any remaining litter may serve as a source of drug exposure to both birds and humans from feces or dropped feed [30]. This could contribute to antimicrobial resistance and possible residues. Nicarbazin has been shown to be stable in litter for prolonged periods and cause persistent residues in the feces and eggs of hens that are kept on unchanged litter after treatment [31].
- If the units for the WDTs are days, a full 24-hour period per day, beginning from the last treatment/dose, must be observed. For example, if the WDT is 2 days, 48 hours must pass after the last treatment/dose before an animal can be slaughtered.
- Proper records and identification of treated animals must be maintained. Inadequate treatment records or failure to identify treated animals lead to insufficient WDTs and violative residues.
- When using rodenticides, bait stations that are inaccessible to birds should be used and dead rodents should be promptly disposed of.
- Label instructions and WDTs should be followed when using pesticides and insecticides. Consult the EPA website for guidance (Table 16.1).

When using medicated water to treat, there are some factors that may affect treatment efficacy. For example, serum concentrations of medications can vary considerably because of differences in water uptake by individual birds. Factors affecting water intake include environmental temperature, feed quality and amount of feed ingested, species, age, health, and circadian rhythm and accessibility [3, 32, 33]. Table 16.7 lists some factors known to affect water consumption.

Characteristics of the water itself, including hardness and pH, should be evaluated when administering medications in water. Tetracyclines form less soluble complexes if the water is hard, reducing bioavailability in the treated birds. Additionally, many drugs have only a certain pH range at which they are stable for any length of time. Therefore, the pH of the water is also an important consideration when determining a drug regimen.

In order to increase the likelihood of achieving therapeutic dosages, a fresh solution of drug should be prepared daily. The solution should be mixed thoroughly and checked to ensure that the drug goes into and remains in solution.

16.9.2 On-Label Drug Use: The Gold Standard for Minimizing Drug Residues

The ideal scenario for minimizing drug residues in gamebird products is to use an approved product according to the label directions and comply with the label WDT as established by the regulatory

Table 16.7 Factors increasing and decreasing water uptake for birds.

Factors increasing water consumption	Factors decreasing water consumption
Soybean meal diet	High-energy diets
High-fiber diet	Nighttime
High environmental temperature	Sickness
Dawn and dusk	Poor palatability
Age	Decreased feed intake
Electrolytes	
Increased feed intake	

Source: Based on [3].

agency. In the United States, a variety of websites also provide the ability to search for approved products (Table 16.1); however, it is the veterinarian's ultimate responsibility to consult the product information contained on the product label or package insert. US veterinary products that are currently approved for various gamebird species can be found in Table 16.8.

In the US, the Office of New Animal Drug Evaluation (ONADE) within the FDA-CVM is responsible for reviewing and approving NDAs. For a drug to be approved, the drug sponsor must demonstrate that the drug is safe in the intended species and is effective for the indication or disease condition that is being treated using the labeled dose and administration route. The sponsor must also demonstrate that the drug is safe for the person administering it, that use of the drug will not harm the environment, and that the drug can be consistently manufactured to standards of strength and purity. If the drug is to be labeled for food-producing animals, human food safety is also a major component of the approval process. In other words, for the product to gain approval, there must be reasonable certainty of no harm occurring to human health from the ingestion of foodstuffs from food-producing animals that are treated with the drug.

Part of the approval process is to estimate a safe time for which the meat, organs, byproducts, or eggs must be withheld before entering the human food chain. This WDT is dependent on the maximum concentration of the drug or its metabolite allowed in the edible tissue that has the longest elimination. In the US, this is known as tolerance, whereas in Europe and other parts of the world, this concentration is known as the maximum residue limit (MRL). Calculations of tolerances or MRLs have been previously described [34, 35].

When WDTs are established by the FDA, they are calculated so that 99% of the animals are below the tolerance when the drug is used according to label directions. This is based on data provided by the sponsor (i.e., a pharmaceutical company or any other entity applying for drug approval in healthy animals). Keep in mind that animals that are systemically compromised, suffering from liver or renal dysfunction, or a septic illness may take longer to eliminate the drug and require an extended WDT even when label directions are followed. Other countries have their own approval processes that are not detailed in this chapter.

16.9.3 Extra-Label Drug Use: Strategies for Minimizing Drug Residues

In the US, the AMDUCA stipulates that it is the legal responsibility of the prescribing veterinarian to make a withdrawal recommendation based on scientific evidence when drugs are used in an extra-label manner. In addition, ELDU must be assigned a substantially "extended" WDT. This

Table 16.8   FDA-approved products for use in gamebirds (as of September 2020).

Active ingredient	Species approved for	NADA
Amprolium	Pheasants	012–350
	Turkeys	012–350, 013–149, 013–663, 033–165, 130–185, 200–463, 200–488, 200–496, 200–630
Bacitracin methylenedisalicylate	Pheasants	141–137, 046–592
	Quail	141–137, 065–470, 046–592
	Turkeys	141–137, 065–470, 046–592, 141–179[a], 141–194[a], 140–937[a], 141–085[a], 140-919[a]
Bacitracin zinc	Pheasants	046–920, 098–452, 200–223
	Quail	046–920, 098–452, 065–313, 200–223
	Turkeys	046–920, 098–452, 200–223, 141–109[a], 141–181[a]
Bambermycins	Turkeys	141–195[a], 140–955[a], 132–448, 130–185[a], 140–918[a], 044–759
Ceftiofur sodium	Turkeys	140–338, 200–420
Chlortetracycline	Ducks	200–510
	Turkeys	200–510
Chlortetracycline (calcium)	Ducks	048–761
	Turkeys	048–761, 092–286, 048–048, 049–287
Chlortetracycline bisulfate	Turkeys	055–020
Chlortetracycline hydrochloride	Turkeys	065–071, 046–699, 065–440, 065–178, 065–256, 065–486, 138–935, 200–295, 200–236, 200–441
Clopidol	Turkeys	034–393
Diclazuril	Turkeys	140–951, 141–195[a], 141–194[a]
Erythromycin phosphate	Turkeys	035–157
Erythromycin thiocyanate	Turkeys	010–092
Fenbendazole	Turkeys	131–675
Gentamicin sulfate	Turkeys	092–523, 101–862, 200–191, 200–147, 200–468
Halofuginone hydrobromide	Turkeys	140-918[a], 140–919[a], 140–824[a], 130–951
Iodinated casein	Ducks	005–633
Lasalocid sodium	Partridges	096–298
	Chukar	096–298
	Turkeys	096–298, 141–181[a], 141–109[a], 141–179[a]
Monensin sodium	Quail	130–736, 038–878
	Turkeys	130–736, 038–878, 140–937[a] 141–301[a], 140–955[a]
Neomycin sulfate	Turkeys	200–050, 200–130, 200–378, 138–939[a], 011–315
Novobiocin	Ducks	012–375
	Turkeys	012–375
Nystatin	Turkeys	012–680
Oxytetracycline	Turkeys	138–938
Oxytetracycline dihydrate	Turkeys	095–143

(Continued)

Table 16.8   (Continued)

Active ingredient	Species approved for	NADA
Oxytetracycline hydrochloride	Turkeys	138-939[a], 130–435, 038–200, 008–622, 008–769, 008–804, 200–144, 200–146, 200–026, 200–066, 200–247
Penicillin G potassium	Turkeys	200–347, 200–372, 200–103, 200–106, 200–122, 055–060
Proparacaine hydrochloride	Turkeys	009–035
Ractopamine hydrochloride	Turkeys	141–290, 141–301[a]
Salinomycin	Quail	128–686, 200–075
Spectinomycin dihydrochloride pentaydrate	Turkeys	200–127, 040–040
Sulfadimethoxine	Turkeys	031–205, 200–258, 200–251, 200–238, 200–192, 200–165, 200–376, 200–443, 200–030, 200–031
Sulfadimethoxine-ormetoprim	Ducks	040–209
	Partridges	040–209
	Chukar	040–209
	Turkeys	040–209
Sulfamerazine sodium	Turkeys	100–094
Sulfamethazine sodium	Turkeys	122–272, 006–084, 200–434
Sulfaquinoxaline	Turkeys	006–391, 006–677, 006–707, 006–891, 007–087, 100–094
Sulfomyxin	Turkeys	031–944
Tetracycline hydrochloride	Turkeys	065–123, 065–140, 065–410, 065–496, 200–136, 200–234, 200–374, 200–049
Thiabendazole	Pheasants	015–875
Tylosin tartrate	Turkeys	013–076, 200–455, 200–473
Zoalene	Turkeys	011–116, 013–747, 141–085[a]

a) Combination products.

"extended" withdrawal time is referred to as the withdrawal interval or WDI in this chapter. The WDI must be longer than the FDA-approved WDT, regardless of the dose, duration/frequency of treatment, or dosing frequency, even if any of these dosing factors are less than those listed on the FDA-approved label. For example, if a hypothetical drug label dosage is 10 mg/kg, the corresponding FDA-approved WDT is 5 days, and so if the drug is administered in an extra-label manner at 5 mg/kg, then the WDI must be longer than 5 days.

A US program that provides advice regarding on-label and ELDU and provides WDIs based on scientific data is the Food Animal Residue Avoidance and Depletion Program (FARAD). FARAD was previously known as the Food Animal Residue Avoidance Databank, but because the program serves many more functions besides data banking, the program's name was changed in 2011. A similar program exists in Canada (Canadian gFARAD), but it is a separate entity from the US program. Any comments in this chapter regarding FARAD are specific to the US program.

US FARAD is a national, congressionally funded, USDA-administered, cooperative program, with a primary mission to prevent or mitigate illegal residues of drugs, pesticides, and other chemicals in foods of animal origin. FARAD collects, analyzes, and evaluates scientific data to provide withdrawal intervals when drugs are used in an extra-label manner. FARAD also advises on pesticide exposure and accidental contaminations When veterinarians prescribe drugs according to the label or in an extra-label manner, they can contact FARAD for WDTs or WDI recommendations, respectively, via the telephone hotline (1-888-873-2723) or submit withdrawal requests online at www.farad.org. Withdrawal recommendations are provided to the prescribing veterinarian on a case-by-case basis. FARAD does not recommend generation of WDI "lists," as these lists can become outdated as a result of new information in the literature changing a WDI, tolerances being changed, or FDA-approved WDTs being modified.

Strategies and techniques for estimating WDIs when drugs are used in an extra-label manner in livestock have been previously published [36, 37]. Additionally, factors or information that FARAD takes into consideration for estimating a WDI for gamebirds and other food-producing animals when they are treated with veterinary products in an extra-label manner have been previously published [38, 39]. Some of these factors include pharmacokinetic parameters in plasma and tissue/eggs, conditions that might impact drug absorption and elimination, physiological factors or compromised health conditions that impact pharmacokinetics, established US tolerance or foreign approvals and foreign MRL, and analytical testing methods and limits of detection.

16.9.4 General Factors Impacting Pharmacokinetic Parameters and Drug Residues

When recommending a WDI after ELDU or a contamination incident, FARAD takes into account conditions that might impact drug absorption and elimination. Some treatment conditions include dose, duration of treatment, and administration route.

Egg withdrawal recommendations can be difficult to estimate, as the variables involved in residue deposition in eggs have not been fully elucidated. Systemic administration of medications generally results in exposure of the ovary, follicle, and oviduct, potentially leading to egg residues. It has been reported that with some medications, egg white concentrations mirror plasma concentrations, with higher doses resulting in higher residue concentrations [40]. Imaging studies have found that during yolk formation, drugs are incorporated into the yolk through daily layering of yolk material. Consequently, drug exposure in early stages of yolk development results in drug residues in the inner rings of the yolk, while exposure in the later stages of development results in residues in the outer portion of the yolk [41, 42]. This means that even drugs with short elimination times may still cause detectable egg residues for prolonged periods as a result of exposure of early-stage egg yolks [41, 43]. Physical–chemical properties of the drug itself, including lipophilicity, hydrophilicity, protein binding, pKa, drug dose, and treatment length, influence the extent of drug transfer to the yolk or albumin [40, 43].

Two excellent review articles addressing the issues of modeling drug residues in edible poultry tissues and eggs have been published [44, 45] and a literature review of scientific studies with egg and tissue residue data in poultry is also available [46, 47].

16.9.5 Physiological Factors/Compromised Health Conditions Impacting Pharmacokinetic Parameters and Drug Elimination

Drug clearance can be affected by the clinical condition of the patient receiving the treatment. Dehydration might impact how the drug is absorbed, especially if the drug is administered subcutaneously. If the drug has an extended absorption time, then this could lengthen the elimination time. Another important factor to consider when estimating a WDI is the overall function of the slowest organ to eliminate the drug. Most antibiotics are excreted via the kidney so any clinical condition affecting the kidney could also impact drug elimination. For example, renal failure could result in prolonged drug elimination of most antibiotics including beta-lactams. Liver failure affects drugs that require hepatic activation, undergo biotransformation, or are affected by hypoproteinemia (i.e., highly protein-bound drugs). As a result, avian-unique characteristics in drug metabolism and clearance should always be considered [3]. Similar to mammals, gastrointestinal diseases in birds may limit drug absorption because of altered intestinal absorption [3]. Physiologic-based pharmacokinetic models, used to help estimate WDIs, have more commonly been created for chickens [48–54]. One model in chickens for midazolam has been extended to pheasants, quail, and turkeys [48].

16.9.6 Pharmacokinetic Parameters: Drug Residue in Serum, Tissue or Egg – Data from Published Studies

FARAD commonly uses published data (especially time versus concentration data) to calculate pharmacokinetic parameters that are subsequently used for recommending WDIs following ELDU. The principal pharmacokinetic parameters of a veterinary drug that are useful for predicting the concentrations of residues after a drug has been administered have been described [55].

In order for FARAD to deem published data to be useful, the time versus concentration data must derive from live animal studies, all the dosing information must be provided, and the matrix analyzed, that is, serum, plasma, tissue, egg, and so on, must be clearly identified. Tissue or egg concentration data are more helpful than serum or plasma data as they represent the edible products that would be consumed by humans. In addition, plasma or serum data may or may not reflect residue concentrations in the tissues or eggs [36, 56, 57]. In some published studies, authors report that residues were still detectable on the last sampling day, thus FARAD is conservative when estimating a withdrawal recommendation, especially if no tolerance exists. Even if residues were not detected on a sampling day post treatment, FARAD would compare the assay's limit of detection with the tolerance for the drug, species, and matrix (i.e., tissue type, egg component, serum or plasma, etc.). If the assay's limit of detection is higher than the tolerance, then violative residues could still be present in the edible products. According to the AMDUCA, following ELDU in the United States, if there is no approved tolerance, no residues (i.e., the tolerance would be deemed to be 0) should be detected in products intended for human consumption. Therefore, if the analytical method is extremely sensitive, an extended WDI is necessary.

16.9.7 Established Tolerance or MRL

Another factor that FARAD takes into account when recommending a WDI is whether a tolerance has been established for the marker residue and matrix of interest for the bird species that was treated. A marker residue is the residue the concentration of which maintains a known relationship to the concentration of total residue in an edible tissue [58]. When the concentration of the marker residue is below the tolerance in the target tissue, the total residues in all the edible tissues are less than their respective safe concentrations [35].

In certain countries, MRLs are the focus. The USDA Foreign Agricultural Service MRL database is a searchable international database for pesticide and veterinary drug MRLs for various commodities and markets. Website URLs for online resources listing tolerances or MRLs can be found in Table 16.1. The Food and Agriculture Organization (FAO) and World Health Organization (WHO) have a joint program known as the Codex Alimentarius Commission that publishes international food standards and guidance documents. The Codex Committee on Residues of Veterinary Drugs in Foods (CCRVDF) is responsible for establishing MRLs for veterinary drugs in foods and related details. Efforts related to international harmonization of MRLs are of interest to countries participating in trade of food animal products and to pharmaceutical companies that wish to market their products in multiple countries [59].

If a drug is not approved in a species, then a tolerance probably does not exist. If no tolerance exists, any detectable residue would be deemed violative following ELDU. Therefore, the WDI needs to be long enough to allow for residue depletion below the limit of detection for analytical methods used by regulatory authorities. This concept can result in a significantly extended WDI recommendation by FARAD in some cases.

16.9.8 Analytical Testing Method and Limits of Detection

Limits of detection for analytical methods that are used to measure residues are an important consideration when FARAD estimates WDIs, especially when there is no established tolerance. As mentioned previously, the WDI may need to be extended to achieve residue concentrations below the detection capability of the analytical method. The FSIS publishes the results of the NRP on a yearly basis, known as the Red Book, which describes the analytical methods used by FSIS and their limits of detection (Table 16.1).

16.9.9 Foreign Drug Approval Data

In some cases, a drug might lack US FDA approval but be approved in another country. In these circumstances, FARAD may use foreign WDTs as a guide for recommending a WDI after ELDU. However, one should be mindful that the WDT or withdrawal period for the drug with an approved foreign label would be based on an MRL that was established by that country, while there would be no FDA-approved tolerance for the drug in the United States. Therefore, when foreign labels are used to estimate WDI recommendations following ELDU in the US, the WDI must always be conservatively longer to allow the drug residues to deplete below the FSIS analytical methods' limit of detection. Table 16.1 includes a listing of international drug databases that have foreign-approved drug label information, including dose and WDTs.

16.10 Testing for Drug Residues

The analytical methods for detecting drug residues have a wide spectrum of needs when it comes to equipment, personnel expertise, reagents, and so on. Some analytical methods are cost-efficient, do not require highly skilled personnel, have simple equipment needs, and offer advantages of rapid testing. The opposite end of the spectrum includes sophisticated expensive techniques that are labor and equipment intensive. Sample preparation and drug residue analysis in poultry products have been previously described [60].

If a practitioner or producer/owner wants to confirm that gamebird products (i.e., meat or eggs) are at or below the tolerance, they can consider submitting a limited number of flock-representative birds for drug residue testing. Age range, disease status, and gender representation are just a few things to consider when choosing birds to be representative of the flock. Samples or carcasses can be submitted to a commercial laboratory for residue testing. Another option for sample submission would be a state veterinary diagnostic laboratory. The website URLs for state veterinary laboratories in the United States are listed under AAVLD in Table 16.1.

16.11   Pharmacovigilance: Guidelines for Prudent Antibiotic Drug Use when Medicating Gamebirds

It is of the utmost importance for veterinarians to use careful consideration when selecting antimicrobial therapy for gamebirds because of ongoing concerns regarding antimicrobial use in food-producing animals, the potential for microbial resistance, and growing concerns for protecting human public health. In some cases, especially with extremely resistant organisms, a veterinarian might have to advise whether or not treatment is appropriate or if euthanasia should be considered. This is especially important in households with immunocompromised individuals. In general, prolonged use of antimicrobials in a population should be avoided to prevent the formation of antimicrobial-resistant reservoirs within the birds' normal bacterial flora.

When choosing an antibiotic, one with a narrow spectrum should be selected over a broad-spectrum agent when possible. Use of a broad-spectrum antibiotic can put selective pressure on nontarget bacteria, thus increasing the likelihood of the development of resistance.

Guidelines for prudent antimicrobial use when treating game birds include the following.

1. All antimicrobials (including over-the-counter medications) should be used under the supervision of a veterinarian.
2. Good husbandry practices, including good hygiene, preventive strategies such as vaccination, probiotics, nutrition [61], and routine health monitoring, should be used to reduce the need for antimicrobials.
3. Extra-label use of antimicrobials should be the exception, not the rule, and should only be performed under the supervision of a veterinarian and in compliance with stipulations set forth by the AMDUCA.
4. Antimicrobial therapy should be administered over as short a treatment period as possible at therapeutic doses to ill or at-risk birds only.
5. Culture and sensitivity results should be used when possible to guide antimicrobial selection.
6. Records should be kept of all antimicrobial administration and may be used to evaluate efficacy and treatment protocols.
7. Immunocompetent statuses of humans in direct or indirect contact with the medicated avian patient should be taken into account, especially when targeting highly resistant organisms. In some cases, if immunocompromised humans will be in contact with the bird, a decision as to whether or not to treat the bird may be necessary. In some cases, euthanasia of the bird might need to be discussed.

Antimicrobials that are deemed less important for treating serious infections in humans should be used before more important antimicrobials are used. Canada Health has classified antimicrobials based on their importance for use in humans and the necessity of preserving their effectiveness [62]. These rankings are listed in Table 16.9.

An excellent source of doses for various medications for poultry, including references to research published in the literature, is available in the avian chapter of the *Exotic Animal Formulary*. It includes individual doses, with references to research or anecdotal information, for over 50 antimicrobial medications for ring-necked pheasants, chickens, waterfowl, poultry, Galliformes, quail, and peafowl [63].

Table 16.9   Health Canada's categorization of antimicrobial drugs based on importance in human medicine.

Category I: Very high importance

These antimicrobials are deemed to be of very high importance in human medicine as they meet the criteria of being essential for the treatment of serious bacterial infections and there is limited or no availability of alternative antimicrobials for effective treatment in case of emergence of resistance to these agents. Examples include:

Carbapenems

Cephalosporins – 3rd and 4th generation

Fluoroquinolones

Glycopeptides

Glycylcyclines

Ketolides

Lipopeptides

Monobactams

Nitroimidazoles (metronidazole)

Oxazolidinones

Penicillin-beta-lactamase inhibitor combinations

Polymyxins (colistin)

Therapeutic agents for tuberculosis (e.g., ethambutol, isoniazid, pyrazinamide and rifampin)

Category II: High importance

Antimicrobials in this category consist of those that can be used to treat a variety of infections, including serious infections, and for which alternatives are generally available. Bacteria that are resistant to drugs of this category are generally susceptible to Category I drugs, which could be used as alternatives. Examples include:

Aminoglycosides (except topical agents)

Cephalosporins – 1st and 2nd generations (including cephamycins)

Fusidic acid

Lincosamides

Macrolides

Penicillins

Quinolones (except fluoroquinolones)

Streptogramins

Trimethoprim/sulfamethoxazole

Category III: Medium importance

Antimicrobials in this category are used for treatment of bacterial infections for which alternatives are generally available. Infections caused by bacteria that are resistant to these drugs can, in general, be treated by Category II or I antimicrobials. Examples include:

Aminocyclitols

Aminoglycosides (topical agents)

Bacitracins

Fosfomycin

Nitrofurans

(Continued)

Table 16.9   (Continued)

Phenicols

Sulfonamides

Tetracyclines

Trimethoprim

Category IV: Low importance

Antimicrobials in this category are currently not used in human medicine. Examples include:

Flavophospholipols

Ionophores

Source: Health Canada [62].

16.12   Conclusion

Veterinarians treating individual birds or gamebird flocks have the challenging responsibility of protecting human public health while simultaneously ensuring avian health. It was the intent of the authors of this chapter to provide a comprehensive review of medication use and approaches for judicious and responsible drug use, because veterinarians are professionals who are well suited to the task of educating owners and producers. To aid in this endeavor, readers were provided with information regarding US legislation affecting medication use in gamebirds, guidance recommendations regarding legal and prudent on-label and ELDU, and approaches for establishing withdrawal intervals when drugs are used in an extra-label manner. In addition, resources listing WDTs for approved drugs in gamebird species in the United States and other countries were provided. It is hoped that, after reading this chapter, veterinarians will be more informed about how to better serve their clients and patients while still helping to protect the human food chain.

References

1 FDA (2020). Minor Use/Minor Species. www.fda.gov/animal-veterinary/development-approval-process/minor-useminor-species (accessed February 2022).

2 Amann, D. (2017). Harvesting Wild Game. www.fsis.usda.gov/wps/wcm/connect/fsis-content/internet/main/newsroom/meetings/newsletters/small-plant-news/small-plant-news-archive/volume-5/spn-vol5-no4 (accessed February 2022).

3 Vermeulen, B., De Backer, P., and Remon, J.P. (2002). Drug administration to poultry. *Adv. Drug Deliv. Rev.* 54 (6): 795–803.

4 Riviere, J.E. (2018). Chemical residues in tissues of food animals. In: *Veterinary Pharmacology and Therapeutics* (ed. J.E. Riviere and M. Papich). Newark, NJ: Wiley.

5 21 CFR Part 500.82 (2022). www.ecfr.gov/current/title-21/chapter-I/subchapter-E/part-500 (accessed February 2022).

6 Landy, R.B., Kim, I.S., Lee, Y. et al. (1999). Regulatory approaches for controlling pesticide residues in food animals. *Vet. Clin. North Am. Food Anim. Pract.* 15 (1): 89–107.

7 Paige, J.C., Tollefson, L., and Miller, M.A. (1999). Health implications of residues of veterinary drugs and chemicals in animal tissues. *Vet. Clin. North Am. Food Anim. Pract.* 15 (1): 31–43.

8 Martínez-Navarro, J.F. (1990). Food poisoning related to consumption of illicit beta-agonist in liver. *Lancet* 336 (8726): 1311.

9 Brambilla, G., Loizzo, A., Fontana, L. et al. (1997). Food poisoning following consumption of clenbuterol-treated veal in Italy. *JAMA* 278 (8): 635–635.

10 Cerniglia, C.E. and Kotarski, S. (1999). Evaluation of veterinary drug residues in food for their potential to affect human intestinal microflora. *Regul. Toxicol. Pharmacol.* 29 (3): 238–261.

11 Greenlees, K.J. (2003). Animal drug human food safety toxicology and antimicrobial resistance – the square peg. *Int. J. Toxicol.* 22 (2): 131–134.

12 Cerniglia, C.E. and Kotarski, S. (2005). Approaches in the safety evaluations of veterinary antimicrobial agents in food to determine the effects on the human intestinal microflora. *J. Vet. Pharmacol. Ther.* 28 (1): 3–20.

13 Greenlees, K.J., Friedlander, L.G., and Boxall, A. (2011). Antibiotic residues in food and drinking water, and food safety regulations. In: *Chemical Analysis of Antibiotic Residues in Food* (ed. J. Wang, J.D. McNeil and J.F. Kay). Hoboken, NJ: Wiley.

14 National Research Council (1999). *Drug Residues and Microbial Contamination in Food*. Washington, D.C: National Academics Press.

15 Botsoglou, N.A. and Fletouris, D.J. (2000). *Safety Assessment and Control of Residues. Drug Residues in Foods: Pharmacology, Food Safety, and Analysis*. Boca Raton, FL: CRC Press.

16 United States Government Printing Office (2004). Public Law 108–282. An act to amend the Federal Food, Drug, and Cosmetic Act with regard to new animal drugs, and for other purposes. www.congress.gov/108/plaws/publ282/PLAW-108publ282.pdf (accessed February 2022).

17 Tell, L.A., Oeller, M., Marmulak, T. et al. (2018). Considerations for treating minor food-producing animals with veterinary pharmaceuticals. In: *Veterinary Pharmacology and Therapeutics*, 10e (ed. J.E. Riviere and M. Papich). Hoboken, NJ: Wiley.

18 21 CFR 530.3a (2022). www.ecfr.gov/current/title-21/chapter-I/subchapter-E/part-530 (accessed February 2022).

19 Oeller, M. (2017). Veterinary Feed Directives for Gamebird Farmers. How Did we Get Here? And What Do We Do Now? North American Gamebird Association Annual Meeting, Gulfport, MS.

20 Davis, J.L., Smith, G.W., Baynes, R.E. et al. (2009). Update on drugs prohibited from extralabel use in food animals. *J. Am. Vet. Med. Assoc.* 235 (5): 528–534.

21 Lathers, C.M. (2001). Role of veterinary medicine in public health: antibiotic use in food animals and humans and the effect on evolution of antibacterial resistance. *J. Clin. Pharmacol.* 41 (6): 595–599.

22 Nelson, J.M., Chiller, T.M., Powers, J.H. et al. (2007). Fluoroquinolone-resistant campylobacter species and the withdrawal of fluoroquinolones from use in poultry: a public health success story. *Clin. Infect. Dis.* 44 (7): 977–980.

23 Parry, J. (2005)). Use of antiviral drug in poultry is blamed for drug resistant strains of avian flu. *Br. Med. J.* 331 (7507): 10.

24 He, G., Qiao, J., Dong, C. et al. (2008). Amantadine-resistance among H5N1 avian influenza viruses isolated in northern China. *Antivir. Res.* 77 (1): 72–76.

25 US Food and Drug Administration (2006). Limited FDA Survey of Compounded Drug Products. www.fda.gov/drugs/guidancecomplianceregulatoryinformation/pharmacycompounding/ucm155725.htm (accessed February 2022).

26 21 CFR 530.13 (2022). www.ecfr.gov/current/title-21/chapter-I/subchapter-E/part-530 (accessed February 2022).

27 CVM (2012). CVM Guidance for Industry #209. The Judicious Use of Medically Important Antimicrobial Drugs in Food-Producing Animals. www.fda.gov/media/79140/download (accessed February 2022).

28 CVM (2013). CVM Guidance for Industry #213. New Animal Drugs and New Animal Drug Combination Products Administered in or on Medicated Feed or Drinking Water of Food-Producing Animals: Recommendations for Drug Sponsors for Volunatrily Aligning Product Use Conditions with GFI #209. www.fda.gov/regulatory-information/search-fda-guidance-documents/cvm-gfi-213-new-animal-drugs-and-new-animal-drug-combination-products-administered-or-medicated-feed#:~:text=with%20GFI%20%23209-,CVM%20GFI%20%23213%20New%20Animal%20Drugs%20and%20New%20Animal%20Drug,with%20GFI%20%23209%20December%202013 (accessed February 2022).

29 Chernos, R.,.I. and T., Martin, J. ((ed.) (2008). *The Responsible Use of Health Management Products for Poultry Production: A Home Study Course for Alberta Producers*, 169–170. Edmonton, Alberta: Spotted Cow Press.

30 Safefood (n.d.). A Revew of Coccidiostat Residues in Poultry. www.safefood.net/getattachment/b71aeec2-cc86-419a-b788-4fec3449642e/AReviewOfCoccidiostatResidueinPoultry-ResearchReport.pdf?lang=en-IE (accessed February 2022).

31 Kan, C.A. (2005). Chemical residues in poultry and eggs produced in free-range or organic systems. In: XVII European Symposium on the Quality of Poultry Meat and the XI European Symposium on the Quality of Eggs and Egg Products, Doorwerth, NL.

32 Wise, D.R. and Connan, R.M. (1979). Water consumption in growing pheasants. *Vet. Rec.* 104 (16): 368–370.

33 Altine, S., Sabo, N., Muhammad, N. et al. (2016). Basic nutrient requirements of the domestic quails under tropical conditions: a review. *World Sci. News* 49 (2): 223–235.

34 IPCS (2009). Maximum residue limits for pesticides and veterinary drugs. Environmental Health Criteria 240: Principles and Methods for the Risk Assessment of Chemicals in Food. https://apps.who.int/iris/bitstream/handle/10665/44065/WHO_EHC_240_eng.pdf (accessed February 2022).

35 Martinez, M., Berson, M., Dunham, B. et al. (2009). Drug approval process. In: *Veterinary Pharmacology and Therapeutics* (ed. J.E. Riviere and M. Papich). Ames, IA: Wiley.

36 Baynes, R.E., Martín-Jiménez, T., Craigmill, A.L. et al. (1999). Estimating provisional acceptable residues for extralabel drug use in livestock. *Regul. Toxicol. Pharmacol.* 29 (3): 287–299.

37 Martín-Jiménez, T., Baynes, R., Craigmill, A. et al. (2002). Extrapolated withdrawal-interval estimator (EWE) algorithm: a quantitative approach to establishing extralabel withdrawal times. *Regul. Toxicol. Pharmacol.* 36 (1): 131–137.

38 Riviere, J.E., Webb, A.I., and Craigmill, A.L. (1998). Primer on estimating withdrawal times after extralabel drug use. *J. Am. Vet. Med. Assoc.* 213 (7): 966–968.

39 Riviere, J.E., Tell, L.A., Baynes, R.E. et al. (2017). Guide to FARAD resources: historical and future perspectives. *J. Am. Vet. Med. Assoc.* 250 (10): 1131–1139.

40 Kan, C.A. and Petz, M. (2001). Detecting residues of veterinary drugs in eggs. *World Poult.* 17: 16–17.

41 Donoghue, D.J. (2001). Mechanisms regulating drug and pesticide residue uptake by egg yolks: development of predictive models. *World Poult. Sci. J.* 57 (4): 373–380.

42 Donoghue, D.J. and Myers, K. (2000). Imaging residue transfer into egg yolks. *J. Agric. Food Chem.* 48 (1): 6428–6430.

43 Kan, C.A. and Petz, M. (2000). Residues of veterinary drugs in eggs and their distribution between yolk and white. *J. Agric. Food Chem.* 48 (12): 6397–6403.

44 Hekman, P. and Schefferlie, G.J. (2011). Kinetic modelling and residue depletion of drugs in eggs. *Br. Poult. Sci.* 52 (3): 376–380.

45 Goetting, V., Lee, K.A., and Tell, L.A. (2011). Pharmacokinetics of veterinary drugs in laying hens and residues in eggs: a review of the literature. *J. Vet. Pharmacol. Ther.* 34 (6): 521–556.

46 Patel, T., Marmulak, T., Gehring, R. et al. (2018). Drug residues in poultry meat: a literature review of commonly used veterinary antibacterials and anthelmintics used in poultry. *J. Vet. Pharmacol. Ther.* 41 (6): 761–789.

47 Donoghue, D.J. (2005). Modelling risks from antibiotic and other residues in poultry and eggs. *Food Safety Control Poult. Ind.* 8 (1): 83–100.

48 Cortright, K.A., Wetzlich, S.E., and Craigmill, A.L. (2009). A PBPK model for midazolam in four avian species. *J. Vet. Pharmacol. Ther.* 32 (6): 552–565.

49 Maclachlan, D.J. (2010). Physiologically based pharmacokinetic (PBPK) model for residues of lipophilic pesticides in poultry. *Food Addit. Contam. Part A Chem. Anal. Control. Expo. Risk Assess* 27 (3): 302–314.

50 Yang, F., Yang, Y.R., Wang, L. et al. (2014). Estimating marbofloxacin withdrawal time in broiler chickens using a population physiologically based pharmacokinetics model. *J. Vet. Pharmacol. Ther.* 37 (6): 579–588.

51 Yang, F., Sun, N., Liu, Y.M. et al. (2015). Estimating danofloxacin withdrawal time in broiler chickens based on physiologically based pharmacokinetics modeling. *J. Vet. Pharmacol. Ther* 38 (2): 174–182.

52 Henri, J., Carrez, R., Méda, B. et al. (2017). A physiologically based pharmacokinetic model for chickens exposed to feed supplemented with monensin during their lifetime. *J. Vet. Pharmacol. Ther.* 40 (4): 370–382.

53 Zeng, D., Lin, Z., Zeng, Z. et al. (2019). Assessing global human exposure to T-2 toxin via poultry meat consumption using a lifetime physiologically based pharmacokinetic model. *J. Agric. Food Chem.* 67 (5): 1563–1571.

54 Lautz, L.S., Nebbia, C., Hoeks, S. et al. (2020). An open source physiologically based kinetic model for the chicken (*Gallus gallus domesticus*): calibration and validation for the prediction residues in tissues and eggs. *Environ. Int.* 136: 105488.

55 Ludwig, B. (1989). Use of pharmacokinetics when dealing with drug residue problem of food-producing animals. *Dtsch. Tierarztl. Wochenschr.* 96 (5): 243–248.

56 Donoghue, D.J., Hairston, H., Henderson, M. et al. (1997). Modeling drug residue uptake by eggs: yolks contain ampicillin residues even after drug withdrawal and nondetectability in the plasma. *Poult. Sci.* 76 (3): 458–462.

57 Afifi, N.A. and Abo El-Sooud, K.A. (1997). Tissue concentrations and pharmacokinetics of florfenicol in broiler chickens. *Br. Poult. Sci.* 38 (4): 425–428.

58 CVM (2015). VICH GL48 R Studies to Evaluate the Metabolism and Residue Kinetics of Veterinary Drugs in Food-Producing Animals: Marker Residue Depeletion Studies to Establish Product Withdrawal Periods. www.ema.europa.eu/en/vich-gl48-studies-evaluate-metabolism-residue-kinetics-veterinary-drugs-food-producing-animals (accessed February 2022).

59 Thompson, S.R. (1999). International harmonization issues. *Vet. Clin. North Am. Food Anim. Pract.* 15 (1): 181–195.

60 Hagren, V., Peippo, P., and Lövgren, T. (2005). Detecting and controlling veterinary drug residues in poultry. In: *Food Safety Control in the Poultry Industry* (ed. G.C. Mead), 44–82. Cambridge, UK: Woodhead Publishing.

61 Abbas, R.Z., Colwell, D.D., and Gilleard, J. (2012). Botanicals: an alternative approach for the control of avian coccidiosis. *World Poult. Sci. J.* 68 (2): 203–215.

62 Health Canada (2009). Categorization of Antimicrobial Drugs Based on Importance in Human Medicine. www.canada.ca/en/health-canada/services/drugs-health-products/veterinary-drugs/antimicrobial-resistance/categorization-antimicrobial-drugs-based-importance-human-medicine.html (accessed February 2022).

63 Hawkins, M.G., Guzman, D.S.-M., Beaufrère, H. et al. (2018). Birds. In: *Exotic Animal Formulary*, 5e (ed. J.W. Carpenter and C.J. Marion). Philadelphia, PA.: W.B. Saunders.

17

Guineafowl

Jacqueline Jacob and Anthony Pescatore

The term *guineafowl* is the common name for six species of gallinaceous birds of the family Numididae. The six species of guineafowl include the white-breasted, helmeted, black, plumed, crested and vulturine. Guineafowl were first discovered in the Guinea coast of West Africa, from which the name derives. Guineafowl are endemic to Africa where temperature and rainfall appear to have played important roles in their ecology and evolution.

The domesticated strains were developed from the helmeted guineafowl (*Numida meleagris*). Guineafowl are said to have been domesticated by the ancient Egyptians about 1475 BCE, the Greeks about 400 BCE, and the Romans by 72 CE. These strains later died out in Europe. The ancestors of the domesticated guineafowl we know today were introduced into Europe during the late fifteenth century. From there, they spread to the rest of the world, including North America. As in the past, guineafowl are valued for their taste and nutritional value [1].

Guineafowl come in color varieties rather than breeds. The original color is referred to as pearl which has a purplish-gray plumage that is "pearled" with white spots on the entire body (Figure 17.1). Breeding has led to the development of at least 25 different colors, but not all colors are recognized by official standards. The American Poultry Association recognizes three varieties: lavender, pearl, and white. The Australian guineafowl standards set by the Victorian Poultry Fanciers Association include those three plus the cinnamon and pied varieties.

Landrace strains are those that have been developed by local traditional agricultural methods and in different countries. Industrial strains have been developed in France, Belgium, and Italy and are exported worldwide. The birds are easily recognized by their distinctive head features (Figure 17.2).

In most developing countries, poultry production is based primarily on scavenging systems which are a traditional component of smallholder farmers. Poultry production is the most common economic activity practiced by 80% of the resource-poor households across southern Africa [2]. For most households, guineafowl complement village chickens by utilizing spaces and feeds that are not accessible to the chickens. Compared to scavenging chickens, scavenging guineafowl produce more eggs.

Guineafowl is a poultry species whose production is increasing worldwide. Commercial production of guineafowl is similar to that of broiler chickens, with the species raised for meat since the consumption of guineafowl eggs is not very popular [3]. In developed countries, most guineafowl meat is served in restaurants. The pearl guineafowl is the dominant variety raised commercially for meat production because they grow twice as fast as nonselected guineafowl, and the carcass is leaner than that of the French industrial strain [4].

Gamebird Medicine and Management, First Edition. Edited by Teresa Y. Morishita and Robert E. Porter, Jr.

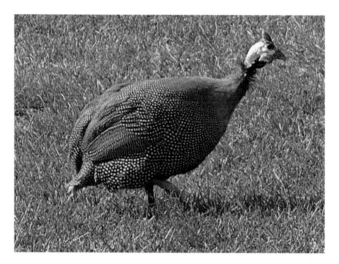

Figure 17.1   Pearl guineafowl. Source: Photo courtesy of Dr Jacqueline Jacob, University of Kentucky.

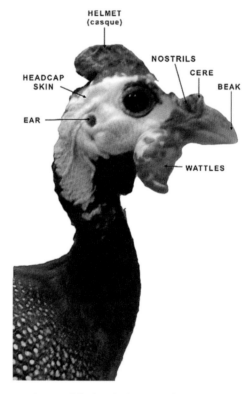

Figure 17.2   Anatomical nomenclature of the head of a guineafowl. Source: Photo courtesy of Dr Jacqueline Jacob, University of Kentucky.

In the United States and Europe, guineafowl meat is seen as an alternative to chicken and is preferred for its gamey flavor [5]. In addition, guineafowl meat is higher in protein and lower in fat compared to broiler chickens [6]. With increasing consumer interest in healthful products and animal-friendly production systems, guineafowl may fill a niche market for alternative poultry species [7].

Guineafowl have a small skeletal frame, and their carcass yield a large amount of meat [8]. Guineafowl breast meat contains more protein and less fat and is darker in color, redder, and less yellow than chicken breast meat [9]. As guinea fowl age, the meat color becomes darker, redder, and yellower. Shear force increases with age, while cooking loss decreases. Different cuts of guineafowl vary in their nutrient content, which in turn is affected to varying degrees by the cooking method used [10]. As with chickens, the thigh meat has a higher fat content than the breast. The open-roasting method has been shown to result in higher protein content in the breast compared to cooking in foil wrap. Moisture content of thigh and drumstick was not affected by cooking method, while breast meat retained the most moisture when open-roasted. Cooking loss is higher in guineafowl than chickens. The higher meat yield of guineafowl suggests that they can be produced as an additional or alternative protein source to the traditional chicken [9].

An American consumer preference study evaluated acceptance of guineafowl as a poultry meat [11]. The study recruited 40 families which prepared supplied guineafowl carcasses. Participants selected a cooking method of their choice, with most choosing either baking or roasting. After consuming the prepared product, they evaluated the product. They reported the meat as being moderate to mild in flavor, tender to very tender, and juicy to slightly juicy. No participants said they disliked the product. Most said that the guineafowl was at least equal to chicken and they would purchase guineafowl if they were available at an economical price.

17.1 General Behavior and Preferred Habitat

Guineafowl are characterized by their harsh cry and are easily agitated. Research has shown that guineafowl keets display acoustic imprinting [12]. Apparently seeing the imprinted object is not necessary as long as it can be heard. A recording of the sound is sufficient.

Guineafowl are less docile than other poultry species [13]. Although a very sociable species, guineafowl do not like confinement [13, 14]. In backyard flocks, guineafowl can be housed with other poultry species since they tend to keep to themselves and occupy different parts of the poultry house. However, aggression between guineafowl and roosters has been reported and is a concern (Figure 17.3).

Many of the behaviors characteristic of wild guineafowl are displayed in domesticated birds. The helmeted guineafowl is a common component of the African landscape. Its wide distribution is partly due to its ability to adapt to varying ecological conditions. Habitats for wild guineafowl include open forests, savannas, and grasslands. Analysis of the crop contents of hunted guineafowl revealed diets consisting of grass seeds, insects, *Cyperus* bulbs, fruits of flowering plants, leaves, and other vegetable matter [15]. As with other poultry species, guineafowl consume pebbles to help with the grinding of feed in the gizzard. With the encroachment of humans into the natural habitat of guineafowl, small maize fields, waste grain, and fallow lands now form important components of their range [16].

Like most poultry species, guineafowl like to dust bathe and in the wild will do so in the sandy soils along riverbeds [17]. Wild guineafowl nest under the canopies of bushes and utilize the trees as roosting sites. In the wild, guineafowl stay in flocks of 7–10 [18]. They appear to establish a pecking order among the males, although the frequency of agonistic actions within the flock is low. The highest-ranking male dictates the movement of the flock, including which direction to travel to forage. Adult females routinely stay between the dominant male and the juveniles to minimize victimization. During the breeding season, the dominant male guineafowl will leave temporarily with his favored female to mate. The second highest male then takes center stage and the rest of the

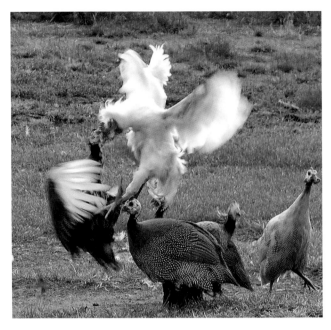

Figure 17.3   Fighting between guineafowl and a rooster. Source: Photo courtesy of Dr Jacqueline Jacob, University of Kentucky.

flock cluster around him to maintain cohesion in the flock. Most adults assist with the brooding of the chicks of the highest-ranking male [18].

17.2   Health Considerations

17.2.1   Infectious Diseases

Guineafowl are said to be resistant to many poultry diseases [19], but they can still be spreaders of many diseases so a good biosecurity program is essential. Globally, there is concern about the introduction of the Asian-origin, highly pathogenic avian influenza subtype H5N1 and its effects on the local commercial poultry industry. In 1999, an epidemic of low-pathogenicity H5N1 avian influenza (LPAI) occurred in intensively reared poultry in north-eastern Italy. Many poultry flocks were affected, including guineafowl. After the LPAI virus circulated through the flocks, highly-pathogenic (HPAI) viruses emerged. HPAI caused similar mortality rates in chickens, turkeys, and guineafowl.

Newcastle disease is a contagious disease of poultry with a wide range of avian hosts worldwide. Guineafowl are susceptible to Newcastle disease (ND) and natural infections have been reported in various countries. In a natural outbreak of Newcastle disease in Nigeria, the affected guineafowl showed paralysis of the legs and wings, coughing, sneezing, white diarrhea, and complete cessation of egg production [20]. Newcastle disease viruses have also been isolated from apparently healthy guineafowl [21, 22]. In many developing countries, control of Newcastle disease is by vaccination, but this applies largely to commercial poultry. Unfortunately, the large population of rural poultry, including guineafowl, remains largely unvaccinated and susceptible to Newcastle disease infection, with continuous shedding of the virus. Domesticated guineafowl should be vaccinated against ND to reduce shedding and spread of virulent ND [22]. It appears guineafowl may not be susceptible to infectious bronchitis virus [23].

Guineafowl have been shown to be naturally infected with mycoplasmas, including *M. synoviae* (MS) and *M. gallisepticum* (MG) [24]. Guineafowl naturally infected with MS showed clinical signs of synovitis. Experimental infection with the MS isolated from the natural infection showed clear pathogenicity for guineafowl, and to a lesser degree for chickens. In guineafowl, the strain was more likely to result in synovitis and amyloidosis when inoculated by the intravenous route and to produce sinusitis after intrasinusal inoculation.

For decades, guineafowl production in France has been affected by fulminating enteritis of unknown origin [25]. Fulminating disease of guineafowl is an acute enteritis that is characterized by intense prostration and a very high death rate. An infection can lead to almost complete destruction of a flock. Lesions are generally limited to severe enteritis, although some guineafowl show pancreatic degeneration. It is suspected to be of viral origin. Liais et al. used metagenomics and identified a novel avian gamma-coronavirus associated with the disease that is distantly related to turkey coronaviruses [25].

17.2.2 External Parasites

Guineafowl can be infested with the same external parasites that infest most poultry species, including mites, fleas, lice, and ticks [26]. Wild guineafowl can be infested with 7–13 species of parasites on any one bird. External parasite infestations in intensively reared guineafowl can led to feather damage, reduced feed intake, and even death. In Africa, scavenging guineafowl flocks host more species of external parasites than those raised under intensive management, but free-ranging guineafowl appear to be not as badly affected by the infestations. This may be due to behavior activities of free-ranging guineafowl which are often not seen in those raised intensively. This includes communal pecking of each other to remove foreign bodies, ritual sexual dancing behavior, play, and sand bathing. Each of these activities could dislodge ectoparasites and thus reduce the parasite buildup that resulted in the clinical signs noted in the guineafowl raised intensively [26].

17.2.3 Internal Parasites

The most important intestinal parasites are coccidiosis (*Eimeria* sp.), roundworms (*Ascaridia galli*), cecal worms (*Heterakis* sp.), and hairworms or threadworms (*Capillaria caudiflata*) [27].

Common hosts of cecal worms (*Heterakis gallinarum*) include the chicken, turkey, guineafowl, ring-necked pheasant, partridge, and many other gallinaceous birds [28]. *Heterakis gallinarum*, however, thrives best in the guineafowl and ring-necked pheasant. The chicken is the third most suitable host. The parasite is unable to reproduce sufficiently in other hosts, including the turkey, to maintain populations. *Heterakis gallinarum* has a direct life cycle and does not require an intermediate host to complete development. The parasite itself typically only causes mild pathology and does not significantly affect bird performance. However, the ovum of *H. gallinarum* serves as the vector for the protozoal parasite *Histomonas meleagridis* which causes histomoniasis in poultry [28]. Treating and preventing *H. gallinarum* infections is complicated by the low efficacy of anthelmintics for eradicating the worm from infected birds and because of the low efficacy of disinfectants for destroying the *H. gallinarum* ova on contaminated farms.

A natural outbreak of toxoplasmosis was reported in a backyard flock of guineafowl in northern Mississippi [29]. The flock was infected with *Toxoplasma gondii* which is a coccidian parasite that can infect many species of warm-blooded animals, including birds. It can also infect some cold-blooded animals. The life cycle is indirect and requires both definitive and intermediate hosts. Both wild and domestic cats are the only definitive hosts and at least 141 different species can serve as intermediate hosts. Natural outbreaks in chickens and turkeys have only been sporadically reported, although infections have been reported to occur naturally in chickens, turkeys, ducks, and many wild birds. The infected guineafowl in Mississippi exhibited lethargy prior to death. On necropsy, there were no gross lesions, but intralesional protozoan cysts were observed microscopically. The diagnosis of toxoplasmosis was confirmed with immunohistochemistry and PCR [29].

A similar outbreak occurred in a mixed backyard poultry flock in Brazil [30]. Both chickens and guineafowl were affected. Clinicals signs were lethargy, anorexia, and neurologic signs over a course of 24–72 hours. Of the 22 birds showing clinical signs, 15 died. There were no gross lesions on necropsy, but histopathologic findings included inflammatory infiltrate of macrophages, lymphocytes, and plasma cells. There was necrosis in several tissues associated with intralesional *Toxoplasma gondii*. Immunohistochemistry for *T. gondii* was positive.

17.3   Pharmacology Considerations

Although the anatomy and physiology of guineafowl are similar to those of chickens, there are some differences in digestive tract morphology that could cause different drug absorptions. The doses of drugs used are often extrapolated from the amount used for chickens or other poultry species. When guineafowl are raised in confinement, bacterial infections such as colibacillosis, mycoplasmosis, or fowl cholera may occur, and antibiotic treatment may be necessary. The pharmacokinetics in quail and guineafowl are similar but show some differences from pheasants [31].

There are limited choices for antibiotics when raising guineafowl and limited information on their use. As an example, for the antibiotic danofloxacin, there is information on pharmacokinetics for chickens, turkeys, and ducks. Danofloxacin, a synthetic fluoroquinolone that is not approved for poultry in the US, is an antibacterial agent that exhibits bactericidal activity against numerous Gram-positive and some Gram-negative bacteria, mycoplasmas, and intracellular pathogens such as *Brucella* and *Chlamydia* species [31]. According to the data for these poultry species, danofloxacin penetrates the tissues. Tissue concentrations are higher and persist longer compared to blood. Danofloxacin is eliminated mainly unchanged and relatively slowly. The oral bioavailability for these species is high without significant interspecies differences [31]. For pheasants, danofloxacin showed lower distribution and clearance values and longer half-life than other galliform species. This resulted in a longer presence of the drug in the organism and high area under the curve (AUC) values. The opposite was seen in guineafowl that demonstrated a relatively short persistence of danofloxacin. While 10 mg/kg bodyweight was effective for Japanese quail and pheasants, the authors recommended a higher therapeutic dose for efficacy in guineafowl [31].

Flubendazole is not approved for use in the US but it is used in many other parts of the world, as reflected in corresponding research. When used as prescribed for gamebirds, flubendazole is very active against gastrointestinal roundworms, gapeworms, and tapeworms in guineafowl [32]. Residues of flubendazole and its major metabolites were detected in breast muscle, thigh muscle, and liver of guineafowl treated at 56 or 86 mg/kg bodyweight for 7 successive days. Maximum residue limits (MRL) are based on the sum of the parent flubendazole molecule and its hydrolyzed metabolites. Based on the MRLs established by the European Union for other poultry species, a minimum 3-day withdrawal period prior to slaughter is recommended [32]. After 3 days, the residues were very low and far below the established safe MRL. However, after an 8-day withdrawal period, flubendazole-derived residues were still found in both muscle tissues and liver. The levels of residues in the breast and thigh meat were comparable.

Ten hours after guineafowl were treated with a subcutaneous injection of a commercial ivermectin product at 0.14 mg/kg body weight, fecal droppings contained both adult and larval stages of the roundworm *A. galli*, the cecal worm *Heterakis gallinarum*, the roundworm *Subulura suctoria*, and fragments of the tapeworm *Raillietina* spp. Drug efficacy was rated as 100% [33]. It is important to remember, however, that ivermectin is not an approved drug for poultry in the US and its use would be off-label and require a veterinarian's prescription.

17.3.1 Probiotics

Probiotics are live microbial feed supplements given to promote the growth and health of the animal. This is achieved by minimizing nonessential and pathogenic microorganisms from the recipient's digestive tract. The microbial profiles of guineafowl and chickens are sufficiently different that the design of effective probiotics for guineafowl would be different [34]. One of the main differences observed was the presence of Verrucomicrobia (mucin-degrading bacteria) and Lentisphaerae (bacteria closely related to Chlamydiae and Verrucomicrobia) in the guineafowl digestive tract that were not present in the chicken.

Guineafowl, like their chicken counterparts, have been shown to be reservoirs of antibiotic-resistant *Salmonella*, *Campylobacter jejuni*, *Camplyobacter lari*, *Escherichia coli*, and *Klebsiella* spp [35]. There is the potential, therefore, for these antibiotic-resistant pathogens to be transferred to humans through contaminated guineafowl products. This reinforces the need for more prudent use of antibiotics by poultry producers, and continued development of methods to reduce the risk of foodborne pathogens is critical.

17.3.2 Anesthetic Compounds

Although surgery is not typically performed on commercial poultry, situations may arise that require the use of anesthesia. This could be the case if surgery is needed, or a broken bone needs to be reset. Isoflurane inhalation anesthesia is typically used for most avian species, but its use may not be feasible in the field. Injectable anesthetics are used in animals, such as birds, in which venous access is difficult [36]. Such anesthetics have the benefit of rapid administration, low cost, and minimal equipment requirements. Ketamine can be administered intramuscularly or intravenously but its use can result in poor muscle relaxation, muscle tremors, myotonic contractions, opisthotonos (spasm of the muscles causing backward arching of the head, neck, and spine), and a rough recovery. To counter these problems, ketamine is rarely used alone but instead is paired with another drug. Ketamine-xylazine combinations have been evaluated in several avian species and have been associated with increased blood pressure, decreased heart rate, and hypoxemia. Intermuscular administration of midazolam improved the anesthetic quality of ketamine and xylazine in guineafowl without adversely affecting safety. The midazolam may improve the quality of anesthesia induced by a ketamine-xylazine combination in guineafowl and also reduce the dosages required [36].

17.4 Reproduction

17.4.1 Anatomy

The reproductive organs of vertebrates typically arise as bilateral primordia and this symmetry usually persists into adulthood. In most avian species, however, there is a failure of one ovary and its corresponding oviduct to develop. The result is normally the presence of the left ovary and oviduct reaching functional development in the adult. This is the case with guineafowl, as with most poultry species [37]. The presence of a right oviduct has been reported in some poultry species, including guineafowl, but it is rare. Typically, if there is a right oviduct, it is underdeveloped with no opening into the cloaca. There is also no corresponding ovary [37].

As with other avian species, guineafowl males have paired testes and highly convoluted vas deferens. The testes and vas deferens are not discernible until about 4 weeks of age [38]. Puberty is said to occur at 12 weeks of age, with sexual maturity around 16–20 weeks. There will, of course, be some variability between varieties and strains in the timing of sexual development [39].

The ovary and oviduct of guineafowl were discernible and measurable at hatching [38]. Sexual maturity in guinea hens appears to occur around 27–28 weeks of age with the onset of egg production, although there are reports of egg production starting as early as 21 weeks of age [38]. Higher oviduct and ovary weights have been reported for guinea hens kept on range versus those on deep litter or in battery cages [40]. This may be an indication of accelerated rate of reproductive development on range. The hens on free range also had higher liver weights which corresponded to follicle recruitment. The liver is the main source of egg proteins and yolk materials.

Compared to the domestic chicken, guineafowl eggs are smaller, but eggs of domestic guineafowl are larger and heavier than eggs of their wild counterparts [41]. Guineafowl eggs are typically yellow to brown in color with varied mottling [41]. Guineafowl eggs have a greater shell thickness than most other birds. Eggshells represent 14% of the egg weight in guineafowl and only 10% in the chicken [42]. This increased eggshell mass is related to differences in the timing of eggshell deposition. The rapid phase of calcium carbonate deposition is initiated about 3 hours earlier in the guineafowl [43]. The developing egg spends about 15.4 hours in the shell gland of guineafowl, compared to 13.3 hours in chickens. The rate of shell deposition, however, is similar in both species at about 0.37 g/h. The longer duration of shell deposition in the guineafowl results in greater eggshell mass. The increased time spent in the shell gland for guineafowl does not modify the interval between ovipositions [43]. The mean interval between egg laying is 24 hours for both species.

Ovulation occurs in guineafowl about 15 minutes after the previous egg is laid. This is similar to that of chickens. In guineafowl, the ovum arrives in the shell gland in less than 4 hours. The time spent in the magnum for albumen deposition is shorter in guineafowl, which may be the reason that their eggs have smaller amounts of albumen compared to chickens [43].

Eggshell color appears to influence eggshell thickness [44]. Although eggshells are thicker in guineafowl, shell thickness does not appear to affect hatching rates [45]. Eggshell thickness appeared to influence weight loss during incubation but had no effect on hatchability [44]. The higher shell thickness in guineafowl eggs is compensated for by a greater density of pores for gas exchange [41]. The area density of pores decreased from the blunt to the pointed end of the egg.

17.4.2 Reproductive Performance

Egg fertility, hatchability, and keet survival rates have been found to be significantly higher in free-living flocks of guineafowl compared to their domesticated counterparts. Low egg fertility appears to be a key limiting factor in the reproductive success of guineafowl kept in semi-confinement [14]. Fertility and hatchability rates are considerably lower in guineafowl compared with other poultry species. Fertility levels of 60% have been reported for flocks of guineafowl breeders. This may be due to sexing difficulties, the narrow sex ratio required, and the seasonality of breeding [46, 47]. Although guineafowl are monogamous in the wild, a sex ratio of one male for every four females has been shown to give relatively good fertility [27].

Hatchability is a complex, age-dependent trait involving both genetic and environmental factors arising from multiple sources [48]. Both sire and dam genetic components are important for overall hatchability. Both the paternal and maternal genetic effects have been shown to vary with the

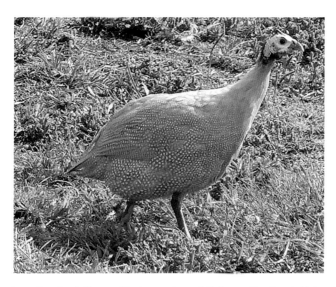

Figure 17.4 Lavender guineafowl. Source: Photo courtesy of Dr Jacqueline Jacob, University of Kentucky.

age of the flock [48]. Hatchability of guineafowl eggs has been found to vary among the different varieties, so a genetic component is definitely involved [49, 50]. Selection for lower dead in-germ and dead-in-shell phenotypic traits can improve overall fertility and hatchability of guineafowl eggs [49].

In the US, domesticated guineafowl come in color varieties and not breeds. The most popular varieties are pearl, lavender (Figure 17.4), black, and white [1]. Semen volume has been shown to be less for males of the white variety compared to the pearl and lavender varieties [51]. While there were no differences in sperm motility or live counts among the varieties, there were a higher number of dead sperm observed in collections from the white variety males. This higher number of dead sperm was linked to a higher number of morphologically abnormal spermatozoa. As a result, hatchability was higher in pearl and lavender varieties compared to the white.

Confinement of guineafowl has been shown to lower fertility rates [14]. Investigating the causes of low hatchability requires a thorough examination of unhatched eggs. It is important to be able to differentiate a live from a dead embryo and a fertilized from an unfertilized germinal disc. This will help determine if the problem lies with fertility or embryo mortality. This requires detailed descriptions of the normal course of morphogenetic development of the embryo. There are variations in the developmental stages of the blastoderm when the eggs are laid between species and within varieties [52]. While the temporal rate of development differed, the external features of any embryo in any given stage were found to be nearly identical for chickens and guineafowl. It appears, therefore, that the normal tables of embryo development described for chickens can be used for guineafowl [52].

Different poultry species tend to lay at different times of the day. The domesticated chicken lays most of her eggs in the morning or early afternoon, and rarely after 2 pm. Domesticated ducks lay most of their eggs very early in the morning while pigeons lay early afternoon. Domesticated turkeys lay mostly around midday while Coturnix quail lay most of their eggs in the late afternoon. Domesticated guineafowl can lay their eggs any time between 6 am and 8 pm but the majority are laid in the evenings (3–8 pm) [53].

The term *clutch size* when used with poultry species refers to the number of eggs laid on consecutive days without a break. Clutch size is used to describe the individual laying pattern and is considered a trait that can be used for genetic selection. For guineafowl, a sequence length of four eggs has been reported [53].

17.4.3 Artificial Insemination

The low fertility rates normally achieved with guineafowl breeder flocks has led to research on the use of artificial insemination. Poultry spermatozoa are fragile compared to other animals [54]. Comparing fresh sperm viability and normality, it is highest in chickens and lowest in guineafowl, with turkeys intermediate [55]. Two semen extenders have been shown to be effective in maintaining at least 80% guineafowl sperm viability with 6 hours of storage: the Beltsville Poultry Semen Extender and the Instruments for Veterinary Medicine Poultry semen preservation media [54–56]. It is recommended, however, that semen collections be used within 3 hours after collection. While natural mating has been shown to result in a 66% fertility rate, artificial insemination has been shown to achieve over 90%. Vaginal douching has been shown to increase the fertility slightly more [54].

For semen collection, abdominal massage is used [54]. Feathers around the vent region are periodically trimmed for easy semen collection. Collection twice a week from any one guinea cock is recommended. Sides of the soft part of the abdomen and bilateral region of the pygostyle are massaged rapidly and continuously until the guinea cock responds by protruding the papillae. On protrusion, the thumb and index fingers of the hand are positioned to gently squeeze out the semen. The pearly white drop of ejaculate coming out of the papillae is aspirated into sterile glass tuberculin syringes. Semen samples are kept in water baths at 18–20 °C for further dilution.

To inseminate the female, pressure is applied over the soft abdominal region to evert the oviduct. Any adhering dirt or fecal particles should be removed by cotton swabs. The glass tuberculin syringe containing the appropriate volume of semen is then inserted to a depth of 3 cm. Pressure is then released over the abdomen and the oviduct returns inside the body cavity. In order to minimize the bacterial load in and around the vagina, vaginal douching is sometimes recommended. Gentamicin diluted with 0.9% sodium chloride solution is used; 1 mL of douching solution is sprayed over the lumen of the vaginal opening of the oviduct using a sterile syringe.

France practices pedigree selection of guineafowl for meat production similar to that used for other commercial poultry species. Concerns related to line extinction due to sanitary or breeding failures led to research into reproductive cell cryopreservation. The ability to survive cryopreservation varies in spermatozoa from different avian species [55]. A cryopreservation method was developed for guineafowl that combines biophysical (cryoprotectant agents, freeze/thaw rate) and zootechnical (artificial insemination frequency) features [57]. The method developed results in 70% fertility with frozen–thawed sperm and is now available for guineafowl gene bank conservation and male reproductive management.

17.4.4 Seasonality

Wild guineafowl are seasonal breeders. The breeding season lasts about 2 months and the timing varies from year to year, depending on environmental conditions [58]. The breeding season usually starts a month after insect numbers have reached their yearly peak. In chickens and turkeys, the onset of sexual maturity can be manipulated using lighting programs. They come into sexual maturity with the increasing number of daylight hours. Guineafowl, however, have not responded to artificial lighting during the winter months. Instead, they appear to respond to changes in temperature [59]. Guineafowl kept at 21.1–26.7 °C have quicker onset of egg and semen production than those kept at 15.6 °C. Those kept at the lower temperature do eventually increase production to the levels achieved by those exposed to higher temperatures. It is possible to initiate sexual maturity in guineafowl by exposure to a warm environment and then reduce the temperature after egg and semen production with no significant differences in overall fertility and hatchability [59]. The use of warm temperature may be beneficial in bringing guineafowl into sexual maturity in the winter.

Although guineafowl do not respond to increasing day length as a stimulation for sexual maturity, recent research has shown that guineafowl production and reproductive performance can be improved by increasing the day length [60, 61]. Study results show that reproductive performance is enhanced by using artificial light to increase day lengths to 14–16 hours per day. A lighting program of 16 L (light) : 8 D (dark) during the laying period has been shown to maximize hen day egg production, fertility, and hatchability.

Different energy-efficient lamps have been used in poultry houses, including compact fluorescent lamps and light-emitting diodes (LEDs). There has been some research with poultry to indicate that the use of blue LEDs has a calming effect on poultry flocks [62]. This has not been shown to be the case with guineafowl. Guineafowl on blue light were more restless and had lower performance compared to those on compact fluorescent and white LED lights [62].

17.4.5 Sexing

One of the main issues with breeding domesticated guineafowl is sexing the birds. One method for sexing adult guineafowl is through their vocalizations. Males have a one-syllable harsh cry while the female's cry is two syllable. It is difficult, however, to sex immature birds.

Guineafowl are monomorphic birds showing little sexual dimorphism [63]. That is, for most guineafowl varieties, it is not easy to determine the sex. There are some varieties where females are darker in color than males, but for most, the plumage is the same. While males have larger values for cere, body mass, helmet length, helmet width, wattle length and wattle width than do females, no single attribute or combination of attributes can be used to sex guineafowl with certainty [64].

Several methods have been employed for sexing monomorphic birds, each with specific advantages and disadvantages. Vent sexing is one method, which involves everting the cloaca of the bird to examine the phallus size. In guineafowl, phallus size in the two sexes can be distinguished from 8 weeks of age with the males having longer and thicker phalli than the females [65]. Some researchers have shown that by combining the two variables of length and thickness, it is possible to separate males from females with about 98% accuracy. Others, however, have had only 48.7% accuracy at detecting males but 81% accuracy at detecting females. Vent sexing, therefore, is not a reliable method for sexing guineafowl prior to breeding season [63].

The inheritance of the sex-linked trait of wing feather development (rapid vs slow) has been shown to occur in chickens [66] and turkeys [67] and is determined by a single pair of sex-linked alleles. The sex-linked trait has been used commercially in these industries to allow for feather-sexing of day-old hatchlings. The same sex-linked trait has been identified in guineafowl keets [68]. Only 85% of the day-old keets (Figure 17.5) show easy-to-define phenotypes. However, 94% accuracy in sexing can be achieved in 10-day old birds. The remaining 6% discrepancy could be the influence of background genes on phenotypic expression. The rapid-feathering keets also showed relatively better developed tail feathers compared to the slow-feathering keets.

The incidence of the rapid-feathering allele was found to be higher in a population of guineafowl selected for high body weight compared to an unselected population. The wing feather development mutation in guineafowl has autosexing potential because male and female keets look alike and sometimes cannot be sexed with certainty even at 20 weeks of age. The breeding would require

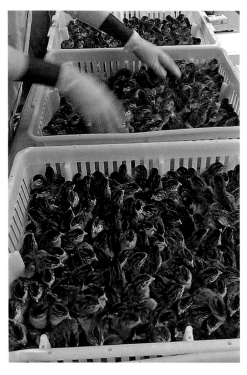

Figure 17.5 One-day-old keets. Source: Photo courtesy of Tennessee State University.

crossing rapid-feathering males homozygous for the fast-feathering allele with slow-feathering females. The slow-feathering offspring would be males and the rapid-feathering ones would be females. In chickens, there has been an association between the slow-feathering allele and the endogenous proviral gene which enhances susceptibility to avian leukosis virus (ALV) infection. It appears, however, that this unwanted gene does not occur in guineafowl [69].

17.4.6 Incubation Parameters

As with all poultry eggs, guineafowl eggs should be incubated small end downwards. Recommended incubation conditions include 37.5–37.8 °C and 60% relative humidity. Water loss during incubation is optimum at 13.3%. The incubation period is 28 days [70].

As with other poultry species, storing guineafowl hatching eggs at 18 °C for more than 7 days negatively affects egg quality and depresses embryo and posthatch growth [71].

17.5 Production Systems

There are three main production systems for guineafowl that have been used worldwide. The first is the extensive system common in rural areas of developing countries where the animals are never confined and must scavenge for feed. They are generally not fed or may receive small quantities of grains. In the semi-intensive system, the animals may have housing provided at night and they are given feed, often to keep them close to the homestead. In the intensive system, the guineafowl are housed in specially designed housing, they receive commercial feed, and a regular health program is followed [72].

There is worldwide interest in intensively raising guineafowl. Their poor docility, however, can create behavior problems in intensive production systems [13]. When comparing semi-intensive and confined production systems, there are significant differences in live weight until the guineafowl reach 14 weeks of age [7]. After that, live weights are similar regardless of housing system. Guineafowl reared in the semi-intensive system consumed more feed than those reared in confinement and had lower feed efficiency. Production system, gender, and slaughter age did not affect the dressing percentage, but the guineafowl raised in the semi-intensive system had significantly less abdominal fat [7].

The effect of floor density on growth performance and carcass characteristics has been studied for both pearl and French guineafowl. For French guineafowl broilers, floor densities of 13.6 birds/m^2 have been found to be most economically feasible [3]. All the guineafowl were raised to 8 weeks in floor pens covered with pinewood shavings. In general, higher feed conversion and lower carcass yields were obtained with higher densities. Average body weight gain for French guineafowl raised at 13.6 birds/m^2 was 1.4 kg with 2.2 kg of feed consumed, giving a feed conversion of 1.6. Mortality was 6%. Carcass yield was 74.7% with 20.3% breast, 12.6% thigh, 8.9% drumstick, and 11.1% wings. For pearl guineafowl replacement pullets, floor densities of 18 birds/m^2 for the first 8 weeks and 12 birds/m^2 for the remaining 8 weeks are recommended in order to achieve the highest possible feed efficiency [73].

Guineafowl raised in tropical environments should have a maximum stocking density of 16 birds/m^2. Higher stocking densities will adversely affect growth performance and welfare of the birds as measured by heterophil to lymphocyte ratios [74].

Battery cages have been used for a variety of different poultry species, most notably chickens and Coturnix quail egg layers. The cage density required for optimal egg production varies by poultry species and is highly variable among varieties and strains. Guineafowl are reported to have superior egg production when raised at a density of 1394 cm^2/bird compared to those reared at 697 or 465 cm^2/bird [75].

Environmental stress in domestic poultry has been shown to increase blood glucose levels. Blood glucose levels for hens on free range were significantly lower than for hens raised in semi-intensive or confinement systems. The poor performance recorded for guineafowl kept in battery cages may be explained by the stress levels of the guinea hens as shown by blood glucose levels. The increased stress level may result in gluconeogenesis in which amino acids are converted to glucose and therefore increase blood glucose levels. This would indicate that the conventional battery cages used for chicken laying hens are not appropriate for housing guineafowl [40].

17.5.1   Label Rouge Production System

Label Rouge guinea is produced according to strictly defined specifications (www.volaillelabelrouge .com/en/guinea-fowl) which include low growth rates, housing size limited to 400 m^2 per poultry house and 1600 m^2 per farm, stocking density limited to 13 guineafowl/m^2, and free access to open space. The birds can be kept on grassy and/or shaded land with a minimum of 2 m^2 per bird, or about 1 hectare per poultry house. Alternatively, the guineafowl can be kept in percheries over 2 m high and at least twice the size of the poultry house. The feed must contain at least 70% cereal grains, no animal products, a restricted number of supplements, and no growth-stimulating additives. Slaughter age is a minimum of 94 days and transport from the farm to the slaughterhouse must be no more than 2 hours or 100 km. The mean weight for guineafowl grown in such systems ranges from 1 kg to 1.4 kg. Fresh, unprocessed whole guineafowl has a shelf-life of 11 days when packaged with shrink film. Shelf-life increases to 15 days maximum when modified atmosphere packing is used.

At slaughter, standard guineafowl are heavier than Label Rouge guineafowl [76]. For both genotypes, females were heavier than males (+5.6%). The skin was thicker for the standard guineafowl (0.84 mm vs 0.77 mm) which could be due to more subcutaneous fat. Label Rouge guineafowl had higher yields of breast and thighs with shanks than standard guineafowl. For both lines, the breast and thigh meat of females was judged more tender and less stringy. Guineafowl raised in the winter when rearing temperatures are lower have decreased growth performance but there is no effect on carcass quality. Females had earlier body and sexual development, explaining the higher carcass fatness when slaughtered at 96 days of age. Their meat was judged more tender and less stringy than their male counterparts. It is recommended that females are slaughtered earlier than males [76].

17.5.2   Feeds and Feeding

A major challenge in guineafowl production has been the establishment of optimum nutritional requirements and the development of feeding programs that maximize growth and minimize the cost of production. Understanding the growth patterns of guineafowl allows for the development of efficient nutritional or feeding regimens. To achieve this end, growth models have been used. Such mathematical models are useful because they summarize time series data into a few parameters that can be used to objectively compare growth efficiencies. When these models are used, irregular fluctuations in weight caused by random environmental effects are eliminated. Growth models, in combination with feed consumption data, can be used in bio-economic studies. It is believed that the mature weight, the rate at which the mature weight is reached, and the standardized age at which an animal achieves the inflection point of the curve can be manipulated by geneticists [77].

With the use of body weight data of pearl guineafowl, the Gompertz model was found to be the most descriptive of the growth pattern [77, 78]. The Gompertz curve is a type of mathematical model for a time series named after Benjamin Gompertz (1779–1865). It is a sigmoid curve which describes growth as being slowest in the beginning and end of a given time period. Laird proposed a modification of the Gompertz equation and today this is more commonly used to fit growth data in poultry and livestock [79]. Nahashon et al. found that the Gompertz–Laird model provided good estimates of growth rate for meat-type French guineafowl broilers [80].

Nahashon et al. used the Gompertz–Laird growth model to estimate nutritional requirements for guineafowl. They recommended feeding 21% and 23% crude protein and 3100 kcal of metabolizable energy per kg feed from hatch to 4 weeks of age [80]. From 5 to 8 weeks of age, they recommended that 19% and 21% crude protein with 3150 kcal of metabolizable energy per kg would be adequate for growth.

In France, where the guinea is a popular meat bird, research has been quite extensive. However, only limited research on the nutritional requirements of French guineafowl has been conducted in the US. Nelson used starter diets with 3100 kcal ME/kg and 23% protein for the first 4 weeks and grower diets 3150 kcal ME/kg and 21% protein for the final 4 weeks [81]. The lysine requirement was determined to be 1.10% for both the starter and grower diets. Eight-week weights were 1.2 kg with feed conversions of 2.3 feed/gain. Using similar diets, Johnson determined the methionine requirement to be 0.45%, and cysteine 0.35% for the first 4 weeks of age [82].

In order to accurately formulate poultry rations, it is important to know the nutrient content of the feedstuffs available for use. This is especially important with dietary energy content since most poultry species eat to meet their energy requirements and the levels of other nutrients in the feed are dependent on that energy level. Most of the nutrient content data on feedstuffs used for poultry are based on research with chickens. When comparing the nitrogen-corrected apparent metabolizable energy (AME_n) content of different feed ingredients, the levels were similar for both young pullet chicks and young guinea keets for maize, soybean meal, peanut meal, dried brewer's yeast, palm kernel meal, and brewer's spent grains. The exceptions were cottonseed meal and wheat bran, for which the AME_n values were significantly higher for guineafowl [83]. Similarly, the AME_n values of low-, medium-, and high-tannin sorghum varieties were similar for both species.

As with other poultry species, guineafowl are susceptible to the effects of aflatoxin in feed [84]. Inclusion of aflatoxin in the diet of day-old keets at levels as low as 0.5 ppm reduced hemoglobin and total plasma protein levels. Increasing levels of aflatoxin (0.5, 1.0, and 1.5 ppm) significantly increased glutamic oxaloacetic transaminase (GOT) and glutamic pyruvic transaminase (GPT) activities. GOT is an enzyme found in the liver, heart, and other tissues. A high level of serum GOT may be a sign of liver or heart damage, cancer, or other diseases. Similarly, GPT is found in the cells of the liver and heart. Serum GPT levels increase when the liver or heart is damaged [84].

Feed particle size can influence poultry performance. In general, fine particles reduce feed intake and growth rates. Pelleting has been well documented to improve poultry performance, but the benefits are only realized if pellet integrity is maintained from the feed mill to consumption. Higher live body weights and feed efficiency were reported when guineafowl were fed 2 mm pelleted diets compared to 4 mm pellets [85].

Care should be taken when changing from one type of feed to another, such as going from crumbles to a meal or pelleted feed [86]. Reports indicate that although guineafowl spent more time near the feeders during a feed change, they actually spent less time pecking at the feed and more time observing. The results were similar to those obtained by observing turkeys under similar conditions.

17.6 Tick Control – Fact or Fiction?

Guineafowl can adapt to different conditions and are good foragers. They are often suggested for biological control of ticks. Ticks have long been a major nuisance pest of humans and animals but have also been recognized as a significant public health threat. Ticks have been shown to be vectors for several human diseases, including Lyme disease and Rocky Mountain spotted fever. The black-legged tick (*Ixodes scapularis*), or deer tick, is the vector for Lyme disease which is recognized as an important infectious disease in North America, Europe, and Asia. Flocks of helmeted guineafowl have been reported to reduce populations of black-legged ticks in penned areas [87]. However, since guineafowl feed on a variety of species, it is unlikely that the impact on tick populations would be significant. In addition, nymphal deer ticks present the greatest risk of transmitting Lyme disease to humans, but they are smaller than adults and may not be captured as easily by guineafowl.

Research has shown that although guineafowl reduce the abundance of adult ticks, they do not affect the levels of nymphal stages [87]. It is the nymphs which transmit the vast majority of Lyme disease cases [88]. There was no correlation between the density of adult ticks and the density of nymphs. It has been hypothesized that providing the guineafowl with feed to keep them in the area attracts small rodents which might import immature ticks onto the property, counteracting the suppression effects of predation by the guineafowl on the adult ticks [89].

Although guineafowl are not effective in controlling Lyme disease, research does show they can be used to control adult tick populations. Guineafowl are inexpensive compared to many pesticide treatments and present less potential for direct environmental damage. However, they have several drawbacks that may make them unsuitable in some situations. They are noisy. Their droppings, while serving as a fertilizer, may not be welcome on lawns used for human recreation. However, the droppings may discourage humans from sitting on the ground and ground sitting has been shown to increase the risk of contracting Lyme disease. Guineafowl are sometimes vulnerable to predation by feral or free-ranging dogs. Guineafowl may be most appropriate as one means of controlling ticks in low-density housing areas and in public parks and school yards where their noise is unlikely to be a problem and where custodial care is available for the flock.

It is important to remember, however, that introduction of guineafowl for tick control can have unintended consequences. When the Turkish government introduced thousands of exotic guineafowl into Turkey for the control of ticks carrying the emerging Crimean-Congo hemorrhagic fever, they discovered that guineafowl are major hosts for the tick vector [90]. The guineafowl ate very few ticks but were excellent nurseries for the young *Hyalomma marginatum* ticks which are vectors for the disease.

17.7 Conclusion

- There is great potential for guineafowl production as a profitable enterprise.
- Guineafowl are resistant to many poultry diseases, but they can still be asymptomatic carriers that can spread these diseases. Guineafowl are susceptible to avian influenza, Newcastle disease, and mycoplasmas, but resistant to infectious bronchitis. Fulminating disease, an acute enteritis, has occurred in commercial guineafowl in France and is characterized by intense prostration and a very high death rate.
- Guineafowl are susceptible to external and internal parasites. The most important intestinal parasites for guineafowl are coccidiosis (*Eimeria* sp.), roundworms (*A. galli*), cecal worms (*Heterakis* sp.), and hairworms or threadworms. Natural infections of *Toxoplasma gondii* have also occurred in guineafowl. Guineafowl can be infested with the same external parasites that infest most poultry species, including mites, fleas, lice, and ticks. External parasite infestations in intensively reared guineafowl can led to feather damage, reduced feed intake, and even death.
- While flubendazole cannot be used in the USA, it has been an effective dewormer in poultry in other parts of the world. When used as prescribed for gamebirds, flubendazole is very active against gastrointestinal roundworms, gapeworms, and tapeworms in guineafowl. For meat birds, a minimum 3-day withdrawal period is necessary.
- The microbial profiles of guineafowl and chickens are sufficiently different that the design of effective probiotics for guineafowl should be different from that for chickens. One of the main differences observed was the presence of Verrucomicrobia (mucin-degrading bacteria) and Lentisphaerae (bacteria closely related to Chlamydiae and Verrucomicrobia) in the guineafowl digestive tract. Guineafowl, like their chicken counterparts, have been shown to be reservoirs of antibiotic-resistant foodborne pathogens including *Salmonella*, *Camplyobacter jejuni*, *Camplyobacter lari*, *E. coli*, and *Klebsiella* spp.
- There are limited pharmaceutical products available for use with guineafowl. The doses of drugs for use with guineafowl are often extrapolated from the amount used for chickens or other poultry species. For some medications, this extrapolation may not be applicable. The lack of effective pharmaceutical products makes the use of effective biosecurity plans extremely important.
- Compared to the domestic chicken, guineafowl eggs are smaller but have thicker eggshells. Guineafowl have a longer incubation period, at 28 days. Fertility and hatchability rates are considerably lower in guineafowl compared with other poultry species. Although guineafowl

are monogamous in the wild, a sex ratio of one male for every four females has been shown to give relatively good fertility. The onset of egg production in guineafowl is not manipulated by increasing light but may respond to changes in temperature. However, production and reproductive performance can be improved by increasing the day length.

- When raising in confinement, stocking densities of 13.6 birds/m² are recommended for French guineafowl. For commercial strains of pearl gray guineafowl replacement pullets, floor densities of 18 birds/m² for the first 8 weeks and 12 birds/m² for the remaining 8 weeks are recommended. Guineafowl raised in tropical environments should have a maximum stocking density of 16 birds/m². Due to the high level of stress, battery cages used for laying chicken hens are not appropriate for guinea hens.
- Nutritional information on guineafowl is limited. The energy content and nutrient availability values for some feedstuffs may not be the same for guineafowl and chickens. For commercial guineafowl broilers, it is recommended that a starter diet containing 3100 kcal ME/kg and 23% protein be fed from hatch to 4 weeks of age. A grower feed with 3150 kcal ME/kg and 21% protein should be fed from 5 to 8 weeks of age. The lysine requirement is 1.10%, methionine 0.45%, and cysteine 0.35%. Eight-week production goals of 1.2 kg body weight with feed conversions of 2.3 are attainable [91]. As with other poultry species, guineafowl are susceptible to the effects of aflatoxin in feed.
- Although guineafowl have been shown to control adult tick populations, they are not an effective control for tickborne diseases such as Lyme disease.
- In backyard flocks, guineafowl can be housed with other poultry species since they tend to keep to themselves and occupy different parts of the poultry house. However, aggression between guineafowl and roosters has been shown to occur.

References

1 Bernacki, Z., Kokoszynski, D., and Bawei, M. (2013). Laying performance, egg quality and hatching results in two guinea fowl genotypes. *Arch. Geflügelk.* 77 (2): S109–S115.

2 Mapiye, C., Mwale, M., Mupangwa, J.F. et al. (2008). A research review of village chicken production constraints and opportunities in Zimbabwe. *Asian-Australasian. J. Anim. Sci.* 21 (11): 1680–1688.

3 Nahashon, S.N., Adefope, N., Amenyenu, A. et al. (2009). The effect of floor density on growth performance and carcass characteristics of French Guinea broilers. *Poult. Sci.* 88 (11): 2461–2467.

4 Nahashon, S.N., Aggrey, S.E., Adefope, N.A. et al. (2006). Modeling growth characteristics of meat-type guinea fowl. *Poult. Sci.* 85 (5): 943–946.

5 Tjetjoo, S.U., Moreki, J.C., Nsoso, S.J. et al. (2013). Growth performance of guinea fowl fed diets containing yellow maize, millet and white sorghum as energy sources and raised under intensive system. *Pakistan. J. Nutr.* 12 (4): 306–312.

6 Madzimure, J., Saina, H., and Ngorora, G.P.K. (2011). Market potential for guinea fowl (*Numidia meleagris*) products. *Trop. Anim. Health Prod.* 43 (7): 1509–1515.

7 Yamak, U.S., Sarica, M., Boz, M.A. et al. (2018). Effect of production system (barn and free range) and slaughter age on some production traits of guinea fowl. *Poult. Sci.* 97 (1): 47–53.

8 Musundire, M.T., Halimani, T.E., and Chimonyo, M. (2018). Effect of age and sex on carcass characteristics and internal organ weights of scavenging chickens and helmeted guinea fowls. *J. Appl. Poult. Res.* 46 (1): 860–867.

9 Musundire, M.T., Halimani, T.E., and Chimonyo, M. (2017). Physical and chemical properties of meat from scavenging chickens and helmeted guinea fowls in response to age and sex. *Br. Poult. Sci.* 58 (4): 390–396.

10 Hoffman, L.C. and Tlhong, T.M. (2012). Proximate and fatty acid composition and cholesterol content of different cuts of guinea fowl meat as affected by cooking method. *J. Sci. Food Agric.* 92 (13): 2587–2593.

11 Hughes, B.L. (1980). Consumer evaluation of guineas. *Poult. Sci.* 59 (3): 543–544.

12 Maier, V. and Scheich, H. (1987). Acoustic imprinting in guinea fowl chicks: age dependence of 2-deoxyglucose uptake in relevant forebrain areas. *Devel. Brain Res.* 31: 15–27.

13 Wumbei, D. (2018). Assessment of the usefulness of heterophil-lymphocyte ratios (H/L ratios) and temperament scores as biomarkers of docility of the local guinea fowl (Numida meleagris) varieties in Ghana. Thesis for Degree in Master of Philosophy in Animal Science at the University for Development Studies. Can be found online at www.udsspace.uds.edu.gh.

14 Kimata, D.M., Mwangi, R.W., and Mathiu, P.M. (2014). Confinement lowers fertility rate of helmeted guinea fowl (*Numida meleagris*). *African Zool.* 49 (1): 153–156.

15 Ayeni, J.S.O. (1983). The biology and utilization of helmeted guineafowl (*Numida meleagris galeate* Pallas) in Nigeria. II. Food of helmeted guineafowl in Kainji Lake Basin are of Nigeria. *Afr. J. Ecol.* 21 (1): 1–10.

16 Ratcliffe, C.S. and Crowe, T.M. (2001). Habitat utilization and home range size of helmeted guineafowl in the midlands of KwaZulu-Natal province, South Africa. *Biol. Conserv.* 98: 333–245.

17 Ayeni, J.S.O. (1984). The biology and utilization of helmeted guineafowl (*Numida meleagris galeate* Pallas) in Nigeria. I. the habitat and distribution of guineafowl in the Kainji Lake Basin area, Nigeria. *Afr. J. Ecol.* 22 (1): 1–6.

18 Van Niekerk, J.H. (2010). Social organization of a flock of helmeted guineafowl (*Numida meleagris*) at the Krugersdorp game reserve. *South Africa. Chin. Birds.* 1 (11): 22–29.

19 Saina, H. (2005). Guinea fowl (*Numidia meleagris*) production under smallholder farmer management in Guruve District, Zimbabwe. Master of Philosophy Thesis, University of Zimbabwe, Harare, Zimbabwe.

20 Haruna, E.S., Shamaki, D., Echeonwu, G.O.N. et al. (1993). A natural outbreak of Newcastle disease in guinea fowl (*Numida meleagris galeata*) in Nigeria. *Rev. Sci. Tech. Off. Int. Epiz.* 12 (3): 887–893.

21 Mathivann, B., Kumanan, K., and Mahalinga Nainar, A. (2004). Characterization of a Newcastle disease virus isolated from apparently normal guinea fowl (*Numida melagridis*). *Vet. Res. Commun.* 28 (2): 171–177.

22 Solomon, P., Bisschop, S., Joannis, T.M. et al. (2013). Phylogenetic analysis of Newcastle disease viruses isolated from asymptomatic guinea fowl and Muscovy ducks in Nigeria. *Trop. Ani. Health Produc.* 45: 53–57.

23 Ayim-Akonor, M., Owusu-Ntumy, D.D., Ohene-Asa, H.E. et al. (2018). Serological and molecular surveillance of infections bronchitis virus infection in free-range chickens and guinea fowls in the Ga-east district of Ghana. *J. Vet. Med.* 2018: 4949580.

24 Pascucci, S., Maestrini, N., Govoni, S. et al. (1976). *Mycoplasma synoviae* in the guinea fowl. *Avian. Pathol.* 5 (4): 291–297.

25 Liais, E., Croville, G., Mariette, J. et al. (2014). Novel avian coronavirus and fulminating disease in Guinea fowl. *France. Emerg. Infect. Dis.* 20 (1): 105–108.

26 Okaeme, A.N. (1988). Ectoparasites of guinea fowl (*Numida meleagris galeata* Pallas) and local domestic chicken (*Gallus gallus*) in southern Guinea savanna. *Niger. Vet. Res. Commun.* 12 (4–5): 277–280.

27 Nwagu, B.I. and Alawa, C.B.I. (1995). Guinea fowl production in Nigeria. *World Poult. Sci. J.* 51 (3): 261–270.

28 Cupo, K.L. and Beckstead, R.B. (2019). *Heterakis gallinarum*, the cecal nematode of gallinaceous birds: a critical review. *Avian. Dis.* 63 (3): 381–388.

29 Jones, K.H., Wilson, F.D., Fitzgerald, S.D. et al. (2012). A natural outbreak of clinical toxoplasmosis in a backyard flock of guinea fowl in Mississippi. *Avian. Dis.* 56 (4): 750–753.

30 Vielmo, A., Pena, H.F.J., Panziera, W. et al. (2019). Outbreak of toxoplasmosis in a flock of domestic chickens and guinea fowl. *Parasitol. Res.* 118 (3): 991–997.

31 Dimitrova, D.J., Haritova, A.M., Diney, T.D. et al. (2014). Comparative pharmacokinetics of danofloxacin in common pheasants, guinea fowls and Japanese quails after intravenous and oral administration. *Br. Poult. Sci.* 55 (1): 120–125.

32 De Ruyck, H., Daeseleire, E., Grijspeerdt, K. et al. (2004). Distribution and depletion of flubendazole and its metabolites in edible tissues of guinea fowl. *Br. Poult. Sci.* 45 (4): 540–549.

33 Okaeme, A.N. (1988). Ivermectin in the control of helminthiasis in guinea fowl *Numida meleagris galeata* Pallas. *Vet. Quart.* 10 (1): 70–71.

34 Bhogoju, S., Nahashon, S., Wang, X. et al. (2018). A comparative analysis of microbial profile of guinea fowl and chicken using metagenomic approach. *PLoS One* 13 (3): e0191029.

35 Kilonzo-Nthenge, A., Nahashon, S.N., Chen, F. et al. (2008). Prevalence and antimicrobial resistance of pathogenic bacteria in chicken and guinea fowl. *Poult. Sci.* 87 (9): 1841–1848.

36 Ajadi, R.A., Kasali, O.B., Makinde, A.F. et al. (2009). Effects of midazolam on ketamine-xylazine anesthesia in guinea fowl (*Numida meleagris galeata*). *J. Avian. Med. Surg.* 23 (3): 199–204.

37 Onyeanusi, B.I., Oja, S.A., Ema, A.N. et al. (1986). Occurrence of the right oviduct in the guinea fowl (Numida meleagris). *Br. Poult. Sci.* 27 (3): 481–482.

38 Abdul-Rahman, I.I., Jeffcoate, I., and Obese, F.Y. (2018). Age-related changes in the gross anatomy of the reproductive organs and associated steroid profiles in male and female guinea fowls (*Numida meleagris*). *Vet. Anim. Sci.* 6: 41–49.

39 Abdul-Rahman, I.I., Obese, F.Y., and Jeffcoate, I.A. (2017). Developmental changes in the histological structure of the testes, and testosterone profiles in male guinea fowls (*Numida meleagris*). *Theriogenology* 101: 114–122.

40 Oke, O.E., Adejuyigbe, A.E., Idowu, O.P. et al. (2015). Effects of housing system on reproductive and physiological response of guinea fowl (*Numida meleagris*). *J. Appl. Anim. Sci.* 8 (1): 47–55.

41 Ancel, A. and Girard, H. (1992). Eggshell of the domestic guinea fowl. *Br. Poult. Sci.* 33 (5): 993–1001.

42 Petersen, J. and Tyler, C. (1967). The strength of guinea fowl (*Numida meleagris*) egg shells. *Br. Poult. Sci.* 7 (4): 291–296.

43 Panheleux, M., Kalin, O., Gautron, J. et al. (1999). Features of eggshell formation in guinea fowl: kinetics of shell deposition, uterine protein secretion and uterine histology. *Br. Poult. Sci.* 40 (5): 632–643.

44 Eleroğlu, H., Yıldırım, A., Duman, M., and Okur, N. (2016). Effect of eggshell color on the egg characteristics and hatchability of guinea fowl (Numida meleagris) eggs. *Braz. J. Poult. Sci.* 18 (Special Issue): 61–68.

45 Yamak, U.S., Boz, M.A.I., Ucar, A.I.I. et al. (2016). Effect of eggshell thickness on hatchability of guinea fowl and pheasants. *Braz. J. Poult. Sci.* 18 (Special Issue 2): 53–58.

46 Hudson, G.H., Omprakash, A.V., and Premavalli, K. (2016). Effect of semen diluents, dilution rates and storage periods on live and abnormal spermatozoa of pearl guinea fowls. *Asian J. Anim.Vet. Adv.* 11 (7): 411–416.

47 Premavalli, K. (2013). Influence of strain, age and system of management on the productive and reproductive performance of guinea fowl. PhD Thesis, Tamil Nadu Veterinary and Animal Sciences University, Chennai.

48 Wolc, A. and Olori, V.E. (2009). Genetics of hatchability and egg quality from the perspective of a chick. 6th European Poultry Genetics Symposium, Bedlewo, Poland.

49 Obike, O.M., Nwachukwu, E.N., and Ukewulonu, I.E. (2014). Effect of strain and associations of some fertility and hatchability traits of indigenous guinea fowls raised in the rain-forest zone of south-East Nigeria. *Global J. Anim. Breed. Genet.* 2 (7): 98–102.

50 Aryee, Z.G. (2016). Effects of strain and non-genetic factors on growth and reproduction, egg quality, and carcass characteristics of indigenous guinea fowl (*Numida meleagris*). Master Thesis in Animal Science (Animal breeding and genetics), University of Education, College of Agriculture Education, Department of Animal Science Education, Winneba, Ghana.

51 Mohan, J., Sharma, S.K., Kolluri, G. et al. (2016). Semen quality characteristics and seasonality in different varieties of male guinea fowl. *Adv. Anim. Vet. Sci.* 4 (6): 320–325.

52 Sellier, N., Brillard, J.-P., Dupuy, V. et al. (2006). Comparative staging of embryo development in chicken, turkey, duck, goose, guinea fowl, and Japanese quail assessed from five hours after fertilization through seventy-two hours of incubation. *J. Appl. Poult. Res.* 15 (2): 219–228.

53 Ogwuegbu, S.O., Aire, T.A., and Adeyemo, O. (1988). Egg laying pattern of the semi-domesticated helmeted guinea fowl (*Numida meleagris galeata*). *Br. Poult. Sci.* 29 (1): 171–174.

54 Hudson, G.H., Omprakash, A.V., Premavalli, K. et al. (2017). Quantifying sperm egg interaction to assess the breeding efficiency through artificial insemination in guinea fowls. *Br. Poult. Sci.* 58 (2): 192–199.

55 Blesbois, E., Grasseau, I., and Seigneurin, F. (2005). Membrane fluidity and the ability of domestic bird spermatozoa to survive cryopreservation. *Reproduction* 129 (3): 371–378.

56 Keerthy, A.J., Omprakash, A.V., Churchill, R.R. et al. (2016). Effect of semen diluents, dilution rates, and storage periods on spermatozoa motility of different varieties of guinea fowl. *J. Vet. Sci. Technol.* 7 (6).

57 Seigneurin, F., Grasseau, I., Chapuis, H. et al. (2013). An efficient method of guinea fowl sperm cryopreservation. *Poult. Sci.* 92 (11): 2988–2996.

58 Njiforti, H.L. (1997). The breeding performance of wild helmeted guineafowl (*Numida meleagris galeata* Pallas) in the Waza national park, North Cameroon. *Rev. Ecol. (Terre Vie)* 52 (2): 173–186.

59 Hughes, B.L. (1986). Effects of temperature on reproduction in guinea fowl. *Poult. Sci.* 65 (1): 186–189.

60 Kyere, C.G., Korankye, O., Duodu, A. et al. (2020). Effect of different lighting regime on growth and reproductive performance of the guinea fowl (*Numida meleagris*). *World J. Adv. Res. Rev.* 7 (2): 294–302.

61 Okyere, K., Kagya-Agyemang, J.W., Annor, S.Y. et al. (2020). Influence of season and day length on production and reproductive traits and egg characteristics of the guinea fowl (*Numida meleagris*). *Asian J. Res. Zool.* 3 (1): 26–34.

62 Keïta, A., Mangart, J.M., Oizel, J.M. et al. (2015). Effects of different lighting sources on the performance and carcass quality of guinea fowl broilers (Effets du type de source lumineuse sur les performances et la qualite de carcasse chez la pintade). Conference poster at Actes des 11èmes Journées de la Recherche Avicole et Palmipèdes à Foie Gras, Tours, France. March 25–26.

63 Ahiagbe, K.M.J., Kayang, B.B., Naazie, A. et al. (2018). Comparison of vent sexing and polymerase chain reaction for reliable sex determination in guinea fowls. *Ghana J. Agric. Sci.* 52: 17–23.

64 Prinsloo, H.C., Harley, V., Reilly, B.K. et al. (2005). Sex-related variation in morphology of helmeted guineafowl (Numida meleagris) from the Riemland of the northeastern Freestate, South Africa. *S. African J. Wildlife Res.* 35 (1): 95–96.

65 Abdul-Rahman, I.I., Awumbila, B., Jeffcoate, I.A. et al. (2015). Sexing in guinea fowls (*Numida meleagris*). *Poult. Sci.* 94 (2): 311–318.

66 Warren, D.C. (1925). Inheritance of rate of feathering in poultry. *J. Heredity* 16 (1): 13–18.

67 Asmundson, V.S. and Abbott, U.K. (1961). Dominant sex-linked late feathering in Turkey. *J. Heredity* 52 (3): 99–104.

68 Pal, S.K. and Singh, H. (1997). Inheritance of wing feather development rate in guinea fowl (*Numida meleagris*). *Br. Poult. Sci.* 38 (3): 245–248.

69 Resnick, R.M., Boyce-Jacino, M.T., Fu, O. et al. (1990). Phylogenetic distribution of the novel avian endogenous provirus family. *J. Virol.* 64 (10): 4640–4643.

70 Ancel, A., Armand, J., and Girard, H. (1994). Optimum incubation conditions of the domestic guinea fowl egg. *Br. Poult. Sci.* 35 (2): 227–240.

71 Kouame, Y.A.E., Nideou, D., Kouakou, K. et al. (2019). Effect of guinea fowl egg storage duration on embryonic and physiological parameters, and keet juvenile growth. *Poult. Sci.* 98 (11): 6046–6052.

72 Kouassi, G.F., Koné, G.A., Good, M. et al. (2019). Factors impacting guinea fowl (*Numida meleagris*) production in Ivory Coast. *J. Appl. Poult. Res.* 28 (4): 1382–1388.

73 Nahashon, S.N., Adefope, N., and Wright, D. (2011). Effect of floor density on growth performance of pearl grey guinea fowl replacement pullets. *Poult. Sci.* 90 (6): 1371–1378.

74 Oke, O.O., Oso, A., Iyasere, O.S. et al. (2020). Growth performance and physiological responses of helmeted guinea fowl (*Numida meleagris*) to different stocking densities in humid tropic environment. *Agricult. Trop. Subtrop* 53 (1): 5–12.

75 Nahashon, S.N., Adefope, N.A., Amenyenu, A. et al. (2006). Laying performance of pearl gray guinea fowl hens as affected by caging density. *Poult. Sci.* 85 (9): 1682–1689.

76 Baeza, E., Juin, H., Rebours, G. et al. (2001). Effect of genotype, sex and rearing temperature on carcase and meat quality of Guinea fowl. *Br. Poult. Sci.* 42 (4): 470–476.

77 Nahashon, S.N., Aggrey, S.E., Adefope, N.A. et al. (2006). Growth characteristics of pearl gray guinea fowl as predicted by the Richards, Gompertz and Logistic Models. *Poult. Sci.* 85 (2): 359–363.

78 Sales, J., Du Preez, J.J., and Van Niekerk, S.A. (1997). Chemical composition of the pearl grey guinea fowl. *Br. Poult. Sci.* 38 (2): 223–224.

79 Laird, A.K. (1964). Dynamics of tumor growth. *Br. J. Cancer* 13 (3): 490–502.

80 Nahashon, S.N., Aggrey, S.E., Adefope, N.A. et al. (2010). Gompertz–Laird model prediction of optimum utilization of crude protein and metabolizable energy by French guinea fowl broilers. *Poult. Sci.* 89 (1): 52–57.

81 Nelson, K. (2013). Evaluation of lysine requirement of the French guinea fowl broiler. Master Thesis at Tennessee State University.

82 Johnson, D. (2015). Evaluation of methionine and cysteine requirements of the French guinea fowl broiler. Master Thesis at Tennessee State University.

83 Nwokolo, E. (1986). A comparison of metabolizable energy content of eight common feed ingredients determined with young guinea fowls (keets) and pullet chicks. *Anim. Feed Sci. Technol.* 15 (1): 1–6.

84 Bedi, P.S., Bedi, S.P.S., Singh, H., and Agarwal, R.K. (1998). Biochemical effects of dietary aflatoxin in guineafowl. *Toxicol. Lett.* 95 (suppl 1): 180.

85 Tufarelli, V., Khan, R.U., and Laudadio, V. (2011). Feed intake in guinea fowl, layer hen and pheasant as influenced by particle size of pelleted diets. *Int. J. Poult. Sci.* 10 (3): 238–240.

86 Chagneau, A.M., Quentin, M., Lescoat, P., and Bouvarel, I. (2011). How guinea fowl react during feed change-over? Poster presented at the Actes des 9èmes Journées de la Recherche Avicole, Tours, France, March 29–30.

87 Price, A.K. (2004). The use of biological controls for vector-borne diseases: The case of guinea fowl and Lyme disease. Undergraduate Ecology Research Reports. www.caryinstitute.org/sites/default/files/public/reprints/Price_2004_REU.pdf (accessed February 2022).

88 Barbour, A.G. and Fish, D. (1993). The biological and social phenomenon of Lyme disease. *Science* 260 (5114): 1610–1616.

89 Duffy, D.C., Downer, R., and Brinkley, C. (1992). The effectiveness of helmeted guineafowl in the control of the deer tick, the vector of Lyme disease. *Wilson Bull.* 104 (2): 342–345.

90 Şekercioğlu, C.H. (2013). Guinea fowl, ticks and Crimean-Congo hemorrhagic fever in Turkey: the perfect storm? *Trend. Parasitol.* 29 (1): 1–2.

91 Bhogoju, S., Nahashon, S.N., Donker, J. et al. (2017). Effect of varying dietary concentrations of lysine on growth of pearl grey guinea fowl. *Poult. Sci.* 96 (5): 1306–1315.

18

Exhibition Galliformes
Abigail Duvall

The bright colors and flashy breeding displays of pheasants have long attracted interest in keeping them in captivity. Peacocks have likely been kept for thousands of years in India, with records of an Indian Emperor living in 320 CE coming from a family of "peacock tamers." There are records of both peacocks and ring-necked pheasants being kept in medieval times in Europe [1]. Other Asian pheasant species appear to have arrived in Europe in the mid eighteenth century, with golden pheasants arriving by 1740. The same species was later kept in the United States at Mount Vernon by George Washington around 1787 [1]. By the Victorian era, pheasants were popular in avicultural collections and treatises on their care and management were written with a mix of natural history and husbandry [2]. They continue to be popular in aviculture today.

Pheasants are almost entirely Asiatic in origin, with species inhabiting a diverse array of habitats ranging from lush tropical forests to frigid, sparsely vegetated montane slopes [3]. There is a single African species, the Congo peafowl (*Afropavo congensis*). Human movements and translocations of species have led to stable feral populations of Indian peafowl worldwide. In the United Kingdom, there are feral populations of Reeves's and golden pheasants.

Ornamental pheasants are generally those other than the ring-necked pheasant, which is raised as a gamebird in the United States. Ornamental pheasant species kept in aviculture can be paradoxically common in captivity but rare in the wild – the Edwards's pheasant (*Lophura edwardsi*) is likely extinct in Vietnam yet is easily obtained in aviculture. In contrast, blood pheasants (*Ithaginis cruentis*) are not uncommon in the wild yet are rare in aviculture. There are 16 total genera of pheasants, but not all are commonly kept.

Ruffed pheasants are extremely common in captivity and include the Lady Amherst (*Chrysolophus amherstiae*) and the golden pheasant (*Chrysolophus pictus*) (Figures 18.1 and 18.2). In the yearly census performed by the World Pheasant Association, the golden is generally the best represented species of pheasant behind the Indian peafowl. This brightly colored species is quite hardy, and has several color morphs which have been attained through captive breeding [4].

The genus *Gallus* contains the junglefowl, of which there are four species. The ancestor of the domestic chicken, the red junglefowl (*Gallus gallus*) is considered an ornamental pheasant and is kept in many collections. In individuals not genetically contaminated with domestic chickens, the males undergo a molt into a drabber "eclipse" plumage outside the breeding season.

Gamebird Medicine and Management, First Edition. Edited by Teresa Y. Morishita and Robert E. Porter, Jr.
© 2023 John Wiley & Sons, Inc. Published 2023 by John Wiley & Sons, Inc.

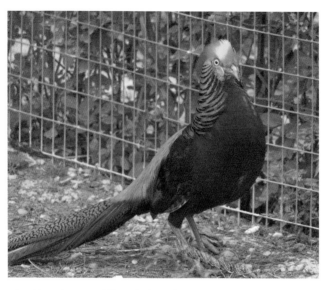

Figure 18.1   Male red golden pheasant (*Chrysolophus pictus*).

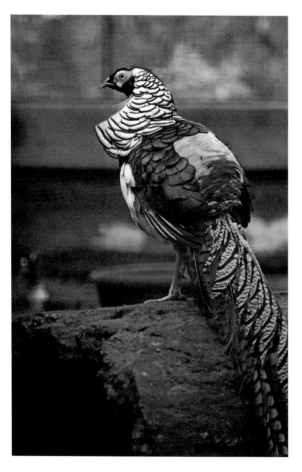

Figure 18.2   Male Lady Amherst's pheasant (*Chrysolophus amherstiae*). Source: Photo courtesy of Katie Lubbock.

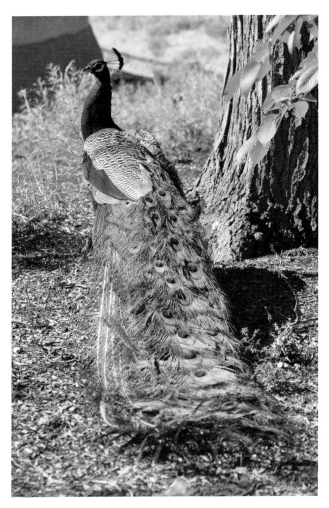

Figure 18.3   Free-roaming adult male Indian peafowl (*Pavo cristatus*).

There are three species of peafowl within two different genera. The Indian peafowl (*Pavo crista-tus*) is likely the most commonly kept ornamental pheasant species worldwide (Figure 18.3). There are many different color and pattern mutations that have been developed, and the United Peafowl Association recognizes an impressive 225 such varieties. Birds which are descendants of hybrids between Indian peafowl and green peafowl (*Pavo muticus*) are called Spalding. The green peafowl is much less commonly kept in captivity than the Indian peafowl. The Congo peafowl (*A. congensis*) is primarily kept within zoological collections.

Other common species include the silver pheasant (*Lophura nycthemera*), Reeves's pheasant (*Syrmaticus reevesii*), Temminck's tragopan (*Tragopan temminkcii*), and gray peacock pheasant (*Polyplectron bicalcaratum*) (Figures 18.4–18.6).

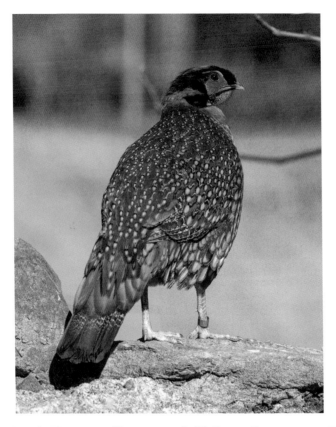

Figure 18.4   Male Temminck's tragopan (*Tragopan temminckii*). Source: Photo courtesy of Katie Lubbock.

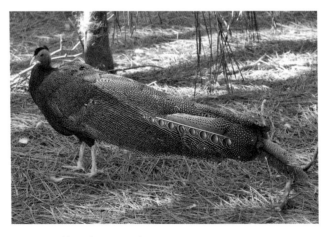

Figure 18.5   Male great argus (*Argusianus argus*).

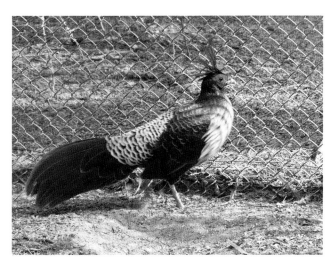

Figure 18.6   Male kalij pheasant (*Lophura leucomelanos*).

18.1   Husbandry

Many ornamental pheasant species are inexpensive, easily obtained, and somewhat hardy. All are generally kept in large, planted aviaries, the layout of which may vary depending on the temperament of the species. Indian peafowl are an exception and are often allowed to free roam. It is common for many different species to be kept at a single facility. A visual barrier is often placed from the ground to about 18–24 in. in height between adjacent aviaries to prevent fighting between pens and reduce pacing.

In designing aviaries, the hardiness of the species being kept is generally taken into account. Many species of pheasants do well even in extremely low temperatures, but species with tropical distributions such as the crested fireback (*Lophura ignita*), peacock pheasants (*Polyplectron* spp.), and argus (*Argusianus argus*) are sensitive to cold and must be offered heated shelter in winter to prevent frostbite or death [5].

Some pheasant species may be destructive in a planted aviary, as they tend to dig. The eared pheasants (*Crossoptilon* spp.), cheer (*Catreus wallichii*), and monals (*Lophophorus* spp.) are especially well known for this [5]. The use of wire mesh close to the floor of the aviary may help protect grass from destruction.

Hybridization is a significant concern in ornamental pheasant species and care should be taken that members of closely related species are not kept together as hybrids within and between different genera are reported. The most common hybrid is likely that of the golden and Lady Amherst pheasants (*C. pictus x Chrysolophus amherstiae*) and many individuals presented as representatives of these species may carry genes of the other from past hybridization. Silver pheasants (*L. nycthemera*) have been reported to hybridize with other *Lophura* and the Swinhoe's pheasant (*Lophura swinhoii*) has been reported to hybridize with the copper pheasant (*Syrmaticus soemmerringii*) and cheer (*C. wallichii*) [4]. The Reeves's pheasant (*S. reevesii*) has hybridized with the cheer, silver, ring-necked (*Phasianus* spp.) and golden pheasant [4].

Specific research into the dietary requirements of ornamental pheasants is generally not available and captive diets may vary widely between aviculturalists. Aviculturalists will base captive diets upon inferences drawn from the natural history of the species and recommendations from others who have successfully kept the same species. Most captive pheasants are maintained on diets based around pelleted feeds designed for poultry, with a seasonal rotation of the type of pellet offered. Breeder pellets of 17–20% protein may be offered during the breeding season, while a maintenance pellet of 13–15% protein may be used outside this season. Chicks are generally started on a high-protein crumble of 28–30% protein, which is dropped to a grower ration of 20–24% protein when about 1 month old and eventually they are placed on a maintenance pellet by the fall, along with the adults [5].

Some species may have a greater preference for fresh greens and vegetables or insects and this can serve as good dietary enrichment. In a study evaluating the impact of the consumption of fresh green vegetables on golden pheasant egg production, egg yolk antioxidants and fecal corticosterone, diets containing 5.0% greens led to higher egg production and egg yolk antioxidant content and lower fecal corticosterone compared to diets containing 1.4% or 2.7% greens [6]. A similar study revealed that 5.0% greens in the diet led to increased retention of carotenoids, nitrogen, calcium, and zinc in golden pheasants compared to those eating diets with a lower percentage of greens [7].

18.2   Breeding and Rearing of Ornamental Pheasants

It is important to take the natural history of any exotic pheasant species into account when attempting to breed them. In some species, the male may be aggressive toward the hen and it is important to offer the hen the ability to hide from the male to prevent injury or death. Pheasants of the genus *Syrmaticus* and some from the genus *Lophura* are especially known for this (Figure 18.7) [5]. Well-planted aviaries help the hen to seek shelter from the cock, and some breeders advise clipping the primary feathers of one wing on the male prior to the breeding season. Aggression can also extend toward human keepers and care should be taken when entering an aviary with breeding males of some species.

In most avicultural collections, eggs are pulled for artificial incubation rather than allowing incubation by the adults. In part, this is because pairs are rarely separated following laying and for most species the continued presence of the male during incubation is not part of their natural history

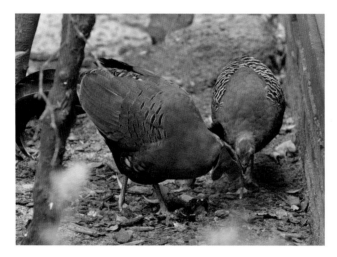

Figure 18.7   A pair of Siamese firebacks (*Lophura diardi*) in a planted aviary. Many male *Lophura* pheasants can become aggressive toward females.

and can lead to accidental injury of an incubating hen or newly hatched chicks. Cheer pheasants and many *Lophura* species may be the exception to this, as males will help brood chicks. In addition, in well-planted aviaries the status of the chicks cannot easily be monitored, and hazards such as vermin and bad weather can lead to the loss of chicks. If parent birds are allowed to rear chicks, it is important to ensure that the aviary is made as safe as possible for them. Restricting access to portions of the aviary, creating "ladders" to roosting perches, and modifying food and water sources may be necessary [8].

It is important to carefully store eggs in a clean environment prior to incubation. The use of a dedicated incubation room is recommended to allow the temperature and humidity inside the room to be held constant. Many different models of incubators are available, with standard forced-air incubators being most commonly used. More recently, contact incubators which distribute heat through a warm air-filled membrane in contact with the dorsal surface of the egg have also become available and their use is increasing (Figure 18.8). Incubation is generally similar to that of domestic chicken eggs, but incubation times vary between species. This difference should be taken into account when setting eggs to ensure that eggs are moved to a hatcher at an appropriate time, especially when eggs from multiple species are being incubated in the same incubator. Some eggs may lose weight at variable rates, especially when those from montane and tropical species are set at the same time. Some breeders may keep several incubators with higher or lower humidity settings to move eggs among these incubators as needed to adjust for rates of weight loss from the eggs during incubation.

The use of broody bantam chicken hens to start pheasant eggs prior to placement in an incubator or allowing the hens to hatch out the eggs is not uncommon and should be considered when evaluating the health of a collection. Broody hens can unintentionally transmit infectious disease to the pheasants being hatched under them.

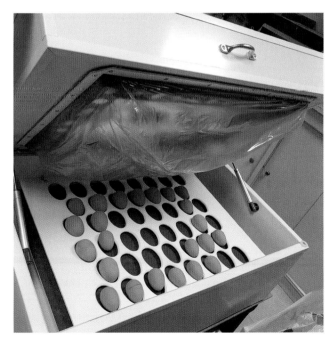

Figure 18.8 A contact incubator with thin air-filled membrane in the upper lid which becomes filled with warm air when closed.

Pheasant chicks are precocial, yet chicks of some species may be difficult to start eating. Use of a "teacher chick," usually a slightly older pheasant chick or domestic chicken chick, aids in the prevention of loss from starvation of maladapted chicks. In some species, such as peacock pheasants, the female usually feeds the chick directly from the beak and they can therefore be especially difficult to get started eating [8]. Most chicks are generally reared in wire-floored brooders to allow them to easily be kept clean. Food items offered to chicks can vary widely between species and between aviculturalists. In more difficult species, addition of crumbled egg yolk, live insect larvae, finely chopped greens, and a "teacher chick" may be used to start chicks on a poultry crumble.

18.3   Medical Concerns

Peer-reviewed reports of disease in exotic galliform species are relatively rare, but as the domestic chicken is itself a pheasant species and many infectious diseases of poultry have been reported in peafowl and other pheasants, they should be considered susceptible to the same. Most aviculturalists will generally request food- or water-based medications as catching individual pheasants for daily treatment is generally not practical and can cause excessive stress in sensitive species. However, water-based medication may deter some birds from drinking. If there is a known food item readily accepted by the individual pheasant as a treat, medication can be hidden within it [8].

Sinusitis is especially common in species which tend to dig, including the eared pheasants, monals, and cheer. *Mycoplasma gallisepticum* has been reported as a cause of sinusitis in ornamental pheasants and clinical signs included coughing, sneezing, infraorbital swelling, rales, muscle wasting, and death [9]. Various Gram-negative bacterial pathogens, including an *Escherichia coli* sinusitis in several Reeves's pheasants, have been cultured from ornamental pheasants with sinusitis by the author.

Peafowl may be particularly susceptible to infection by *Mycobacterium* spp. In contrast to other species, they may display more respiratory signs when infected rather than gastrointestinal signs [10, 11]. However, cachexia without respiratory signs has also been reported [12]. Due to difficulty in treatment and concerns for zoonosis, strongly suspected or confirmed cases are generally euthanized.

Ornamental pheasants may have variable susceptibility to *Histomonas meleagridis.* Experimental infections in peafowl suggest they may be particularly susceptible [13]. Clinical signs in infected peafowl were nonspecific and included apathy, anorexia, yellow or pale stool, bruising of the head, and death. Necrotizing typhlitis and hepatitis were found on postmortem examination. It is not recommended to keep chickens with ornamental pheasants to help reduce spread of this parasite. Birds in grass-floored aviaries are most susceptible to infection by consumption of earthworms.

Other internal and external parasites common in domestic chickens can accidentally be spread to ornamental pheasants. Scaly leg mites can be of particular concern when broody hens are used to rear young pheasant chicks. Some breeders will preventively deworm pheasants once or twice yearly with water-based poultry medications.

Monals or impeyan pheasants (*Lophophorus impeyanus*) may be particularly susceptible to West Nile virus. In a compilation of species of dead birds in which West Nile virus has been detected in the United States from 1999 to 2016, only the monal, blue-eared and ring-necked pheasants are reported among hundreds of species (www.cdc.gov/westnile/resources/pdfs/BirdSpecies1999-2016.pdf). Anecdotally, aviculturalists report them to be susceptible to this virus. West Nile virus was the cause of an acute mortality event which killed 15 juvenile monals in 2 weeks, with necropsy revealing cecal ulcers and hemorrhage at the gastric isthmus [14]. Preventive vaccination for West Nile virus may be worthwhile in this species.

Monals are also the only pheasant species in which natural infection with avian bornavirus has been reported [15]. The affected individual developed weakness, chronic wasting, and ataxia before dying. Postmortem findings included degenerative encephalopathy, nonsuppurative encephalitis, and lymphoplasmacytic myenteric ganglioneuritis. The source of the infection was believed to be an infected caique living within the same collection. Mixing monals with psittacines in mixed enclosures is not recommended.

There is concern that those pathogens that cause mild or asymptomatic infections in domestic poultry could cause illness in ornamental species. In one collection, eight mountain peacock pheasants (*Polyplectron inopinatum*), three Malayan peacock pheasants (*Polyplectron malacense*), and one Congo peafowl were found to have died from a phasianid herpesvirus most closely related to gallid herpesvirus 3, a nonpathogenic virus commonly used as a vaccine against gallid herpesvirus 2, or Marek disease [16]. The close genetic relation of the newly identified herpesvirus to one commonly used in vaccination raises concern for potential accidental morbidity or mortality from vaccination strains used in domestic species, though this has not yet been observed.

In young pheasants, bent or curled toes are not uncommon and can be corrected by splinting if caught early [8]. Perosis developed in an entire clutch of golden pheasants raised by the author following a change in the starter diet used and was believed to be nutritional in origin. Attempts at conservative management were unsuccessful.

Pheasants are generally long-lived and many individuals may approach 20 years of age. There is limited information about the care of geriatric individuals available. Normal electrocardiograms have been described in the red golden and silver pheasant and may be of use when cardiac disease is suspected [17]. Neoplasia is poorly reported in ornamental pheasants, but the order Galliformes has a relatively high prevalence of neoplasia compared to other orders. There is a single report of a leiomyosarcoma on the wing of a geriatric Vieilott's fireback (*Lophura rufa*) [18].

18.4 Aviculture in Conservation

Captive ornamental pheasants may be useful in serving as genetic reservoirs for those species which are endangered or extinct in the wild. However, genetic analysis of some captive populations of such threatened species has revealed loss of genetic diversity compared to wild populations [19–21]. To prevent loss of captive diversity, studbooks have been established for several species to help guide breeding. Individuals in zoological collections are generally given breeding recommendations under species survival plans.

Of extant pheasant species, there is one critically endangered species, the Edwards's pheasant (Figure 18.9). This species is believed to be extinct in the wild, making captive breeding critical to its continued survival. The green peafowl (*P. muticus*), crested argus (*Rheinardia ocellata*), Bornean peacock-pheasant (*Polyplectron schleiermacheri*), and Hainan peacock pheasant (*Polyplectron katsumatae*) are all considered endangered. Captive populations of all these species exist, though some are more numerous than others. Many other pheasant species are considered vulnerable.

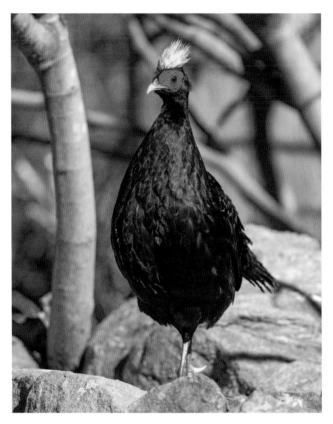

Figure 18.9 The Edward'ss pheasant (*Lophura edwardsi*) is likely extinct in the wild, making captive breeding essential to its conservation. Source: Photo courtesy of Katie Lubbock.

Threats to wild pheasants generally relate to hunting, habitat loss, degradation, or fragmentation. Increased human activity not directly altering the environment, such as seasonal mushroom harvesting, may also play a large role in decreasing nesting success in some sensitive species [22]. Hybridization can also be an important cause of decline and is of special concern in the red junglefowl, where hybridization with domestic chickens is common. Tropical species are at special risk for habitat loss, especially in island species.

18.5 Further Resources

There are many organizations which have been developed to help share information related to the captive husbandry and wild conservation of pheasants. In the USA, there are many smaller regional pheasant and/or wildfowl breeding associations, especially on the East Coast. Such organizations are an important source of information on captive husbandry and breeding of ornamental pheasants, and surplus breeding stock is often exchanged among members of these groups.

- World Pheasant Association: www.pheasant.org.uk
- American Pheasant and Waterfowl Society: https://apwsbirds.com.
- United Peafowl Association: https://unitedpeafowlassociation.org

References

1 Svanberg, I. (2007). Golden pheasants (*Chrysolophus pictus*) in Sweden in the 1740s. *Zool. Garten. NF* 77 (1): 24–28.

2 Tegetmeier, W.M. (1881). *Pheasants: Their Natural History and Practical Management*. London: Horace Cox.

3 Delacour, J. (1951). *The Pheasants of the World*. London: Country Life Ltd.

4 Brown, D. (1998). *A Guide to Pheasants and Waterfowl, their Management, Care and Breeding*. South Tweed Heads, NSW: ABK Publications.

5 Howman, K.C.R. (1996). *Introduction to Ornamental Pheasants*. Blaine, WA: Hancock House.

6 Kullu, S.S., Das, A., Bajpai, S.K. et al. (2017). Egg production performance, egg yolk antioxidant profile and excreta concentration of corticosterone in golden pheasants (*Chrysolophus pictus*) fed diets containing different levels of green vegetables. *J. Anim. Physiol. Anim. Nutr.* 101 (5): e31–e42.

7 Kullu, S.S., Das, A., Saini, M. et al. (2016). Increasing the dietary supply of carotenoids through forage supplementation: effect on nitrogen and mineral retention in captive golden pheasants (*Chrysolophus pictus*). *Zoo Biol.* 35 (6): 522–532.

8 Corder, J. (2011). *Breeding and Managing Pheasants*. Newcastle upon Tyne, UK: World Pheasant Association.

9 De Oliviera, L.G.S., Boabaid, F.M., Lorenzett, M.P. et al. (2017). Outbreaks of Mycoplasmosis and Histomoniasis in a southern Brazilian flock of ornamental birds. *Acta Sci. Vet.* 45 (Suppl 1): 200.

10 Kul, O., Tunca, R., Haziroglu, R. et al. (2005). An outbreak of avian tuberculosis in peafowl (*Pavo cristatus*) and pheasants (*Phasianus colchicus*) in a zoological aviary in Turkey. *Vet. Med. Czech.* 50 (10): 446–450.

11 Ledwon, A., Augustynowicz-Kopec, E., Parniewski, P. et al. (2018). Mycobacteriosis in peafowl: analysis of four cases. *Med. Weter.* 74 (12): 772–776.

12 Oh, Y., Lee, S.-J., Tark, D.-B. et al. (2021). *Mycobacterium genavense* induced mycobacteriosis in an Indian peafowl (*Pavo cristatus*). *Korean J. Vet. Serv.* 44 (2): 119–124.

13 Clarke, L.L., Beckstead, R.B., Hayes, J.R. et al. (2017). Pathologic and molecular characterization of histomoniasis in peafowl (*Pavo cristatus*). *J. Vet. Diagn. Invest.* 29 (2): 237–241.

14 Wunschmann, A. and Ziegler, A. (2006). West Nile virus-associated mortality events in domestic chukar partridges (*Alectoris chukar*) and domestic Impeyan pheasants (*Lophophorus impeyanus*). *Avian Dis.* 50 (3): 456–459.

15 Bourque, L., Laniesse, D., Beaufrere, H. et al. (2015). Identification of avian bornavirus in a Himalayan monal (*Lophophorus impejanus*) with neurological disease. *Avian Pathol.* 44 (4): 323–327.

16 Seimon, T.A., McAloose, D., and Raphael, B. (2012). A novel herpesvirus in three species of pheasants: mountain peacock pheasant (*Polyplectron inopinatum*), Malayan peacock pheasant (*Polyplectron malacense*), and Congo peafowl (*Afropavo congensis*). *Vet. Pathol.* 49 (3): 482–491.

17 Hassanpour, H., Zarei, H., Nasiri, L. et al. (2018). Electrocardiogram analysis of the golden (*Chrysolophus pictus*) and silver (*Lophura nycthemera*) pheasants. *J. Zoo Wildl. Med.* 49 (4): 881–886.

18 Zordan, M.A., Garner, M., Smedley, R. et al. (2017). Leiomyosarcoma of the wing in a Vieilott's Fireback pheasant (*Lophura rufa*). *J. Avian Med. Surg.* 31 (2): 152–155.

19 Thintip, J., Singchat, W., Ahmad, S. et al. (2021). Reduced genetic variability in a captive-bred population of the endangered Hume's pheasant (Syrmaticus humiae, Hume 1881) revealed by microsatellite genotyping and D-loop sequencing. *PLoS One* 16 (8): e0256573.

20 Jiang, P.-P., Lang, Q.-L., Fang, S.-G. et al. (2005). A genetic diversity comparison between captive individuals and wild individuals of Elliot's pheasant (Syrmaticus ellioti) using mitochondrial DNA. *J. Zhejiang Univ. Sci. B* 6 (5): 413–417.

21 Mukesh, M., Garg, S., Javed, R. et al. (2016). Genetic evaluation of ex situ conservation projects of cheer pheasant (*Catreus wallichii*) and Western Tragopan (*Tragopan melanocephalus*) in India. *Zoo Biol.* 35 (3): 269–273.

22 Fuller, R.A. and Garson, P.J. (2000). *Pheasants: Status Survey and Conservation Action Plan 2000–2004*. Cambridge, UK: IUCN.

19

Peafowl

Teresa Y. Morishita, Linda G. Flores, and Steven E. Benscheidt

The peafowl has long been treasured for its great beauty. It is the Indian blue peafowl species, which originated in Asia, that is the most depicted of all the peafowl species in both art and literature. The Indian blue peafowl is also the species most dispersed throughout the world. It was hypothesized that the peafowl was brought to Europe during the March of Alexander the Great [1]. However, during this same time period, the Greek philosopher Aristotle referred to the peafowl as a common bird in Greece so many scientists believe that the peafowl was most likely introduced in 450 BCE [1]. Hence, it is thought that the peafowl became established in the Roman Empire and ancient Greece. Peafowl are also referenced in Biblical times and reports of peafowl being brought in ships to King Solomon demonstrate the trade of this beautiful bird [1, 2]. In ancient Rome, the peafowl was a great delicacy as a roast and served in its own feathers [3]. This trend continued to England and the rest of the European continent.

19.1 Peafowl as a Gamebird

Many individuals would not even imagine that the ornate peafowl was hunted as a gamebird. These ornamental birds with beautiful tail feathers originated on the Asian continent, where they are still admired in many Asian countries. The peafowl is revered as the national bird in India. However, as their distribution spread globally with trade routes, populations of these beautiful and exotic birds became established on many other continents. Some of the earliest records of peafowl being a gamebird were documented in medieval England. Being far from its native habitat, it was considered an exotic creature and was valued by wealthy individuals and considered a luxury item where it was featured and served in elaborate feasts for these wealthy households. The preparation for serving peafowl entailed the freshly killed bird being skinned while keeping intact its head and neck, along with its body feathers and elaborate tail feathers. After the bird was cooked, these parts were replaced on the cooked bird to resemble a live peacock. The dish was referred to as peacock pie and can be viewed in oil paintings such as the 1627 "Still Life with Peacock Pie" by Dutch artist Pieter Claesz (Figure 19.1) at the National Gallery of Art in Washington, DC (USA) [4]. This artwork provided documentation that peafowl were indeed served as a meal.

As one of the authors (TYM) experienced, such a display was recreated in the Bracebridge Dinner, a long-held annual Christmas tradition, at the historic Ahwahnee Hotel in Yosemite National Park (California, USA). This event recreates a seventeenth-century English manor where guests are

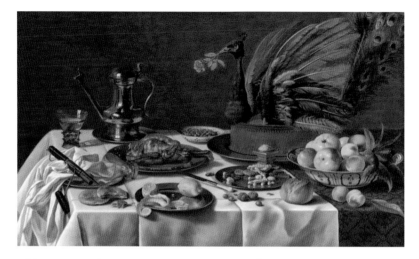

Figure 19.1   Oil painting by Dutch artist Pieter Claesz entitled "Still Life with Peacock Pie, 1627" which depicts a sumptuous feast with some of the most extravagant foods available in the Netherlands in the early seventeenth century [4]. The painting features a large peacock pie decorated with its own feathers, a delicacy, to celebrate a special occasion [4]. Source: Courtesy of the National Galley of Art, Washington, D.C., made possible by The Lee and Juliet Folger Fund.

invited to the Christmas celebration with a menu featuring "peacock pie" [5]. Hence, in medieval Europe, the peafowl was hunted as a gamebird for special feasts. While peacock was not served, the Bracebridge Dinner guests had a live experience of what these magnificent feasts may have entailed as these special dishes were presented in all their natural beauty (Figure 19.2).

Currently, peafowl are not commercially raised in large numbers for hunting purposes, as with other gamebirds. However, some private aviculturists do breed them to develop new color varieties and to help perpetuate more threatened species, like the green peafowl. Other private owners also harvest the feathers and utilize eggs and meat, which can be sold in small-scale gourmet exotic meat markets.

While there are peafowl enthusiasts who raise and breed birds in captivity, most public inter-actions with peafowl are with the free-living birds. In fact, some once captive populations have escaped and have been successful living a semi-feral life. Some populations have been overly suc-cessful, and with no predators in neighborhood communities, their populations have increased to nuisance levels. In some of these neighborhoods, relocation programs have been established by local city and county offices to try to reduce the population.

19.2   Taxonomic Relationship to Other Galliformes

Peafowl belong to the order of birds known as Galliformes. Galliformes are characterized as grain-eating ground-dwelling birds that hatch precocial chicks. Within this Galliformes order is the Phasianidae family which are heavy ground-dwelling birds that include pheasants, partridges, junglefowl, chickens, turkeys, Old World quail, and peafowl. This Phasianidae family is further subdivided into two subfamilies: Perdicinae and Phasianinae. The Perdicinae subfamily includes the partridges, Old World quail, and francolins, while the Phasianinae subfamily includes the pheasants, tragopans, junglefowl, and peafowl. Within the Phasianinae subfamily, peafowl belong to either the *Pavo* or *Afropavo* genera. There are two species in the genus *Pavo*: the Indian blue

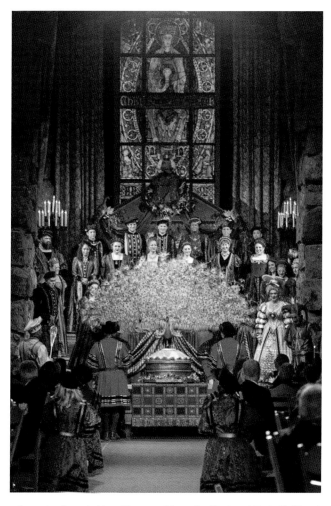

Figure 19.2   A scene from the Bracebridge Dinner at Yosemite National Park (California, USA) where the Lord of the Manor is presented with the "Peacock Pie" before it is served to the invited guests. Source: Courtesy of Bracebridge Dinner/Andrea Fulton Productions.

peafowl (*Pavo cristatus*), also known as the common blue or Indian peafowl, and the green peafowl (*Pavo muticus*), also known as the green-necked peafowl or Java green peafowl. The Congo peafowl (*Afropavo congensis*), also known as the African peafowl, is the only species within the genus *Afropavo* and is the only peafowl species not originating from Asia but rather from Africa.

19.3   Peafowl Terminology

Peafowl is the general term used to refer to birds of the *Pavo* or *Afropavo* genera. The males are referred to as peacocks and have ornate elongated tail (or train) feathers that end in iridescent eye-like patterns (ocelli). Both males and females possess a crest of feathers on the head. While in colloquial language, the term *peacock* is used when referring to all members (male or female) of the genus, the term should only be used when referring to the male. Females are called peahens, and the chicks are known as peachicks. A group of peafowl is known as an ostentation or a muster.

19.4   Peafowl Behavior

Peafowl congregate in small social groupings. These groupings usually include one peacock with 2–5 hens and their peachicks [6]. In captive settings, one peacock is usually paired with two or three hens. While peafowl can be kept with other avian species, it is important to introduce them at the same time and at a young age. The Indian blue peafowl, of all the peafowl species, are more likely to tolerate other poultry species [6]. However, it should be noted that peafowl tend to be more aggressive than other poultry species and can dominate the feeders due to their larger size, especially when feed supply or feeder space is limited.

Besides being known for their beautiful tail feathers, *Pavo* peafowl are also known for their distinct male vocalizations that are especially prominent in the mating season. The calls of the green peafowl are slightly less shrieking (lower pitched) than the Indian blue peafowl, which are likened to the call of a shrieking cat's meow. Green peafowl tend to be more aggressive toward other birds and possibly their human caretakers as well. Males of the green peafowl should be kept separate if they are kept in total confinement. Their sharp spurs can cause injury to other males so caution must be taken when working with this species.

Lukanov [1] referenced the ancient Hindu description of the peafowl as follows: "A peacock has the feathers of an angel, the voice of the devil, and the walk of a thief." The "walk of a thief" demonstrates the ever-observant behavior of the peafowl in its environment and this is based on a unique physiological feature of the peafowl.

Peafowl tend to be active in the early morning, then take shelter during the mid-day sun. As evening approaches, they will tend to congregate before seeking shelter in higher branches at night. It has been reported that wild peahens can carry their peachicks on their back as they fly to higher branches at night.

19.5   Unique Anatomical and Physiological Features

Peafowl are characterized by their crested head feathers and, in the male, the colorful elongated tail (train) feathers terminating in eye-like structures known as ocelli. During the mating season, male peacocks will fan their tail in the hope of attracting a female. Peafowl also have long necks and strong legs, and are one of the largest and heaviest flying birds on earth. While peafowl possess similar anatomical and physiological features to some of the most common Galliformes like the chicken and turkey, they do have unique anatomical and physiological features. Figure 19.3 depicts some of the anatomical parts of the peafowl.

It should be noted that peafowl show a near-absence of the vestibuloocular reflex which allows them to move their heads as quickly as their eyes [7]. Hence, when their gaze shift is greater, their head movement is more substantial than eye movements, as when scanning the environment for predators. However, for small gaze shifts, it is more efficient for the peafowl to utilize only eye movements. This finding accounts for some of the characteristic behavior and movements noticed in peafowl and allows them to be successful in the feral state by being alert to predator presence. Their quick head movements allow them to effectively scan the environment for potential danger.

The tail feathers are one of the unique features of the peafowl and the main feature when one imagines the species. In fact, the commonly used expression "proud as a peacock" arose because the peacock was a symbol of vanity and ostentation as they display their fanned-out tail feathers. This expression was used as early as the fourteenth century when the English poet Geoffrey Chaucer wrote in his work *The Reeve's Tale* that "As any peacock he was proud" in 1387 [8]. Burgess [9]

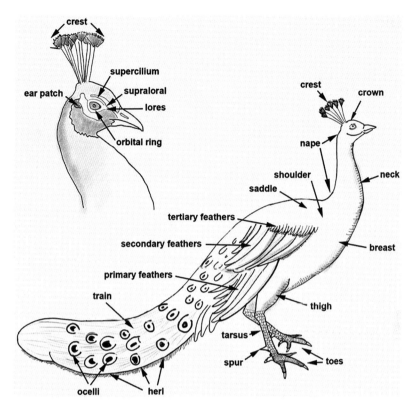

Figure 19.3 Illustration highlighting some of the terminology used in describing the external anatomy of the peafowl. Source: Courtesy of Dr Josep Rutllant-Labeaga.

reported that the peacock tail feathers do not function in flight or in thermoregulation but have the sole purpose of providing an attractive display. This was a great puzzle to evolutionist Charles Darwin who struggled with the thought that the elaborate long train feathers of the peacock appeared to be a handicap for survival [10]. However, the display of the tail feathers plays an important role in peafowl courtship and ultimately, the success of the individual to propagate its genes.

In the courtship dance, peacocks will raise their upper tail covert feathers to frame themselves and quiver their fanned tail feathers to attract potential peahens. There is evidence that the larger and/or more elaborate the male train, the more it may signal high genetic quality and good genes [11]. The fanning and subsequent vibrations of the male tail feathers is one of the unique behavioral aspects of the peacock. It should be noted that not only the tail feathers but the crest feathers may also signify the conditioning of the peacock [12]. Kane et al. [13] reported that in the crest feathers on the Indian Blue peafowl were coupled to filoplumes, the small feathers known to function as mechanoreceptors, and that the vibrational resonant frequencies of peafowl crests were closely related with the frequencies used during the male train-rattling and female tail-rattling displays. This unique feature of the peafowl's crest feathers was not observed in other feathers of similar length on the peafowl or in the other bird orders with crest feathers (Victorian crowned pigeon, Himalayan monal, golden pheasants, and yellow-crested cockatoo) [13]. Thus, the movements of the peafowl crest are well matched to the train's mechanical sound. When the tail feathers are not erected into a fan, this train trails behind the bird.

An adult peacock has an average of 200 tail feathers that are shed and regrown annually. What appears to be the ocelli-laden tail is really the upper tail coverts. The true tail feathers only number around 20 and all end with ocelli. All these iridescent feathers can influence mating success [14]. Burgess [9] reported that of these 200 upper tail covert feathers, about 170 are "eye" feathers. The remainder of the tail feathers are known as "T" feathers based on the shape they form. The "T" feathers complement the "eye" feathers because the "T" feathers' profile is the inverse of the shape of the "eye" feather and the "T" feathers form a beautiful border to the fanned-out "eye" feathers [8].

For the tail feathers, in the Indian blue peacock, the second-year male resembles the adult male except the tail is shorter and lacks ocelli. These tail feathers continue to increase in size until the fourth year. In the green peacock, like the Indian blue peacock, second-year males are like the adult males, but their train feathers lack ocelli.

19.6   Species, Subspecies, and Hybrids

In the *Pavo* genera, there are two species: the Indian blue peafowl and the Java green peafowl. The Indian blue peafowl is the most common worldwide and is a species of least concern for conservation purposes. However, the green peafowl is considered a threatened species, and the majority are held in zoological institutions or private collections [15].

The Indian blue peafowl (*P. cristatus*), also known as the common blue peafowl or Indian peafowl, is the most common peafowl held in captivity and in feral populations. In its original distribution, it has been reported in Pakistan, India, Sri Lanka, and Bangladesh but has been established throughout the world in a semi-feral state [15]. The Indian blue peafowl has a very distinctive crest, composed of fanned-out wire-like feathers topped with bluish flattened ends. Males have a blue head, neck, and chest feathers with tan and black barred shoulders and green and bronze feathers throughout their bodies (Figure 19.4). There is sexual dimorphism and, unlike the male, the female is brown in coloration, has some green feathers in its neck, and a

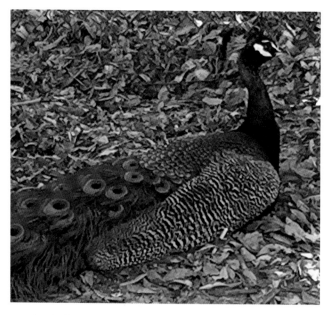

Figure 19.4   A free-roaming Indian blue peacock outside the Los Angeles Arboretum (California, USA). Note the characteristic barred shoulders and the distinctive fanned-out crest feathers. The barred pattern allows the bird to camouflage against vegetation. Source: Courtesy of Dr Teresa Y. Morishita.

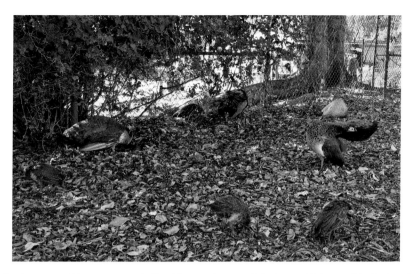

Figure 19.5   A muster of free-roaming Indian blue peahens and their peachicks outside the Los Angeles Arboretum (California). The drab colors of the peahens and peachicks allow them to camouflage in vegetation. Note that most birds are preening themselves which is one of their main activities. The peacock of this muster (featured in Figure 19.4) is away from the group but does keep a vigilant eye on them. Source: Courtesy of Dr Teresa Y. Morishita.

characteristic white belly [15]. The drab color of Indian blue peahens allows them to blend into the environment as they tend to rest in the shade during the hot midday sun (Figure 19.5).

From beak to tail-head, peafowl males are approximately 3.5–4 ft in body length (100–130 cm) [15]. The smaller females lack a long tail (train). In males, these long tail feathers can be up to 5–6 ft in length (150+ cm) [15]. Females have a brown head ornament (noodle) while the male's head ornament color is the same as its tail (blue and green) [15].

Color mutations have been reported in the Indian blue peafowl. *Pavo cristatus nigripennis*, known as the black-shouldered ("black-winged") color mutation, is a subspecies of the Indian blue peafowl (Figures 19.6a,b). Males will be melanistic in color whereas the females are creamy white in color (Figure 19.6c). Other color mutations of the Indian blue peafowl include pied and white (eyed) varieties. Interbreeding of these color and/or pattern mutations has resulted in many color and pattern variations (Figure 19.6d).

The Indian blue peafowl has been interbred with the Java green peafowl, which is a threatened species, to produce a fertile hybrid known as the Spalding peafowl. It was named after a breeder in California (USA) who first interbred these two species, the hardier Indian blue, which was more tolerant of cold weather, and the Java green peafowl. The resulting hybrid has a more defined green metallic color around the neck. The original cross was a Java green peacock and a black-shouldered peahen to form the first Spalding peafowl [16]. It should be noted that the male Spalding peacock is similar in color to the Java green peacock but has a much lighter but larger body with slightly longer legs than the Indian blue peacock. The Spalding peahen is more colorful with a green metallic color around the neck and darker body feathers compared to the drab Indian blue peahen [16]. As with the Indian blue peafowl, Spalding peafowl can have multiple color variations. Since they are a hybrid, a Spalding hybrid bred to another Spalding hybrid has characteristics dependent on the percentage of Java green peafowl genes present in the hybrids used.

The green peafowl (*Pavo multicus*), also known as the Java green peafowl or green-necked peafowl, originated in Asia and is the largest species of pheasant (Figures 19.7). There are three

(a)

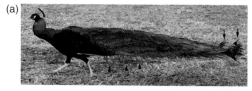

(b)

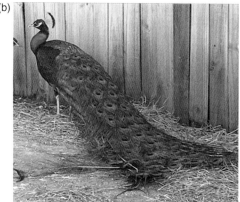

Figure 19.6 (a) The long train of the Indian blue peafowl. Note the prominent fan-shaped crest of this species. Arrows highlight the T-feathers. Source: Courtesy of Bridgett Addy. (b) A black-shouldered peacock. Source: Courtesy of Bridgett Addy. (c) A trio of variations (from left to right) of an Indian blue pied (pattern mutation), black-shouldered (pattern mutation) peacock, an Indian blue black-shouldered (pattern mutation) peahen (note that the black-shouldered mutation in the peahen results in a cream coloration rather than the melanistic coloration seen in the males), and an Indian blue peahen. Source: Courtesy of Keldon Howard. (d) An example of variation in the color and pattern of the Indian blue peafowl. This peacock is classified as a peach (color mutation), black-shouldered (pattern mutation), white-eyed (pattern mutation) split pied (pattern mutation) Indian blue peafowl. Source: Courtesy of Nikola Stella Hadar.

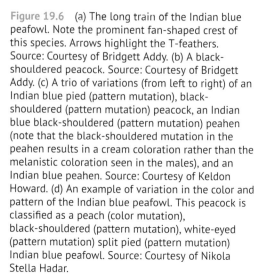

(c)

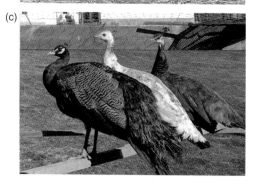

(d)

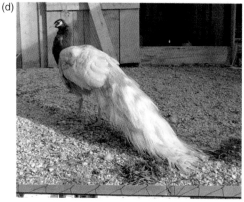

reported subspecies of the green peafowl: Burmese peafowl (*Pavo multicus spicifer*), which was originally reported in India, Bangladesh, and Burma and is thought to be extinct in the wild; Indo-Chinese peafowl (*P. m. imperator*), which was originally reported in Burma, Thailand, China, Vietnam, and Laos; and Java peafowl (*P. m. multicus*), which was originally reported in Java, Indonesia [15]. The green peafowl is listed as endangered by the IUCN [14]. Its population decline

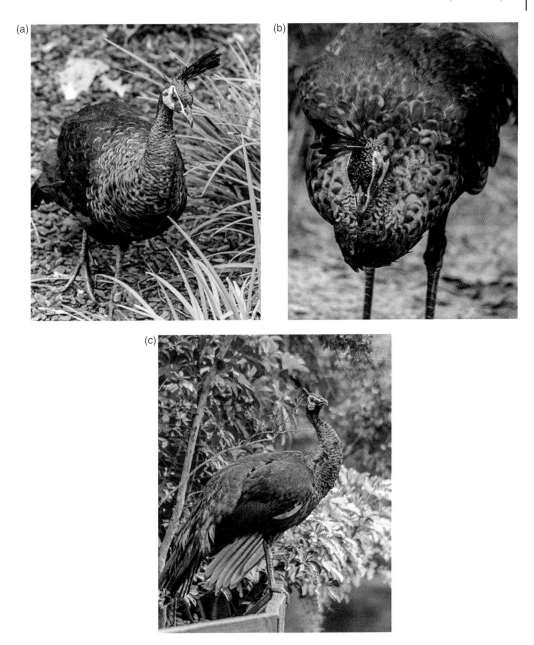

Figure 19.7   (a) The prominent yellow-orange ear patch and shafted crest feathers that are characteristic for the green peafowl. (b) The prominent white to light blue facial skin markings seen in the green peafowl. (c) The metallic green head and neck of the green peafowl. Source: Courtesy of Travis Kay, Busch Gardens.

in the wild is attributed to habitat destruction as a result of the increase in palm oil plantation development on their habitats [17]. This peacock has yellow and blue skin on the face. Its head and neck are metallic green with most of the body contour feathers in a bluish-green and some bronze coloration and a dark green belly [15]. Unlike the sexual dimorphism between the sexes in the Indian blue peafowl, green peafowl are similar in coloration. The female has the same

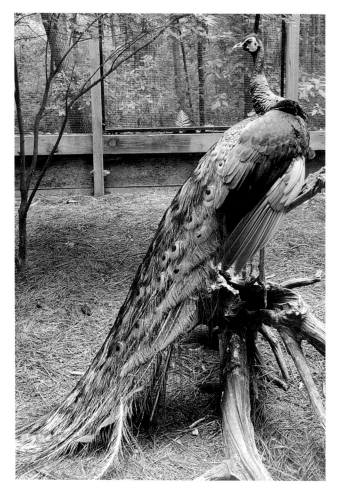

Figure 19.8 A male green peafowl with the prominent shafted crest feathers. Green peacocks have slightly longer upper tail coverts (train feathers) than the Indian blue peacock. Source: Courtesy of Gen Anderson/Sylvan Heights.

color pattern as the male but is more muted in color (Figure 19.8). The female does not have dark bars on the tail feathers. Peachicks are darker gray-brown in color compared to Indian blue peachicks [15]. While the Indian blue peafowl is more tolerant of colder temperatures, the Java green peafowl prefers warm weather and is prone to frostbite [18].

The green peafowl differs from the Indian blue in two distinct features. Green peafowl have crest feathers that are shafted rather than fanned out. In addition, there is a white stripe above the eye and a crescent-shaped white patch below the eye. The facial skin has a characteristic double striped pattern that blends from white to light blue with a crescent-shaped ear skin patch of orangish yellow. There is a dark triangular feathered patch in the cranial antorbital areas that is blue green in the male but brown in the female [15]. Compared to the Indian blue peafowl, green peafowl are slightly lighter but their tail covert feathers are longer. Males range from 5 to 9 ft in length (including trains) while the female is about 3 ft in length from beak to tail [15]. A quick way to differentiate between the Indian blue peafowl and green peafowl is to observe the crest feather shape and the facial coloration.

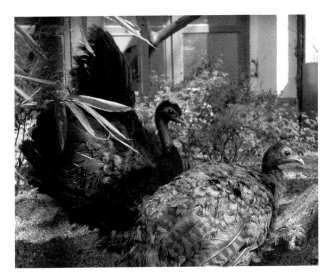

Figure 19.9   Male (left) and female (right) Congo Peafowl in captivity. As observed in other peafowl species, there is sexual dimorphism between male and female plumage coloration.

The Congo peafowl (*A. congensis*), also known as the African peafowl, is the only peafowl species originating in Africa (Figure 19.9). The Congo peafowl is listed as vulnerable by the IUCN [14, 17]. It is rare to view these birds in the wild due to their elusive nature and they were only first described in the early twentieth century [17]. Information on their natural history is still scarce. They are vulnerable due to their use in the bush meat trade and the destruction of their habitat due to agriculture and political conflicts [17]. The Congo peafowl is usually found in zoological collections and is usually housed in pairs. Birds found in zoos are the descendants of the original pair that was obtained in the wild and first housed at the Antwerp (Belgium) Zoo in 1962 [17].

19.6.1   Varieties and Genetic Mutations

Since the peafowl has been domesticated for centuries, people have been intrigued with the multiple patterns and/or color variations that are possible. Extensive breeding studies have been performed to explain these variations, which are all reported as originating in the Indian blue peafowl. There are no current reports of any mutations in the wild-type Java green peafowl or the Congo peafowl.

There are three main mutations in the feather pattern described in peafowl and all are reported in the Indian blue peafowl [3, 19, 20]. One mutation is the black-shoulder (black-winged) mutation in which the barred pattern found on the wings of peacocks are not present but are melanistic [20]. Other pattern mutations are the pied and white (eyed) mutations [3, 19]. A pied mutation is when the peafowl's colored feathers are replaced by white feathers [3, 19]. Whether there are just a couple of white feathers or many (up to 50% white), it is a pied mutation pattern. For this pied color pattern, the whiter, the more desirable. Finally, in the white eyed mutation, the center of the ocelli is white [3, 19].

The white and pied peafowl colors were probably the first and second color and pattern mutant types described in the peafowl, respectively [3, 19]. In 1868, Charles Darwin mentioned the 1850 report by Dixon of a large flock of blue, white, and pied peafowl [3, 19]. To better understand the terminology behind peafowl color pattern variation and their genetics, it is necessary to define the Indian blue peafowl phenotype as a genetic wild type for *P. cristatus*. Phenotype refers to the pattern and/or color of what is visually seen. The nonwild-type phenotypes observed for the Indian blue peafowl are caused by mutations to the genes, i.e., genetic material. This would be the genotype or genetic make-up of the bird [20]. The white mutation is a color mutation, and the pied mutation is a pattern mutation (Figures 19.10–19.12).

When examining the pied, dark pied, white, and blue white flight plumage color phenotypes and their relationship to each other and to the wild-type blue, it was determined that a single autosomal locus was responsible for all these observed phenotypes. The white mutant allele (W), when homozygous, produced an all-white plumage [3, 19]. When a peafowl is heterozygous (Ww), with

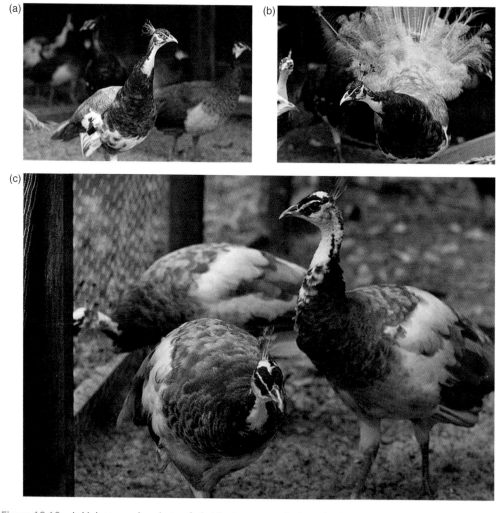

Figure 19.10 (a,b) A composite photo of pied (pattern mutation) peafowl with the purple coloration. Note the fanned crest feathers of the peafowl of this captive flock, indicating that the Indian blue peafowl is the predominant genetic presence. (c) The peahens show variations in the number of white feathers. Source: Courtesy of Jennifer Pike.

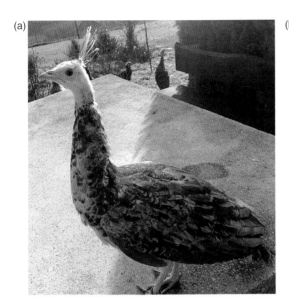 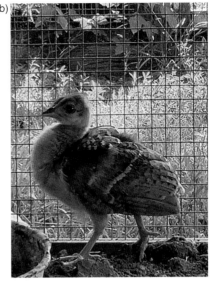

Figure 19.11 (a) European violet black juvenile male. Source: Courtesy of Nikola Stella Hadar. (b) An Indian Blue peachick. Source: Courtesy of Veronica Little.

the wild-type allele (w), that individual will have the blue white flight plumage. The pied pheno-type does not breed true but rather produces birds with phenotypes of white, pied, and dark pied in a 1 : 2 : 1 ratio [3, 19]. Dark pied peafowl when bred to white phenotype produce all pied plumage. Thus, the white allele is the most dominant and the dark pied allele the most recessive [3, 19]. The white mutation and the pied pattern mutation are from two mutant alleles on the same locus, with an allele being defined as one of two or more alternative forms of a gene that arise by mutation and are found on the same place on a chromosome [3, 19].

Somes and Burger [20] reported the inheritance of peafowl plumage color and described the third and fourth plumage color and/or pattern mutations documented in peafowl. These mutations included the cameo (color) mutation, which resulted in a peafowl that, instead of its colorful wild-type appearance, was now tan in coloration [20]. The other mutation was the black-shoulder (pattern) mutation which was due to an autosomal recessive gene which showed excessive sexual dimorphism in the adult plumage. Details on the crosses and color variations have been reported [3, 20]. Currently, the United Peafowl Association (https://unitedpeafowlassociation .org/breeders) recognizes over 225 variations in color and/or pattern and is an excellent source for additional information and description on these variation patterns. Years of dedicated work by peafowl breeders have yielded a multitude of peafowl phenotypic variations that can be available for purchase. Genetics has played an important role in the development of these variations.

Peafowl are often maintained in a free-living state and are provided only with supplemental feed-ing to complement their own foraging. Feeding is necessary to ensure that they return to their original "home" location although they will tend to roam. If they are kept free range, it is crucial to ensure that there are nearby trees with at least lower branches that allow the birds to perch at night out of the range of potential predators. Of course, these free-ranging birds should not be wing-clipped so they can fend for themselves in the environment.

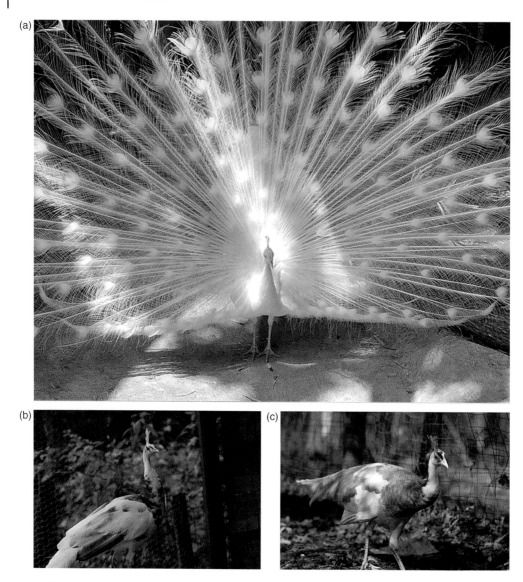

Figure 19.12 (a) A leucistic (white) peacock. A leucistic phenotype carries the (WW) mutatoin; leucistic peafowl are not albino. Source: Courtesy of Amanda Johnson, Zoo Atlanta. (b) An example of a Spalding silver pied peacock. The Spalding is a hybrid of the green peafowl and Indian blue cross. Just looking at the color variation, one might think that this was a variation of the Indian blue peafowl. However, this is a Spalding. A tell-tale sign is the shafted crest feather which is characteristic of the green peafowl which indicates that this individual is a hybrid. Source: Courtesy of Jennifer Pike. (c) A cameo (color mutation) pied (pattern mutation) Indian blue peacock. Source: Courtesy of Jennifer Pike.

Peafowl can be kept in captive conditions, especially for breeding and/or for developing new color/pattern variations. However, due to their large size, they would need to have very spacious captive pens. Vigran [6] recommended pen sizes of 12 ft by 60 ft, although they could be kept in smaller pens of 24 ft by 30 ft if housing multiple bird species. However, many individuals may not have the acreage for these dimensions. There is a dearth of scientific studies documenting the space requirements and their impact on peafowl growth and reproduction. Many of the recommendations are based on personal experience and the trial and error of individual peafowl breeders. The main concern is that these pens should provide enough space for normal bird activities such as preening, walking, eating, and perching. In addition, the males should be able to fan their tails as part of the mating ritual [6]. There should also be perches available to allow the males to perch without damaging their tail feathers on the ground since the trains can reach approximately 7 ft long. The more birds held in a confined space, the larger the space requirements needed to avoid fighting. Pen sizes less than 100 sq ft will result in fighting so captive peafowl owners need to assess their land and determine if they have the space to house peafowl [6]. It should be noted that green peafowl do not do well in cold environments and the Indian blue peafowl is more tolerant to cold weather and this fact should be taken into consideration when constructing peafowl housing for captive populations.

Hybrid housing can also be used for peafowl. For owners who choose to have their birds in a free-living state, in regions where the temperature may drop, owners may need to provide housing to protect peafowl from the rain and cold. This could be a barn or other open structure that allows the birds to enter if they need protection from inclement weather.

It should be noted that green peafowl cannot be housed at liberty like many Indian blue peafowl as they do not establish a home range and will tend to fly off [6].

19.7   Feeding Peafowl

If peafowl are kept in captivity, food and clean, fresh water should be provided daily. Peafowl are omnivorous and are voracious eaters of insects and are good at keeping pest levels down. In the natural state, their diet ranges from grains to green crops to insects, small reptiles, mammals, and snakes. Free-ranging peafowl in neighborhood communities have been reported to destroy vegetable and flower gardens. Free-ranging peafowl can obtain their own feed, so supplemental feeding is needed primarily to retain the birds to a local area.

In contrast, peafowl kept in total captivity should be provided commercially prepared feed to ensure that they receive a balanced nutritional diet. While there is no dedicated diet specifically formulated for the different life stages of the peafowl, many captive peafowl owners utilize commercial feed prepared for pheasants and other gamebirds. Biggs [21] stated that peafowl need high protein levels to maintain their feathers which are comprised of approximately 90% protein. Biggs recommends three primary diets for peafowl depending on age and life stage [21]. For young peachicks from 0 to 6 weeks of age, a 30% crude protein/2.5% crude fat/6.5% crude fiber diet (Purina® Gamebird & Turkey Startena®) is recommended. After this starter phase, peafowl can be maintained on a diet of 19% crude protein/2.0% crude fat/12.0% crude fiber (Purina Game Bird Flight Conditioner) or a 20% crude protein/3.5% crude fat//5% crude fiber diet (Purina Flock Raiser® Crumbles). It should be noted that protein levels decrease significantly from 30% to 18–20% during the maintenance phase [21].

As with other poultry, peahens that are going to be in lay or are laying should be provided a diet with additional calcium. Biggs recommends diets made for laying hens that contain a minimum of 2.5% calcium to a maximum of 3.5% [21]. As a comparison, the levels for gamebirds in lay or for laying chickens are 3.25–4.25%. It should be noted that diets used for peahens should only be used during the laying season [21]. Once laying is over, the peafowl must go back to the maintenance diet where calcium levels range from 0.80% to 1.35%. Leftover feed from laying peahens should not be fed to young peachicks, which only require 1.0–1.5% calcium [21]. Providing a laying diet to peachicks can cause kidney damage,

Parveen et al. [22] reported that peafowl prefer grains like corn or millet over poultry feed. However, commercial feed is preferred to homemade diets to ensure the proper balance of nutrients. While peafowl prefer grains over prepared poultry feed, grains and scratch feed should not be considered a complete diet and, as in chickens, can be used as periodic treats. Hence, diets formulated for gamebirds like pheasants followed by turkey diets are recommended [6]. In addition, use of the appropriate life stage diet – grower, maintenance, or layer – is of the utmost importance. While Sikander et al. [23] recommended also feeding greens and oil seeds to captive birds to improve their health, half to two-thirds or more of their diet should be a complete, commercial mix [18]. As with any bird, oil seeds, such as sunflower seeds and peanuts, should be kept to a maximum of 5–10% of their diet to avoid nutritional deficiencies [18].

A nutritious diet is important when understanding the time budget of peafowl. While Jun and Lan [24] reported that captive green peafowl spend much of their time maintaining feathers, Parveen et al. [22] reported that there were no species behavior differences when it came to the time budgets of peafowl. On average, captive peafowl are active, spending approximately 20% of the day walking; 19% feeding or pecking the ground and foraging; 18% feather pecking and preening; 13% standing and observing the environment; 11% resting; 6% flying; 5% displaying train; 4% vocalizing; 2% drinking; and 2% demonstrating aggressive behavior. Hence, peafowl are highly active birds, with many activities related to the maintenance or displaying of feathers so high-protein diets are required.

Feed has been used to attract peafowl to remain at a particular location. This strategy has been used with Indian blue peafowl which tend to have a home range. To entice the peafowl to return to their home range, it is recommended to feed them 1/4 cup of food in the morning, and a larger amount at night. Allowing them to eat what they can in 15–20 minutes twice a day will provide the minimum amount for daily food consumption yet keep them hungry enough so they will want to return at night. Underfeeding peafowl may also cause them to look elsewhere for food so that has always been a concern when peafowl are allowed to free roam. Peafowl have adapted quite well to human habitation and their populations have ballooned in some neighborhoods, resulting in complaints and the banning of feeding peafowl [25]. Feeding peafowl is a misdemeanor crime in Los Angeles County (California, USA) punishable by up to 6 months in jail, a $1000 fine or both [26]. The overpopulation of peafowl in neighborhoods has resulted in complaints about their shrieking vocalizations, destruction of gardens, defecation on roofs and cars, and blocking of roads. Ultimately, the "beauty" of the peafowl is in the eye of the beholder.

One of the authors (SB) suggests that if their cries cause a neighbor complaint, then consider making a large custom elevated treehouse, where the doors will close at night (using a photocell) and open in the morning [18]. This battery-operated device is much preferred over the use of household electricity and can be operated manually and/or by a remote transmitter. This night housing should also not have the recommended 110 V heat lamps since these lamps cannot be monitored daily.

As mentioned previously, peafowl prefer to be outside and not inside a house when compared to chickens. However, if the use of a night enclosure is desired, it is recommended that the peafowl become accustomed to the housing during the peachick phase. The birds will need to be fed in this enclosure, which can be accomplished using an extension pole and cup to drop the food into a fixed bowl before dark. Please note that this method may not allow for routine cleaning of the housing as it would be hard to access daily and cleaning would have to occur when the birds are out foraging during the day [18].

If peafowl are housed with other poultry and/or avian species, there can be interspecies conflicts if confinement is less than 100+ sq ft./adult peafowl pair (peacock and peahen) [27]. A much larger space is required if there is more than one sex of each bird in confinement.

As with the housing of any other captive avian species, the housing should be predator proof. Caging wire should be buried at least 2 ft into the ground to prevent predators from digging into an enclosure for those birds that will be housed in total captivity or have a hybrid housing setup, such as enclosure only at night but free roam during the day.

Since peafowl are one of the largest flying terrestrial birds, they prefer a free-roam existence. While larger mammals such as coyotes, foxes, and both domestic and feral dogs can serve as predators for the adult peafowl, the smaller peachicks can be preyed upon by much smaller predators, including rats preying on newborn peachicks. It is fortunate that adult peafowl are large and can be aggressive so predation can be minimized if free-roaming birds have access to a tree where they can perch at night. The trimming or even pinioning of wings is not recommended for free-roaming birds as it will interfere with their flight which will be needed if they are to escape from predators. If wing clipping or pinioning is performed for the sole reason of keeping birds localized in an area, then the peafowl should really be housed in total confinement.

19.8 Reproduction

The most obvious characteristic feature of the peafowl is the ornate tail feathers of the male with their iridescent eyespots or ocelli. The characteristic fanning and vibration of the tail feathers play an important role in reproductive male behavior. Dakin and Montgomerie reported that peahens prefer males with more ocelli and both full and long tail feathers play an important role in mate selection for peahens [28]. Dakin and Montgomerie [29] also reported that peacocks orient their courtship display to the sun as that would enhance their shimmering, iridescent feathers.

Peafowl breeding season starts in the spring, usually around April. At the end of the season, which usually occurs in mid-summer, peacocks will drop their tail feathers. One male typically has a harem of 3–5 females. During the breeding season, the males will have more noticeable vocal cries during all hours of the day.

Peahens will prefer to lay eggs on the ground and will lay a clutch of 4–12 eggs, with six being the average clutch size. Some hens may have two clutches per year [15]. The incubation period is 28 days. Peachicks are precocial when hatched. While peachicks can utilize their yolk sac for the first 1–3 days of life, they should be provided food and water immediately after hatch. Peachicks can be commenced on a starter diet which is the optimum, especially if they are kept in total confinement. It is also recommended for those peachicks that will be raised by the peahen. The peachick will imprint and remain with their mother if eggs are hen-incubated and will stay with her until at least 2 months of age. At 10 months of age, juvenile peafowl can attain adult size. Sexual maturity occurs around 2 years of age [15]. Peafowl breeders are usually recommended to use artificial incubation to increase efficiency in raising numerous peachicks synchronously.

Indian blue peachicks are pale buffy brown with dark brown along the nape and neck and a deep rufous back. It has been reported that it is difficult to sex peachicks but females tend to have darker tan tips on their secondary feathers compared to male chicks whose secondary feathers are more of a cream color [3].

It should be noted that the Spalding hybrids lay much larger and thicker eggs compared to other peafowl. Since the shells are thicker, this can present some issues during hatching so the hatchability rate can be lower compared to other peafowl species [16]. The larger eggs also mean that

Spalding peachicks are larger in size at hatch [16]. Their down is also much darker compared to the Indian blue peachick. Since both Spalding males and females have green metallic coloration of the neck, it may be hard to sex the peachicks but the males do tend to have longer legs compared to the females [16].

19.9 Medical Considerations

19.9.1 Surgical Procedures and Anatomical Manipulations

One of the commonly requested anatomical alterations for peafowl is to alter the wings either temporarily or permanently in order to reduce a bird's flight ability. Wing trimming has often been proposed to make a bird more restricted to a particular area. Trimming of the primary wing feathers to render a bird "flightless" to prevent escape has been proposed. Usually, the first 5–6 feathers are trimmed, no more than half of the total length. This procedure is usually done in one wing so the resultant flight will be ineffective. This is considered a temporary condition as the primary flight feathers will eventually molt and new feathers will grow.

However, there are major concerns with the use of this procedure. First, it is a temporary condition and will require periodic capture of the bird in order to perform this procedure with each set of new feathers. Peafowl that are allowed to free roam will be difficult to capture unless they are housed at night where they can be confined for capture. However, the birds may associate the stress of capture with their housing and may become reluctant to enter the housing in the future. Second, if birds are allowed to free roam, they should not have their wings clipped as this may make them more vulnerable to predator attacks as they may not be able to escape. Moreover, wing trimming has been reported to be ineffective in peafowl as birds that have been wing trimmed can still jump a 6 ft fence or fly onto house roofs [18, 27].

Pinioning of the wing is a more invasive and permanent surgical procedure. In pinioning, the bony tip of the wing which usually carries the primary feathers is removed.

Before one undertakes procedures to limit flight permanently, consider what is the purpose for raising peafowl. If you need to keep them to one location, then they should be held in total captivity. However, if they are allowed to free roam then these procedures should not be performed as they are not only ineffective (wing trimming) but can permanently render a bird unable to protect itself from predators.

Devocalization of peafowl has been conducted in order to reduce the shrieking cries that can irritate the public. The syrinx is that portion of the respiratory system where the voice is produced. The syrinx in peafowl is located at the junction where the trachea bifurcates into the two bronchi that will eventually lead to the lung. The anatomical structure of birds is such that the syrinx is located dorsal to the heart within the coelomic cavity. To devocalize a bird, the muscles surrounding the syrinx need to be severed. One issue that often arises is that tissues in the area heal and voice is still produced although the pitch is altered. Hence, many of these surgeries remain ineffective. The greater concern is that this very invasive surgery will require surgical manipulation near the heart. In essence, it is a highly invasive surgery that is usually ineffective. For animal welfare reasons, this procedure is not recommended. Peafowl should not be kept if there is a concern about their natural behaviors and vocalizations.

19.9.2   Disease Prevention

As with all gamebird species, there should always be a quarantine period whenever new or returning peafowl enter the facility. The ideal quarantine period is 3–4 weeks as this will allow sufficient time to evaluate birds for exposure to common diseases in order to prevent a disease from being introduced to the home location [30]. A minimum of 3 weeks is necessary as many poultry diseases have an incubation time of about 2 weeks. Incubation time is the time from when birds first become exposed to a disease agent to when clinical signs appear that would indicate to the owner that something is not normal in the flock. It is necessary to keep birds in quarantine (and isolation) so that if they are exposed to pathogens and do become infected, they will not infect the entire flock. During this quarantine period, these birds should be kept in isolation and not near or in direct contact with other birds. It is also recommended that birds be evaluated for external parasites via a physical exam and for internal parasites through a fecal flotation exam [30].

Disease prevention is of the utmost importance when raising peafowl. Currently, there are no vaccines routinely used in peafowl to protect them from disease [2]. While many diseases have been documented in Galliformes, peafowl tend to be similar in their susceptibility to the diseases reported in turkeys. These diseases have been discussed in more detail in previous chapters and this chapter will highlight special characteristics of the more frequently observed diseases seen in peafowl.

19.9.3   Viral Diseases

Avian pox has been reported in peafowl and can affect peachicks, especially between 2 and 3 months of age. Al Falluji et al. [31] reported avian pox in a zoological aviary where 45 of 60 Indian blue peafowl had lesions around the beaks and eyes. Morbidity was 75% of the affected flock with a 13% mortality. This isolate was partially purified and precipitated by antisera to fowlpox and pigeon pox viruses. Khan et al. [32] reported cutaneous pox in peachicks with a reported 60% case fatality rate. Affected peachicks, especially those between 9 and 12 weeks of age, had typical dry pox pustular and nodular lesions on the eyelids, beak, legs, and toes. While most poultry species have pox lesions on the head, it should be noted that in this case, lesions were also noted on the legs and toes. Hence, avian pox should be considered a differential for peachicks with scabs on the feet. Mosquito control and mosquito-proofing of aviaries reduced the prevalence of this disease when the flock was followed for successive years in this aviary.

Other respiratory viral infections that can occur in peafowl include Newcastle disease and avian influenza. Both diseases are reportable to state and federal authorities within the USA. These diseases can have clinical signs affecting the digestive, respiratory, and neurological systems along with death loss. Hence, owners of any bird, including peafowl, exhibiting multisystem involvement should consider these two potential diseases.

Kumar et al. [33] reported 145 peafowl with Newcastle disease which exhibited clinical signs of head shaking, torticollis, and paresis. However, a postmortem examination revealed no gross lesions typical of Newcastle disease. The amino acid motif was indicative of the velogenic nature of the isolate and phylogenetic studies demonstrated that the virus belonged to the class II genotype VII and was closely related to the virus isolates originating from outbreaks in western Europe,

Israel, Indonesia, Taiwan, and India. This study highlights the concerns of global disease transmission. Moreover, Designu et al. [34] further described clinical signs of incoordination, tremors, wing paralysis, circling movements, and opisthotonos with Newcastle disease. Necropsy revealed well-nourished carcasses with whitish thick ocular discharge, mild pulmonary congestion, caseous exudates in the palate and choanal region, and hemorrhages on the epicardium. The cecal tonsils were mildly hemorrhagic.

Avian influenza has been reported in both the Indian blue peafowl and Java green peafowl. There is a wide assortment of avian influenza virus subtypes that can occur in peafowl, including highly pathogenic avian influenza (HPAI) virus and H5N1 [35, 36]. Affected birds exhibited depression, anorexia, and white diarrhea. Moreover, low-pathogenicity avian influenza H6N6 was also found in a clinically healthy Java green peafowl in a wildlife park during a surveillance program [37].

Crenshaw and Boyle [38] reported infectious laryngotracheitis in both pheasants and peafowl with clinical signs similar to those reported in chickens. Hence, infectious laryngotracheitis, which is considered primarily a chicken disease, can also occur in peafowl.

Another viral disease that is often reported in turkeys and has also been reported in peafowl is hemorrhagic enteritis caused by a siadenovirus [39, 40]. Affected peafowl have similar clinical gastrointestinal signs as reported for turkeys, including the characteristic hemorrhagic enteritis which results in bloody feces. Schwarz reported that birds between 4 and 13 weeks of age are most susceptible [2]. In a serosurvey conducted in 31 Indian blue peafowl at three zoological institutions, 19.3% were seropositive for adenovirus [41].

19.9.4 Bacterial Diseases

Mycoplasma gallisepticum is a bacterial infection with a wide avian host range. Peafowl are highly susceptible to this bacterium. Willis [42] initially reported this disease in peafowl. One of the most common clinical signs is a swollen antorbital (infraorbital) sinus and increased lacrimation [43]. Cookson and Shivaprasad [43] reported an outbreak in peafowl in a mixed-species gamebird flock where chickens had been introduced. Hollamby et al. [41] conducted a serological test on free-roaming peafowl at a zoological park and reported seropositivity via the serum plate agglutination test for *Mycoplasma meleagridis* and *Mycoplasma synoviae* in 3.2% and 38.7% of 31 peafowl samples, respectively. This same population of birds was seronegative for *M. gallisepticum*. Since *Mycoplasma* are vertically transmitted, peafowl breeders should consider participation in the National Poultry Improvement Plan (NPIP) to ensure MG, MS, and MM-free birds for their breeding stock.

For peafowl breeders, participation in the NPIP (as discussed in Chapter 2) is highly recommended. Many of the major vertically transmitted diseases will be monitored to ensure that the genetic line remains free of these vertically transmitted diseases. Besides *Mycoplasma*, other bacteria that can be transmitted include *Salmonella*, specifically *S. pullorum* and *S. gallinarum*. While *S. pullorum* and *S. gallinarum* are avian-specific *Salmonella*, there are also over 2000+ species belonging to the paratyphoid grouping, which affects a variety of animal and human hosts. One study characterized a paratyphoid *Salmonella* isolate from captive peafowl that contained the *inv* A gene for virulence [44].

Pasteurella multocida, the causative agent of avian (fowl) cholera, was reported as a disease of peafowl as early as the 1940s [45]. In the author's experience, affected peafowl exhibit infraorbital swelling.

As with other Galliformes kept in total confinement, the quality of the flooring is of the utmost importance for disease prevention. Wet litter or abrasive surfaces can lead to infections of the footpad of birds, also known as pododermatitis (bumblefoot). These foot lesions can become contaminated with bacteria normally found on the skin, including *Staphylococcus aureus*. Since these birds also have contact with their feces on the litter, it is not uncommon to have these lesions also contaminated with *Escherichia coli*. Since most peafowl live a free-roaming lifestyle, this disease is more of a concern for those kept in total confinement.

Avian tuberculosis has been documented in peafowl. One case reported an outbreak associated with peafowl and pheasants housed in a zoological park [46]. One peahen had cachexia with granuloma in the lung and smaller granulomas in the spleen. A second peahen had caseous granuloma on the serosal surface of the cecum, cloaca, and lungs. Compared with the pheasants, which did not have lesions in the lungs, it was speculated that the respiratory route was involved in infection in these peafowl of undetermined ages. It should be noted that *Mycobacterium avium avium*, which was isolated in this case, usually affects the gastrointestinal tract of birds. Since the respiratory system was affected, it was suggested that peafowl may be more sensitive to respiratory contamination. Ledwon et al. [47] documented four additional cases in peafowl and reported that unlike other avian species infected with *Mycobacterium avium*, in peafowl the primary clinical signs involved the respiratory system which included severe and sustained dyspnea. In this case report, three of the peafowl, which ranged from 2 to 5 years of age and were from the same location, had *M. a. avium*, while the third peahen, less than 1 year old and housed on a separate farm, had *M. a. paratuberculosis* isolated [47].

19.9.5 Parasitic Diseases

19.9.5.1 Protozoa

Histomonas meleagridis, the causative agent of blackhead, has been reported in peafowl. Clarke et al. performed a retrospective study on submissions of peafowl from two diagnostic laboratories and reported that while experimental infection occurs with *Histomonas*, there are few naturally occurring outbreaks [48]. This study reported that the peafowl had lesions including bilateral, transmural fibrinonecrotic typhlitis and multifocal necrotizing hepatitis but there was no evidence of cecal worms (*Heterakis gallinarum*) infestation in the birds examined. These findings are similar to those reported for other cases in peafowl [49]. *H. meleagridis* was molecularly characterized from these cases and one peafowl had a concurrent infection with *Tetratrichomonas gallinarum* [48]. The authors concluded that peafowl are susceptible to *Histomonas*. They suggest that peafowl should not be housed with chickens and/or pheasants which are more resistant to this disease and may serve as reservoirs for peafowl. While this disease is more commonly seen in poultry in commercial settings, naturally infected peafowl do occur.

While chickens and turkeys are frequently reported with intestinal coccidiosis caused by various *Eimeria* species, it is a well-known fact that *Eimeria* are host specific and certain species are localized to particular regions of the intestinal tract. Hauck and Hafez [50] isolated *Eimeria pavonina* in a peafowl. Other *Eimeria* reported in peafowl include *E. pavonis* and *E. patnaika* as well as the species *Isospora mayuri* and *Cryptosporidium meleagridis* [51].

Crespo et al. [52] reported that peafowl can also be susceptible to trichomoniasis and the protozoan is similar to other bird species.

Blood Protozoans Protozoan blood parasites have been reported in many avian species, but their prevalence depends on the presence of the parasite in the local population and its insect vector. Hollamby et al. [41] performed a serological survey and found no peafowl that were positive for blood-borne protozoa. Laird [53] reported a case of avian malaria present in an introduced peafowl in Nigeria and cautioned about disease transmission from domesticated, introduced birds.

19.9.5.2 Internal Parasites

Teixeira et al. [54] reported the roundworm *Ascaridia galli* in peafowl. Peachicks were reported to be severely affected with signs of diarrhea, dehydration, decreased feed intake, and progressive weight loss. This contrasts with the adults which were also positive on fecal examination but did not demonstrate clinical signs.

Titilincu et al. [51] found multiple infections in peafowl on a single farm which had 60 peafowl, ranging in age from 3 months to 8 years. These peafowl had coinfections with multiple intestinal parasites: *Ascaridia* sp. (59.95%), *Heterakis* sp. (59.9%), *Syngamus trachea* (64.5%), *Capillaria* spp. (35.3%), and *Strongyloides pavonis* (51%). This study demonstrated that numerous nematode species can be found in peafowl. The prevalence is most likely dependent on exposure, population density, and sanitation.

Heterakis gallinarum (cecal worm) plays an important role in transmission of the protozoan *H. meleagridis*. When Lund and Chute [55] experimentally infected young peafowl with the eggs of *Heterakis* containing *Histomonas*, the birds became infected with *Histomonas*. However, the authors reported that the young peafowl were not effective in transmitting *Histomonas* because the cecal worm rarely completes its life cycle in these birds when *Histomonas* is present. This is due to the damage that *Histomonas* causes to the cecal wall which does not make it conducive for *Heterakis* to complete its life cycle. They also added that pheasants and peafowl should not be housed in the same area, especially if peafowl have access to earthworms that have contact with infected pheasants. Aviculturists who raise both ornamental pheasants and peafowl should be aware of this risk. Since blackhead is a disease of turkeys, peafowl, and other gallinaceous birds, Benscheidt [18] recommended that to aid prevention of this disease, peafowl and chickens (or pheasants), if on the same premises, should periodically have their feces examined for parasites.

Subramanian et al. [56] reported that the *Syngamus* sp. isolated from free-ranging peafowl were smaller ($50 \times 50\,\mu m$) than those previously described from domestic fowl, turkey, and guineafowl, which measures $70–100 \times 43–46\,\mu m$. They suggested that this may represent a host-specific species. This study also reported acanthocephalans present which may be due to the insectivorous habits of peafowl since they also feed on beetles which are the intermediate hosts of acanthocephalans.

The threadworm, *Capillaria contorta*, was reported in a peafowl that died after displaying clinical signs of severe chalky white diarrhea with progressive weakness [57]. On necropsy, masses of worms were found in the thickened and rough crop mucosa.

Tapeworm ova have been identified in some surveillance studies, but they have not been speciated [58].

19.9.5.3 External Parasites

Mites and lice are external parasites that can be found on many bird species including peafowl. Mites have a wide host range and common mites include the northern fowl mite and the tropical fowl mite. Mites live on both the bird and in the crevices of the housing structure. If peafowl are raised free-roam, mite infestation may be less likely since the birds are not localized in one setting. Lice tend to be host specific and live solely on the host. Hollamby et al (2003) [31] detected *Goniodes gigas* from free-roaming peafowl at a zoological park in three of 31 birds tested.

19.9.6   Trauma

Peafowl are large and tend to make sudden movements. In many locations, peafowl are often the victims of vehicular trauma, both unintentionally and intentionally. Drozd et al. [59] reported that 32% of 334 necropsy records of peafowl submitted to a diagnostic lab from zoological institutions and private aviculturists died of trauma, followed by 31% that died of infectious causes. While infectious diseases do cause peafowl mortality, it is interesting to note that trauma also plays a major role in the death of peafowl and equals or exceeds the presence of infectious diseases.

19.9.7   Human–Peafowl Interactions

In recent times, there was a fatal case of a man in Thailand being involved in a freak accident where one of his pet peacocks attacked him while he was feeding them. The peacock had mutilated his head region where a puncture wound was found in the region above his ear, causing a subsequent blot clot. As mentioned previously, peafowl, especially the Java green peafowl, are highly aggressive especially during the breeding season [60].

19.10   Conclusion

Peafowl are the most elaborate and easily recognizable galliformes due to their large size and ornamental feathers that play a role in mating. When keeping peafowl, it may be best to raise them free range with free access to the environment while housing, if used, can be provided only at night. Peafowl can also be kept in total confinement to breed threatened species or develop new color or pattern variations. Depending on the individual purpose chosen, these decisions will influence the risks for disease and should be taken into consideration when raising these magnificently beautiful birds.

References

1 Lukanov, H. (2013). Peafowl species and their mutations. *Aviculture Europe* 1–14.

2 Schwartz, D.L. (2021). Diseases of peafowl. United Peafowl Association, https://unitedpeafowlassociation.org/articles/diseases-of-peafowl (accessed February 2022).

3 Somes, R.G. Jr., and Burger, R.E. (1993). Color patterns in the Indian peafowl (*Pavo cristatus*). *J. Hered.* 84: 57–62.

4 Claesz, P. (1627). Still Life with Peacock Pie, 1627. www.nga.gov/collection-search-result.html?artobj_credit=The%20Lee%20and%20Juliet%20Folger%20Fund%0D%0A%0D%0A (accessed February 2022).

5 Yosemite Hospitality LLC, Aramark Yosemite Hospitality (2021). Bracebridge Dinner, Yosemite National Park (California, USA). www.bracebridgedinners.com (accessed February 2022).

6 Vigran, N. (1995). Peafowl in the aviary. *Watchbird* March/April: 31–32.

7 Yorzinski, J.L., Patricelli, G.L., Platt, M.L., and Land, M.F. (2015). Eye and head movements shape gaze shifts in Indian peafowl. *J. Exp. Biol.* 218 (Pt 23): 3771–3776.

8 Anonymous (2021). Origin of: Proud as a Peacock. https://idiomorigins.org/origin/proud-as-a-peacock (accessed February 2022).

9 Burgess, S.C. (2002). The physical structure, optical mechanics and aesthetics of the peacock tail feathers. In: *Design and Nature* (ed. C.A. Brebbia, L. Sucharov and P. Pascola), 435–443. Southhampton, UK: WIT Press.

10 Wade, N. (2009). Darwin's evolving genius. www.nytimes.com/2009/02/09/world/europe/09iht-darwin.4.20058973.html (accessed February 2022).

11 Hale, M.L., Verduijn, M.H., Møller, A.P. et al. (2009). Is the peacock's train an honest signal of genetic quality at the major histocompatibility complex? *J. Evol. Biol.* 22 (6): 1284–1294.

12 Dakin, R. (2011). The crest of the peafowl: a sexually dimorphic plumaje ornament signals condition in males and females. *J. Avian. Biol.* 42: 405–411.

13 Kane, S.A., Van Beveren, D., and Dakin, R. (2018). Biomechanics of the peafowl's crest reveals frequencies tuned to social displays. *PLoS One* 13 (11): e0207247.

14 Dakin, R. and Montgomerie, R. (2013). Eye for eyespots: how irridescent plumage ocelli influence peacock mating success. *Behav. Ecol.* 24 (5): 1048–1057.

15 del Hoyo, J., Elliott, A., and Sargatal, J. (1994). Volume 2: New World Vultures to Guineafowl. In: *Handbook of the Birds of the World*, 551–552. Barcelona, Spain: Lynx Edicions.

16 Anonymous (2021). Spalding peafowl. www.peacocksuk.com/peafowl-breeds/spalding-peacocks (accessed February 2022).

17 Galliformes TAG (2018). *AZA Regional Collection Plan*, 3e. Silver Springs, MD: Association of Zoos and Aquariums.

18 Benscheidt, S.E. (2021). General care of the peafowl (peacock). www.nelsonroadvet.com/articles/livestock/fowl/general-care-of-the-peafowl-peacock (accessed February 2022).

19 Somes, R.G. Jr., and Burger, R.E. (1990). Pied plumage color of the Indian blue peafowl (*Pavo cristatus*), an allele at the white locus. *Poult. Sci.* 70 (suppl. 1): 128.

20 Somes, R.G. Jr., and Burger, R.E. (1991). Plumage color inheritance of the Indian blue peafowl (*Pavo cristatus*), blue, black-shouldered, cameo, and oaten. *J. Hered.* 83: 64–68.

21 Biggs, P. (2021). What Do Peacocks Eat: Raising Peacocks, Quail and Other Game Birds. www.purinamills.cpm (accessed February 2022).

22 Parveen, Z., Sidra, S., and Khan, B.N. (2018). Diet preferences and general behavior of peafowls in captive environment. *Punjab. Univer. J. Zool.* 33 (1): 16–21.

23 Sikander, S.K., Ali, Z., Nemar, A. et al. (2015). Diet provision for zoo animals in captive conditions of Lahore zoo. *Pakistan. J. Animal. Plant .Sci.* 25: 493–499.

24 Jun, Y.X. and Lan, Y. (1996). The observation of time budgets of captive green peafowl (*Pavo multicus*). *Acta. Zool. Sin.* 5: 149–154.

25 Colon, B. and Silverman, H. (2021). Shrieking peacocks roam the streets in LA County, damaging vehicles. Now officials want to ban residents from feeding them. www.cnn.com/2021/06/09/us/los-angeles-peacock-ordinance-trnd/index.html (accessed February 2022).

26 Cosgrove, J. (2021). Feeding peacocks is now a crime in unincorporated L.A. County, some cities.www.latimes.com/california/story/2021-09-01/it-is-now-a-crime-to-feed-peacocks-in-unincorporated-l-a-county-some-cities (accessed 3 February 2022).

27 Reid, J. (1979). Raising peafowl. *Watchbird Magazine* 6 (2).

28 Dakin, R. and Montgomerie, R. (2011). Peahens prefer peacock displaying more eyespots, but rarely. *Anim. Behav.* 82: 21–28.

29 Dakin, R. and Montgomerie, R. (2009). Peacocks orient their courtship displays towards the sun. *Behav. Ecol. Sociobiol.* 63: 825–834.

30 Morishita, T.Y. and Derksen, T. (2021). Biosecurity. In: *Backyard Poultry Medicine and Surgery* (ed. C.G. Greenacre and T.Y. Morishita), 107–116. Hoboken, NJ: Wiley.

31 Al Falluji, M.M., Tantawi, H.H., Al-Bana, A., and Sheikhly, S. (1979). Pox infection among captive peacocls. *J. Wild. Dis.* 15 (4): 597–600.

32 Khan, A., Yousaf, A.Z., Khan, M. et al. (2009). Cutaneous form of pox infection among captive peafowl (*Pavo cristatus*) chicks. *Avian Pathol.* 38 (1): 65–70.

33 Kumar, A., Maan, S., Mahajan, N.K. et al. (2013). Detection and molecular characterization of Newcastle disease virus in peafowl (*Pavo cristatus*) in Haryana state, India. *Indian J. Virol.* 24 (3): 380–385.

34 Desingu, P.A., Singh, S.D., Dhama, K. et al. (2016). Molecular characterization, isolation, pathology and pathotyping of peafowl (Pavo cristatus) origin Newcastle disease virus isolates recovered from disease outbreaks in three states of India. *Avian Pathol.* 45 (6): 674–682.

35 Ismail, M. M., Khan, O. W., Cattoli, G., and Lu, H. (2009). Isolation and identification of highly pathogenic avian influenza virus subtype H5N1 in peafowl (*Pavo cristatus*). *7th International Symposium on Avian Influenza* (Poster Presentation), Athens, GA, April 4–8.

36 Rashid, P., Saeed, N.M., and Dyary, H.O. (2016). Genetic characterization and phylogenic analysis of H5N1 avian influenza virus detected in peafowl in Kirkuk province. *Iraq. J. Med. Virol.* 89 (2): 1179–1185.

37 Fan, Z., Ci, Y., Ma, Y. et al. (2014). Phylogenetic analysis of a novel H6N6 avian influenza virus isolated from a green peafowl in China and its pathogenic potential in mice. *Infect. Genet. Evol.* 28: 107–112.

38 Crawshaw, G.J. and Boycott, B.R. (1982). Infectious laryngotracheitis in peafowl and pheasants. *Avian Dis.* 26: 397–401.

39 Dharma, K., Gowtharman, Y., Karthik, K. et al. (2016). Haemorrhagic enteritis of turkeys – current knowledge. *Vet. Quart.* 37 (1): 31–42.

40 McFerran, J.B. and Smyth, J.A. (2000). Avian adenoviruses. *Rev. Sci. Tech. Off. Int. Epiz.* 19 (2): 589–601.

41 Hollamby, S., Sikarski, J., and Stuht, J. (2003). Survey of peafowl (Pavo cristatus) for potential pathogens at three Michigan zoos. *J. Zoo Wildl. Med* 34 (4): 375–379.

42 Willis, F.K. (1955). Isolation of pleuropneumonia-like organism from a peacock (Pavo cristatus). *Southwest. Vet.* 8: 258–259.

43 Cookson, K. and Shivaprasad, H.L. (1994). Mycoplasma gallisepticum infection in chukar partridges, pheasants, and peafowl. *Avian Dis.* 38 (4): 914–921.

44 Oludairo, O.O., Kwaga, J.K.P., Dzikwi, A.A., and Kabir, J. (2013). The genus *Salmonella*: isolation and occurrence in the wild. *Bio-Genet. J.* 1 (1): 12–14.

45 Hansen, F.W. (1940). Peafowl. *Vet. Med.* 35 (3): 194–195.

46 Kul, O., Tunca, R., Haziroglu, R. et al. (2005). An outbreak of avian tuberculosis in peafowl (*Pavo cristatus*) and pheasants (*Phasianus colchicus*) in a zoological aviary in Turkey. *Vet. Med. Czech.* 50 (10): 446–450.

47 Ledwon, A., Augustynowicz-Kopec, E., Parniewski, P. et al. (2017). Mycobacteriosis in peafowl: analysis of four cases. *Med. Weter.* 74 (12): 772–776.

48 Clarke, L., Beckstead, R.B., Hayes, J.R., and Rissi, D.R. (2017). Pathologic and molecular characterization of histomoniasis in peafowl (*Pavo cristatus*). *J. Vet. Diag. Invest.* 29 (2): 237–241.

49 De Mello Zanim Michelazzo, M., Sasse, J.P., de Souza, M. et al. (2017). Systemic histomoniasis in a leucistic Indian Peafwol (*Pavo cristatus*) from southern Brazil. *Avian Dis.* 61: 325–329.

50 Hauck, R. and Hafez, H.M. (2012). Description of E*imeria pavonina* (coccidia) of peafowl in Germany. *Avian Dis.* 56 (1): 238–242.

51 Titilincu, A., Mircean, V., Bejan, A. et al. (2009). Prevalence of endoparasites in peacocks (*Pavo cristatus*). *Rev. Scient. Parasitol.* 10 (1/2): 101–105.

52 Crespo, R., Franca, M.B., Fenton, H., and Shivaprasad, H.L. (2018). Galliformes and Columbiformes. In: *Pathology of Wildlife and Zoo Animals* (ed. K.A. Terio, D. MCAloose and J. St. Leger), 747–773. St Louis, MO: Elsevier.

53 Laird, M. (1978). *Plasmodium durae* Herman from the introduced common peafowl in northern Nigeria. *Eukaryotic. Microbiol.* 25 (1): 21–24.

54 Teixeira, M., Monteiro, T.P., Silva Catenacci, L. et al. (2012). Ascariasis in peafowl *Pavo cristatus* (Phasianidae) due to Ascaridia galli Schrank, 1788. *J. Zoo Wildl. Med.* 43 (3): 585–587.

55 Lund, E.E. and Chute, A.M. (1972). *Heterakis* and *Histomonas* infections in young peafowl, compared to such infections in pheasants, chickens, and turkeys. *J. Wildl. Dis.* 8 (4): 352–358.

56 Subramanian, K.S., John, M.C., and Raman, M. (2003). Pilot study on parasitic fauna of free-ranging Indian peafowl (Pavo critatus). *Zoos Print J.* 18 (5): 1096–1098.

57 Sujatha, K., Venu, R., Srilatha, C., and Amaravathi, P. (2012). Infection of *Capillaria contorta* in peafowl. *Zoo's Print J.* 27: 21.

58 Costa, L. and Timossi, L. (2009). Peafowl. In: *Handbook of Avian Medicine* (ed. T. Tully, G. Dorrestein and A. Jones). St Louis, MO: Elsevier.

59 Drozd, M., Dominguez, M., Morishita, T.Y., et al. (2022). Causes of morbidity and mortality of peafowl and peafowl pheasants at zoological institutions: A retrospective study. Proceedings of the 2022 Western Poultry Disease Conference, April 4–6, 2022, Vancouver, British Columbia, CANADA.

60 Anonymous (1997). Peacock kills man in Thailand. https://apnews.com/article/ 91333b98d4bb0cdb6c100e24450249c9 (accessed February 2022).

20

Conservation of Gamebirds
Chris Holmes

The Galliformes have captured our imagination and influenced myth, art, and dance for centuries and more than any other bird we have depended on them as a protein source, entertainment, status symbol, and pet. Wild populations of this order play an important role as bioindicators and domesticated species like the chicken have circumvented the globe with us. These domesticated species are an important part of our economy and the chicken has become one of the most numerous birds in the world.

Establishing an exact methodology for the conservation of all species in this order is just not possible because of the varied needs of the birds and the cultures they inhabit. This chapter will instead focus on a social science-based approach to conservation which provides an inclusive and holistic framework. Through this lens, we will evaluate the conservation programs for two subspecies (one extinct and one extant) and one species representing two of the most imperiled birds in this order. This chapter will conclude with an overview of areas where further research and work are needed to advance the success of Galliformes conservation programs.

20.1 Conservation Status

As children, we are all taught that elephants and tigers are endangered, but *endangered* is just one of eight terms used to define the conservation status of a species. These terms describe how urgent conservation action is required to prevent extinction. The International Union for Conservation of Nature (IUCN) was formed in 1948 as a branch of the United Nations and its mission is to "Influence, encourage and assist societies throughout the world to conserve nature and to ensure that any use of natural resources is equitable and ecologically sustainable" [1]. The Red List of Endangered Species was founded in 1964 and is a part of the IUCN.

The Red List ranks all animals at the species level and places them into eight conservation status designations, defining a population status from stable to extinction (data deficient, least concern, near threatened, vulnerable, endangered, critically endangered, extinct in the wild, and extinct). The Red List further defines the status of a population through four population trends from unknown to decreasing (unknown, increasing, stable, and decreasing). A species is placed

Gamebird Medicine and Management, First Edition. Edited by Teresa Y. Morishita and Robert E. Porter, Jr.
© 2023 John Wiley & Sons, Inc. Published 2023 by John Wiley & Sons, Inc.

Table 20.1   Galliformes complete conservation status and population trends.

Complete Conservation Status of the Order of Galliformes	
Total 295 species of Galliformes	
664 subspecies of Galliformes	
176	Least Concern (LC)
38	Near Threatened (NT)
44	Vulnerable (VU)
23	Endangered (EN)
7	Critically Endangered (CR)
1	Extinct in the Wild (EW)
1	Extinct (EX)
5	Data Deficient (DD)
Population Trends for the Galliformes	
9	Increasing
62	Stable
213	Decreasing
9	Unknown
2	Not Evaluated

in these classifications by the IUCN Taxonomic Specialist Groups. [1] These groups comprise expert volunteers on the taxon who evaluate all the species under their purview in conjunction with experts in the country of origin. This system is the accepted international conservation status authority at the species level and can be accessed by the public through the Red List website (Tables 20.1 and 20.2). Of the 295 species in this order, 74 are threatened with extinction and 213 have a decreasing population trend.

Within the 295 species, there are 664 described subspecies of Galliformes and none of these subspecies are currently evaluated on the Red List. The conservation status of a subspecies is important because it represents a portion of a species' range. For example, the ring-necked pheasant (*Phasianus colchicus*) is listed as Least Concern by the IUCN Red List but it has 34 described subspecies, some of which are regionally considered endangered and protected. As genetic analysis is applied more to taxonomy, some of these subspecies may in fact be elevated to full species status.

The risk of extinction to a subspecies is determined by the regional authority of the country (or countries) within its range. The Endangered Species Act (ESA) is the accepted resource for the conservation status of a US subspecies. A species can be listed as Least Concern on the IUCN Red List but can be protected as endangered under the ESA. This Act provides resources for the protection of a species, protects critical habitat and defines the recovery process through a published recovery plan. Foreign species can be listed under the ESA and this protects against imports and exports to or from the United States of America [2].

Table 20.2 Galliformes conservation by family.

Megapodes Conservation Status		Cracidae Conservation Status	
22 Species, 33 Subspecies		54 Species, 54 Subspecies	
10	Least Concern (LC)	29	Least Concern (LC)
0	Near Threatened (NT)	4	Near Threatened (NT)
7	Vulnerable (VU)	8	Vulnerable (VU)
4	Endangered (EN)	8	Endangered (EN)
0	Critically Endangered (CR)	4	Critically Endangered (CR)
0	Extinct in the Wild (EW)	1	Extinct in the Wild (EW)
0	Extinct (EX)	0	Extinct (EX)
1	Data Deficient (DD)	0	Data Deficient (DD)
Megapodes Population Trends		**Cracidae Population Trends**	
1	Increasing	1	Increasing
3	Stable	5	Stable
17	Decreasing	46	Decreasing
1	Unknown	1	Unknown
0	Not Evaluated	1	Not Evaluated
Numididae Conservation Status		**Odontophoridae Conservation Status**	
6 Species, 16 Subspecies		33 Species, 128 Subspecies	
4	Least Concern (LC)	21	Least Concern (LC)
0	Near Threatened (NT)	5	Near Threatened (NT)
1	Vulnerable (VU)	7	Vulnerable (VU)
0	Endangered (EN)	0	Endangered (EN)
0	Critically Endangered (CR)	0	Critically Endangered (CR)
0	Extinct in the Wild (EW)	0	Extinct in the Wild (EW)
0	Extinct (EX)	0	Extinct (EX)
1	Data Deficient (DD)	0	Data Deficient (DD)
Numididae Population Trends		**Odontophoridae Population Trends**	
0	Increasing	3	Increasing
2	Stable	7	Stable
3	Decreasing	23	Decreasing
1	Unknown	0	Unknown
0	Not Evaluated	0	Not Evaluated

(Continued)

Table 20.2 (Continued)

Phasianidae Conservation Status
180 Species, 433 Subspecies
122 Least Concern (LC)
29 Near Threatened (NT)
21 Vulnerable (VU)
11 Endangered (EN)
3 Critically Endangered (CR)
0 Extinct in the Wild (EW)
1 Extinct (EX)
3 Data Deficient (DD)
Phasianidae Population Trends
4 Increasing
45 Stable
124 Decreasing
6 Unknown
1 Not Evaluated

20.2 Social Science Approach

The Holocene, our current geological epoch, is defined by anthropogenic extinctions. To understand anthropogenic extinctions, we must understand more than just the biology of a species, but how our actions cause(d) endangerment. The social sciences (anthropology, sociology, and history) provide a holistic framework within which to define our cultural interactions with a species.

A recent movement in conservation known as ethnoornithology emphasizes cultural knowledge of a species at the forefront of its recovery [3]. This method places the species into its cultural context and defines cultural use, cultural beliefs, and the role a species plays within a culture. Through this process, the factors that have contributed to the endangerment of a species (e.g., trade, hunting, habitat augmentation, etc.) are quantified. Investigating our own cultural beliefs of a species can lend a greater understanding to this concept. The crow of a rooster is associated with waking up the farmer, but it also symbolizes the rising of the sun itself. But what if the rooster goes extinct? Does the sun still rise? How long does this knowledge stay within our culture?

20.3 Conservation Population Management

The paradigm shift of zoos from menageries to conservation organizations in the 1970s ushered in the management of populations as conservation safeguards. In 1980, conservation was the highest priority of the 158 member institutions of the American Association of Zoological Parks and Aquariums (AAZPA), the precursor to the present-day Association of Zoos and Aquariums (AZA). The AZA acts as the professional association and accrediting body for zoos and aquariums in the United

States. In 1981, the Species Survival Plan (SSP) was formed, establishing cooperative management of select species across all AAZPA institutions [4].

Taxonomic Advisory Groups (TAG) were created in 1990 to oversee and create the species survival plans (SSPs). The TAG role is to publish a regional collection plan every five years that provides species recommendations to AZA institutions. An important aspect of the collection plan is ensuring that an SSP can meet its long-term genetic and demographic goals. One of the most important factors for a successful captive breeding program is space to grow the population within AZA to ensure sustainability [5].

In 2000, to aid in the management of SSPs, the Population Management Center was founded at the Lincoln Park Zoo in Chicago. This center employs population biologists who evaluate the genetics of a SSP and recommend transfers to increase genetic diversity and demography. SSPs are managed with the goal of maintaining 90% of a population's genetic diversity for 100 years [6]. This is a lofty goal and one that many populations, especially those that were rescued from the wild, do not meet due to a limited or unknown founder base. This genetic criterion serves as a goal to work toward and a benchmark to compare SSPs across taxa.

20.4   History of the Conservation of the Heath Hen and Attwater's Prairie Chicken

The greater prairie chicken (*Tympanuchus cupido*), Near Threatened on the Red List, had three subspecies, one of which, the heath hen (*Tympanuchus cupido cupido*), is now extinct and another, the Attwater's prairie chicken (*Tympanuchus cupido attwateri*), which is Endangered. These birds have a form of mating display called lekking which is dependent on many males displaying together to attract mates. The male display occurs in spring and consists of inflating brightly colored air sacs on either side of the head, producing a low boom vocalization, accompanied with the rapid drumming/stamping of the feet, and a loud "cackle" vocalization (Figure 20.1a). Copulation occurs

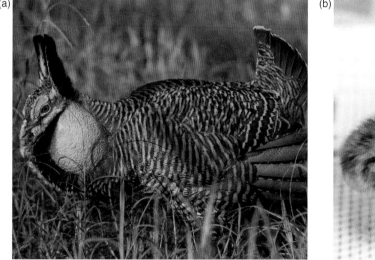
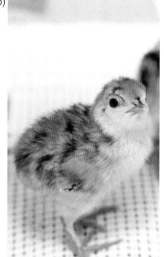

(a)   (b)

Figure 20.1   (a) Adult male Attwater's prairie chicken "booming" or displaying. (b) Attwater's prairie chicken chick. Source: Courtesy of Stephanie Adams, Houston Zoo.

at the lekking site and the hen is solely responsible for the incubation and rearing of the chicks. These grouse have a breeding season restricted to the spring months, making them vulnerable to changes in weather patterns (e.g., late winters, hurricanes, floods). The breeding display of the greater prairie chicken is the inspiration for the "Chicken Dance" or "Prairie Chicken Dance" which is performed by the First Nation cultures of the Cree and the Blackfoot [7].

The heath hen was described to science in 1758 by Linnaeus and ranged along the coastal regions of the Eastern Seaboard from Maine possibly as far south as the Carolinas [8]. The New England region was the site of the first American colonies which experienced rapid human population growth, intense habitat conversion through new agriculture practices, and harvesting of natural resources for both the colonies and export to Europe. Other negative pressures by colonists came in the form of large-scale hunting, farming of Old World domestic fowl (which brought new diseases), introduced predators in the form of pests (rats and mice), and domestic companion animals (dogs and cats). These combined threats all had a negative impact on this bird, quickly limiting its habitat and population [9].

As early as 1791, laws were proposed in Long Island, NY, to prevent the overharvesting of this bird and were one of the first US Galliformes conservation measures. By the 1830s, heath hens had become extremely rare and in 1831, Massachusetts passed legislation that established a hunting season, but enforcement was lax [8]. In 1869, the mainland population of the heath hen had collapsed and gone extinct, with one remaining holdout on the island of Martha's Vineyard, Massachusetts [10]. Martha's Vineyard is approximately 96 square miles (or 61,400 acres) though not all was suitable habitat for the heath hen. A census of the bird in 1890 found that the entire global population totaled only 100–200 birds [10].

A census in 1907 found 77 birds remaining and in that same year, the state of Massachusetts renewed its effort to conserve this bird. It established a 1600-acre refuge on Martha's Vineyard, initiated a yearly census, a captive breeding effort, supplemental feeding of the wild birds, limiting predators, and increased protections against poaching. The captive breeding effort started with a clutch of nine heath hen eggs that were fostered under a domestic chicken broody hen. Only one egg hatched, and the resulting chick was killed by the broody hen [8]. Between the years of 1908 and 1912, the population vacillated before finally rebounding to 300 birds in 1912. This increase was followed by another population milestone in 1914 with an estimated 1000 birds present. In 1916, the population of the heath hen reached its highest at an estimated 2000 individual birds on the island [8]. The 1916 recovery of this population shows how fast a bird in this genus can multiply if conditions are favorable. In only nine years, from 1907 till 1916, the population grew by an estimated 1923 birds.

The population's recovery met with tragedy on May 12, 1916 (during the nesting and chick rearing season) when a wildfire broke out on the island and decimated the population to under 150 birds. To safeguard this bird from extinction, a translocation of adults to the former mainland range on Long Island was attempted; 16 males and 10 females were taken into captivity to establish a captive flock. The translocations failed all the birds taken into captivity died. Harsh late winters followed the wildfire and the population never rebounded. The 1928 census located only one bird, a male who was given the nickname of "Booming Ben". He was last seen on March 11, 1932, and after some unconfirmed sightings, never again was a heath hen seen alive and it was declared extinct [8].

The story of the heath hen illustrates important conservation tools that remain pertinent today (habitat protection, hunting bans, habitat management, translocations, supplemental feeding, captive breeding). It also highlights important early changes that were occurring within American culture with the realization that animals were not an unlimited resource. The heath hen's extinction is regarded as one of the great losses of North American bird biodiversity along with the passenger pigeon (*Ectopistes migratorius*), extinct in 1918, and the Carolina parakeet (*Conuropsis carolinensis*), extinct in 1939.

20.4.1 Attwater's Prairie Chicken Recovery Program

The Attwater's prairie chicken was described to science in 1893 by Major Charles Emil Bendire. A greater prairie chicken (*T. cupido*) subspecies, it inhabits the southernmost area of this species range through the coastal prairies of the Gulf of Mexico in Texas and formerly Louisiana. The extinction of the plains bison (*Bison b. bison*) in the mid-1800s changed the flora of the coastal prairies. These large herbivores prevented the growth of trees in these regions and without them, the plains transitioned into more wooded areas. Domestic cattle took the place of the plains bison with the increase in ranching, but these sedentary herds damaged the habitat by overgrazing [11].

The subtropical Gulf Coast region experienced rapid development of agriculture, oil production, and commercial trade, attracting more people to the region. Today, Houston is the fourth largest city in the US and may soon become the third largest, with an ever increasing urban sprawl. Agriculture practices focused on cotton and rice production further damaged the coastal prairie in the nineteenth century. In Louisiana, rice production increased from 1.5 million pounds in 1864 to more than 40 million pounds by 1877 [12]. By 1903, 376,000 acres in Louisiana and 234,000 acres of the Texas coastal regions had been converted for rice cultivation, producing 99% of the total US crop [13]. Habitat conversion coupled with unsustainable sport hunting practices caused the Attwater's extinction in Louisiana in 1919 and its increasing rarity in Texas.

In Texas, the Attwater's was a focal point for conservation efforts in 1883 with a closed hunting season for five months. This ban was challenged in 1885 and rendered invalid. In 1903, more hunting regulations were imposed but there was little enforcement of this legislation. In 1910, the Texas Game, Fish, and Oyster Commission was formed to oversee hunting restrictions. Although a step forward, this effort was understaffed, and nine years later in 1919, there were only six wardens [14]. In 1941, the most complete study of the Attwater's was published by Valgene W. Lehmann. He estimated that the population was between 8000 and 9000 birds in isolated fragments in 19 Texas counties [14]. For perspective, the historic range included 48 Texas counties and at that time, it had already gone extinct in 29 counties [15].

The population continued to decline and by the late 1960s it only numbered 1000 birds [16]. Due to this rarity and continued decline, this subspecies was one of the first animals to be listed under the Endangered Species Conservation Act of 1967 which was the precursor to the US ESA of 1973. The first captive breeding attempt occurred in 1967 at Texas A&M University. This program resulted in the first captive hatch in 1968 but ultimately failed. Captive breeding was tried a second time in 1970 but sadly, it had the same results as the 1967 program [15].

Out of all the Galliformes species, grouse have been maintained the least and husbandry standards were lacking and had to be developed. In 1972, the Attwater's Prairie Chicken National Wildlife Refuge (APCNWR) was created which today encompasses 10,528 acres of coastal prairie in Colorado County. A renewed captive breeding effort was started in 1992 due to the continued decline of the wild population which at that time was under 500 birds. Eggs and adult birds were collected from the wild and this was the start of the SSP at Fossil Rim Wildlife Center [15].

These collections preserved the genetics for an estimated 19 founders, establishing a genetic diversity of 37.2% for 100 years. It is important to note that genetic diversity at that level is not uncommon in SSPs for species as imperiled as the Attwater's. The captive breeding effort established key demographic data for this bird, providing greater information to underpin understanding of the wild population. A short lifespan and quick sexual maturity allow this species to increase rapidly, but genetic diversity is lost faster due to the quick generation time [17]. The SSP has been able to achieve releases of hand-raised chicks each year from 1995 to the present. The releases are focused on the APCNWR and a private ranch in Goliad County [15].

With all release efforts, initial survivability is often low post release as birds adapt to the wild. After being released, the captive-reared birds were surviving, but chicks (Figure 20.1b) hatched in the wild were not [15]. Investigations into this low survivability found a correlation with the introduced red fire ant (*Solenopsis invicta*). This study determined that the introduction of this ant species in 1970 was not directly responsible for the death of the chicks, but the ants were eating insects, a critical food source for the first 2 weeks of a chick's life. Treatment of the reserve resulted in higher chick survivability [16]. Another invasive species that has been a challenge for the Attwater's is the Chinese tallow tree (*Triadica sebifera*). This tree was prized as an ornamental due to its fall foliage, but its rapid growth and spread quickly create a monoculture forest that overtakes the prairie.

The Attwater's prairie chicken will be delisted and considered recovered when the following two objectives have been met.

> 1. Downlist to Threatened status when the overall population maintains a minimum of 3000 breeding adults annually over a 5-year period and there is sufficient habitat of coastal prairie grasslands (approximately 150 000 acres (60 702 ha)) to support this population. These 3000 breeding adults should be distributed along a linear distance of no less than 50 miles (80 km) to mitigate for environmental stochasticity (e.g., hurricanes) while maintaining genetic flow.
> 2. Delist when the overall population reaches a minimum of 6000 breeding adults annually over a 10-year period occupying approximately 300 000 acres (121 457 ha) of maintained or improved coastal prairie grassland habitat along a linear distance of no less than 100 miles [15].

The Gulf Coast region is vulnerable to hurricanes and tropical storm events which can reduce the population of the Attwater's. In 2017 "Harvey," a category 4 hurricane, decimated the Texas Gulf Coast and the wild population of Attwater's. This storm dropped unprecedented amounts of rainfall on the region and large amounts of flooding occurred. There were 42 wild birds recorded on the APCNWR before the storm and it is estimated that 80% of this population was lost [18]. This storm illustrates the sensitivity of this bird to natural disasters, and one must wonder what historical hurricanes have done to the population (e.g., the Great Galveston Hurricane of 1900). After Harvey, releases have continued and the wild Attwater's population is starting to recover.

The heath hen and Attwater's were early indicators of a then evolving conservation issue of the loss and unhealthy status of the grassland biomes in North America. A recent study by Audubon has found that less than 40% of this biome that once extended from Canada to Mexico remains [19]. It is estimated that since 1970, there has been a decline in the total populations of all North American bird species, resulting in a staggering estimated loss of 3 billion breeding birds, with grasslands being the most endangered of all North American biomes with 74.2% dependent species in decline [20].

The Attwater's Prairie Chicken SSP has been supported through the combined efforts of Abilene Zoo, Caldwell Zoo, Fossil Rim Wildlife Center, George Miksch Sutton Avian Research Center, Houston Zoo, San Antonio Zoo, SeaWorld San Antonio, and Texas A&M University. These institutions have worked valiantly to save this bird from extinction.

20.5   Vietnam Pheasant SSP

The Vietnam pheasant (*Lophura edwardsi*) is a Vietnam endemic, ESA listed Endangered species, and is currently considered Critically Endangered but this species is likely Extinct in the Wild. Extensive searches in the last decade have not located any individuals, making this species the most endangered of all pheasants. The country of Vietnam had long periods of conflict from 1945 till the 1980s. The Vietnam War (1955–1975) resulted in the largest damage to the habitat of this pheasant with the use of the defoliant and herbicide Agent Orange. The current wild population estimate is 50–249 mature individuals.

Previously, this species was thought to be two: *L. edwardsi* was described in 1896 and the now defunct Vietnamese pheasant (*Lophura hatinhensis*) was described in 1975 by Vo Quy [21]. The two birds differed in tail feather coloration – *edwardsi* has blue tail feathers (Figure 20.2a) and *hatinhensis* had white tail feathers (Figure 20.2b). The captive history of this species is one of the most interesting of any species of Galliformes. The original *edwardsi* type birds were collected from the wild by the prominent French ornithologist Jean Delacour in the 1920s. Over four trips between 1924 and 1930, he collected 30 birds from the wild [22]. Delacour gave some birds as gifts to friends in Japan and England. The largest number of birds returned with him to his aviaries in Clères, France. As these populations produced offspring, birds were eventually sent worldwide which is another great mystery of this species as to where current populations originated from (France, England, or Japan). During World War II, Delacour's extensive records and aviaries, including many birds, were destroyed, and valuable information on exports was lost [21].

The Vietnamese pheasant (*L. hatinhensis*) population was founded from four wild caught birds that came into the collection of the Hanoi Zoo in 1990–1991. Offspring from these birds were exported to the European Association of Zoos and Aquaria (EAZA) collections in 1996 [21]. *Hatinhensis* was never imported into the US, but birds bred in the US from *edwardsi* pairs produced white-tailed offspring matching the description of *hatinhensis*. It was determined through a genetic study of *edwardsi* and *hatinhensis* that these two birds are in fact the same species. It is thought now that the *hatinhensis* type coloration represents an isolated population that experienced genetic drift and that the US birds were proof of this, as it is thought genetic diversity in this population is limited. The number of white tail feathers was not consistent between individuals, and in 2012, the two were officially declared one species – *L. edwardsi* [21]. When the two populations are

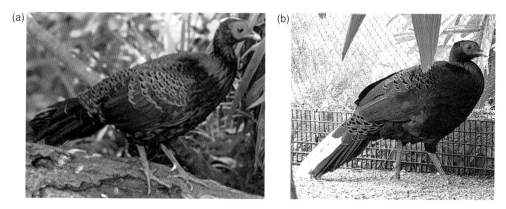

Figure 20.2   (a) Adult male Vietnam pheasant of the *edwardsi* coloration. Source: Courtesy of Sarah Patterson, St. Augustine Alligator Farm Zoological Park. (b) Adult male Vietnam pheasant of the *hatinhensis* coloration. Source: Courtesy of Kelly Pardy, Houston Zoo.

combined, this will be the first supplement to the *edwardsi* genetics since the collection of this species from the wild.

The Vietnam Pheasant was historically rare in AZA collections, but was common in the US private sector. The first bird, a male, was held at the Philadelphia Zoo in 1926, but this species was uncommon until the 1970s [23]. In 2006, there was a large push to increase the representation of this species in AZA collections as there were only 11 individuals at five institutions [24]. Birds were acquired from different US private breeders in the hope of capturing all the genetics represented in the US. The fact that we still have this bird in North America is a credit to dedicated US private aviculturists. Through intensive management in 2020, there are now 63 birds in 22 AZA institutions and the population is continuing to grow (S. Patterson, pers. comm.).

This bird is relatively unknown in its native Vietnam. EAZA and the World Pheasant Association (WPA) are working with Viet Nature to build a breeding center for the eventual translocation of birds from EAZA to Vietnam. Genetic studies supported by the WPA and EAZA have been able to clarify the genetics of the European population [25]. A combined genetic study with EAZA is planned in the future to evaluate birds in AZA and select US private collections to determine the entire genetic diversity of this species. This will be the only way genetic diversity can be supplemented for the survival of this species (S. Patterson, pers. comm.). This study will also address a rumor that has persisted that birds were brought back with returning airmen from the Vietnam War [23].

20.5.1 What's in a Name?

The Vietnam pheasant was formerly called the Edwards's pheasant in honor of the French ornithologist Alphonse Milne-Edwards. This was done with great respect in 1896, but this name placed emphasis on the colonial past of this region and did not reflect the importance of this species to Vietnam. The naming and scientific descriptions of almost this entire order were made by mostly European scientists (see Chapter 3). With the change in species status of the Vietnamese pheasant (*L. hatinhensis*), Vietnam asked that *L. edwardsi* be now referred to as the Vietnam pheasant [25].

Another example of a name not capturing the importance of a species is the Critically Endangered Colombian endemic blue-billed curassow (*Crax alberti*). This bird was described to science in 1852 by Louis Fraser, a British ornithologist, who named it in honor of Prince Albert. This too was done in great respect, but Prince Albert had no association with this species and this name does not reflect the importance of this bird to Colombia. A name more akin to *Crax zenú*, after the Colombian indigenous culture that immortalized this species in gold (see Accession Number: 1979.206.775 in the MET), or *Crax colombina*, to reflect the uniqueness of this species to that country, may in the end be more appropriate. This is not a call to rename the entire order, but to bring attention to developing issues that we as a conservation community will need to be receptive to. Names have power and in the past, naming was used to place emphasis and honor the contributions of an individual. Renaming should be considered as a tool to increase awareness of these imperiled birds and form a link with the present-day culture.

20.5.2 Release

There has been a long history of captive breeding of the species in Galliformes and the birds generally adapt well and increase in number. One of the greatest conservation challenges with this family group has been the release of captive birds back into the wild. Survivability is low and populations rarely become sustainable. In a captive setting, providing optimum welfare is the goal but this can cause maladaptation for release birds. A captive bird experiences a reliable schedule of daily events (e.g., when they are feed, cleaned, etc.) and an abundance of resources as we strive to reduce stress on the birds as much as possible.

Dr Nigel Collar, a British ornithologist, recently reviewed five Galliformes release programs of captive-bred birds and found that all of them failed to establish a sustainable wild population. This review was carried out in preparation for the release of the Vietnam pheasant. Dr Collar concluded that some of the most important aspects in rearing chicks for release are parent rearing, socialization before release, a longer adjustment time in the release pens before release, and training the birds to identify predators. He proposes parent-rearing the Vietnam pheasants for five generations to allow the birds to display more natural behaviors than a hand-reared bird [26]. Hand and foster-reared chicks can result in a greater production in a season. Having more birds for release is seen as a positive factor to ensure better survivability, but the proposed method concentrates on quality over the quantity that is to be released. Determining a successful method for establishing wild populations is one of the greatest areas of research required for the recovery of this order and the Vietnam pheasant will be a model of interest in the future.

20.6   Moving Forward and Conclusion

An emerging and important task for the conservationist is not only returning birds to the wild, but returning birds to the cultures where they range. Previously, conservation was done in a vacuum by foreign institutions and as a result, a species that may have been forgotten was further separated from that culture. In extreme cases, this has caused fear of conservation either through a perceived loss of land or of an occupation which can hinder efforts to return and recover a species. To increase the success of conservation projects, emphasis must be placed on inclusiveness, the cultural connection to, and sense of pride in a species to ensure long-term success.

The extant species/subspecies accounts may seem bleak but unlike the heath hen, these species are still alive. They are not specimens in a museum collection or color plates in a book where we are trying to envision how they sounded or interacted with the environment. The Attwater's prairie chicken and Vietnam pheasant are two of the most imperiled birds in this order and through captive management they have been saved from extinction. The development of their endangerment was a long and complex process and returning them back to the wild will be just as complex. As bioindicator species, they give us the opportunity of understanding at what point these environments that we have damaged have become healthy enough to support them.

Through globalization, the conservation of a species is no longer the responsibility of one country but is now a shared responsibility of the global consumer. Shifts in cultural consumption patterns, changes in agriculture techniques, and climate change have caused extreme and rapid fluctuations in many populations of Galliformes, notably North American grouse and South American curassows. Our recent pandemic has shown us all that conservation needs to begin at home and birds like the Attwater's prairie chicken need to be at the forefront to ensure our environment is healthy as this has major implications for the health of all animal populations, including our own.

References

1 IUCN (2020) www.iucn.org/about (accessed February 2022).

2 United States of America (1983). *The Endangered Species Act as Amended by Public Law 97–304 (the Endangered Species Act Amendments of 1982)*. Washington, D.C.: Government Printing Office.

3 Tidemann, S. and Gosler, A. (ed.) (2010). *Ethno-Ornithology: Birds, Indigenous Peoples, Culture and Society*. London: Earthscan.

4 Hutchinson, M. (1991). Beyond genetic and demographic management: the future of the species survival plan and related AAZPA conservation efforts. *Zoo Biol.* 10: 285–292.

5 Association of Zoos and Aquariums (2020). *Species Survival Plan® (SSP) Program. Handbook*. Silver Spring, MD: Association of Zoos and Aquariums.

6 Association of Zoos and Aquariums (2020). *Taxon Advisory Group (TAG) Handbook*. Silver Spring, MD: Association of Zoos and Aquariums.

7 Dempsey, H.A. (1956). Social dances of the blood Indians of Alberta, Canada. *J. Am. Folklore* 69 (271): 47–52.

8 Cokinos, C. (2009). *Hope Is the Thing with Feathers*. New York: Penguin.

9 Day, D. (1981). *The Doomsday Book of Animals*. New York: Viking Press.

10 Greenway, J.C. Jr., (1967). *Extinct and Vanishing Birds of the World*. New York: Dover.

11 Jordan, T. (1973). Pioneer evaluation of vegetation in frontier Texas. *Southwestern Hist. Q.* 76 (3): 234–254.

12 Benedict, L. and Schultz, B. (2012). Research Soon Follows as Rice Growing Begins. LSU College of Agricultural. www.lsuagcenter.com/portals/communications/publications/agmag/archive/2012/spring/research-soon-follows-as-rice-growing-begins.

13 Dethloff, H.C. (1976). Rice Culture. Handbook of Texas Online. www.tshaonline.org/handbook/entries/rice-culture (accessed February 2022).

14 Lehmann, V.W. (1941). *Attwater's Prairie Chicken its Life History and Management. North American Fauna 57*. Washington D.C.: Government Printing Office.

15 United States Fish and Wildlife Service (2010). *Attwater's Prairie-Chicken Recovery Plan*, Second Revision. Albuquerque, NM: US Fish and Wildlife Service.

16 Morrow, M., Chester, R., Lehnen, S. et al. (2015). Indirect effects of red imported fire ants on Attwater's prairie-chicken brood survival. *J. Wildlife Manag.* 79 (6): 898–906.

17 Bailey, H., Coym, M., and Senner, P. (2019). *Population Analysis and Breeding and Transfer Plan: Attwater's Prairie Chicken*. Houston, TX: Houston Zoo.

18 Elbein, A. (2018). Boom or Bust: The Last Stand of the Attwater's Prairie-Chicken. www.audubon.org/news/boom-or-bust-last-stand-attwaters-prairie-chicken (accessed February 2022).

19 Wilsey, C.B., Grand, J., Wu, J. et al. (2019). *North American Grasslands*. New York: National Audubon Society.

20 Rosenberg, K.V., Dokter, A.M., Blancher, J. et al. (2019). Decline of the North American avifauna. *Science* 366: 120–124.

21 Hennache, A., Mahood, S., Eames, J. et al. (2012). Lophura hatinhensis is an invalid taxon. *Forktail* 28 (2012): 129–135.

22 Hennache, A. (2003). *International Studbook for the Edwards' Pheasant Lophura edwardsi (Update 2002)*. Clères: Publication Parc de Clères.

23 Patterson, S. (2019). *AZA Regional Studbook Edwards's Pheasant Lophura edwardsi*. St Augustine, FL: St. Augustine Alligator Farm Zoological Park..

24 Holmes, C. (2012). *Galliformes TAG Regional Collection Plan*. Houston, TX: Houston Zoo.

25 Dams, J. (2020). *EAZA Best Practice Guidelines Vietnam Pheasant (Lophura edwardsi)*. Antwerp, Belgium: Antwerp Zoo Society.

26 Collar, N. (2020). Preparing captive-bred birds for reintroduction: the case of the Vietnam pheasant *Lophura edwardsi*. *Bird Conserv. Int.* 1–16.

Index

Gamebird Medicine and Management, First Edition. Edited by Teresa Y. Morishita and Robert E. Porter, Jr.
© 2023 John Wiley & Sons, Inc. Published 2023 by John Wiley & Sons, Inc.